The Role of the Patient-Analyst Match in the Process and Outcome of Psychoanalysis

The Role of the Patient-Analyst Match in the Process and Outcome of Psychoanalysis is a compilation of Judy Kantrowitz's previously published papers on the patient-analyst "match" and its effect on the process and outcome of psychoanalysis.

The match between patient and analyst places attention on the dynamic effect of interactions of character and conflict of both participants on the process that evolves between them—a spectrum of compatibility and incompatibility that is relevant to the analytic work. Classical psychoanalysis had been viewed as a "one-person" enterprise, with one analyst interchangeable with another. Analysts' experiences of countertransference reactions were viewed as unresolved conflicts, reasons to return to personal treatment, not inevitable and potentially informative about the current analytic work. This view began to shift in the 1980s, with Judy Kantrowitz's work contributing to the development of the recognition that psychoanalysis was a "two-person" process. In this collection of her most significant papers, Kantrowitz explores the importance of the match, which refers to observable styles, attitudes, and personal characteristics that may be rooted in residual and unanalyzed conflicts, triggered in any patient-analyst pair. *Match* is neither a predictive nor static concept. Rather, it refers to the unfolding transaction that itself may shift and change during the course of analytic work.

Pulling together the history of the shift in theory from the one-person to two-person understanding of the psychoanalytic enterprise, *The Role of the Patient-Analyst Match in the Process and Outcome of Psychoanalysis* will be of great interest to contemporary psychoanalysts.

Judy Leopold Kantrowitz, PhD, is a Training and Supervising Analyst at the Boston Psychoanalytic Society and Institute. She has been an Associate Clinical Professor at Harvard Medical School and is currently a corresponding member. She is the author of three books: *The Patient's Impact on the Analyst* (1996), *Writing about Patients: Responsibilities, Risks, and Ramifications* (2006), and *Myths of Termination: What Patients Can Teach Analyst about Endings* (2014).

"Comprised of papers written over three decades, this volume demonstrates both Kantrowitz's prescience in her early attention to the intersubjective and the gradual evolution and refinement of her thought. Drawing upon the dual perspectives of research and clinical work, these papers provide an organizing structure within which such heterogeneous issues as patient-analyst match, impasse, and the impact of the analyst's own life experiences may be understood. A wealth of detailed clinical examples bring the author's ideas alive for the reader. The book is both a pleasure and an intellectually enriching experience to read."

Lucy LaFarge, Regional Editor for North
America of the *International Journal of
Psychoanalysis*; Clinical Professor of Psychiatry,
Weill Cornell Medical College

"There have always been two people in the treatment room. Judy Kantrowitz, early in her work, corrected the imbalance of a 'one-person' psychology, whereby only the patient's qualities determine the outcome. More recently, Kantrowitz focuses on a new imbalance, where the work may be dangerously analyst-centered. Her clarity about the fundamental analytic responsibility–'to remain inside and outside of the process' – enables her to tell the story of American psychoanalysis over the last fifty years, in a way that is both ardent and balanced, personal and scholarly. The Role of the Patient-Analyst Match is a treasure."

Ellen Pinsky, PsyD, author, *Death and Fallibility
in the Psychoanalytic Encounter: Mortal Gifts*

"Judy Kantrowitz demonstrates a whole new way of looking at an on-going treatment. With clear, comfortable language and vivid vignettes, Kantrowitz follows the configuration of the match not only into the areas we expect, such as impasses and supervision, but also such areas as the changes undergone by both analyst and patient in the course of the treatment, the handling of the frame, and even the impact of shaking events in the analyst's life. Other than supporting the treatment objective, Kantrowitz has no axe of grind, is not a moralizer or a partisan. She is always sympathetic to both parties in treatment, and draws on relevant contributions from all psychoanalytic quarters. What she offers is subtle, experienced psychoanalytic empiricism and a broadened appreciation of what has been an uncomfortable area for practitioners."

Lawrence Friedman, MD, Clinical Professor
of Psychiatry, Weill-Cornell Medical College,
Instructor, Psychoanalytic Association of New York

"Judy Kantrowitz integrates in a unique and admirable way a research perspective in her clinical work as a psychoanalyst. Her work is characterised by originality, courage, scientific care, honesty and relentless self-reflection combined with professional sensitivity, human warmth and a deeply human interest in psychic suffering snd it's complex causes. During her psychoanalytic training in-the 1970's, and against the prevailing zeitgeist of one person psychology she developed the intersubjective concept of the match between psychoanalyst and analysand. In the papers in this unique volume, this concept is constantly further developed, clinically deepened and linked with new experiences, reflections and observations on changing 'zeitgeists' within and outside the psychoanalytic community: a deep source of inspiration for generations of psychoanalysts and researchers!"

Prof Dr. Marianna Leuzinger-Bohleber, Former
Head of the Sigmund Freud Institute in Frankfurt,
Germany; Training Psychoanalyst DPV(IPA)

"In a stunningly discerning report of the ever unique personal aspects of patient-analyst engagements, Judy Kantrowitz offers us one of the most wise and mature overviews of the psychoanalytic process I know. Her open-minded and deep scholarship is wed to a keen clinical sensitivity that transcends pluralistic partiality. As a result, she not only brings together our varied understandings but notably and most movingly extends them.

This is a master class in serious thinking about psychoanalysis as a therapy, about analytic inquiry as a personally touching study of how hard it is to be a person. It is also a pleasure to read. Reading this, I learned much, but I also was moved to hear the richness of the music of psychoanalysis freed from the static of partisanship. Kantrowitz is a maestro, and this work is a profound contribution."

Warren S. Poland, author, *Intimacy and
Separateness in Psychoanalysis*

Psychoanalysis in a New Key Book Series

When music is played in a new key, the melody does not change, but the notes that make up the composition do: change in the context of continuity, continuity that perseveres through change. Psychoanalysis in a New Key publishes books that share the aims psychoanalysts have always had, but that approach them differently. The books in the series are not expected to advance any particular theoretical agenda, although to this date most have been written by analysts from the Interpersonal and Relational orientations.

The most important contribution of a psychoanalytic book is the communication of something that nudges the reader's grasp of clinical theory and practice in an unexpected direction. Psychoanalysis in a New Key creates a deliberate focus on innovative and unsettling clinical thinking. Because that kind of thinking is encouraged by exploration of the sometimes surprising contributions to psychoanalysis of ideas and findings from other fields, Psychoanalysis in a New Key particularly encourages interdisciplinary studies. Books in the series have married psychoanalysis with dissociation, trauma theory, sociology, and criminology. The series is open to the consideration of studies examining the relationship between psychoanalysis and any other field—for instance, biology, literary and art criticism, philosophy, systems theory, anthropology, and political theory.

But innovation also takes place within the boundaries of psychoanalysis, and Psychoanalysis in a New Key therefore also presents work that reformulates thought and practice without leaving the precincts of the field. Books in the series focus, for example, on the significance of personal values in psychoanalytic practice, on the complex interrelationship between the analyst's clinical work and personal life, on the consequences for the clinical situation when patient and analyst are from different cultures, and on the need for psychoanalysts to accept the degree to which they knowingly satisfy their own wishes during treatment hours, often to the patient's detriment. A full list of all titles in this series is available at: https://www.routledge.com/series/LEAPNKBS

The Role of the Patient-Analyst Match in the Process and Outcome of Psychoanalysis

Judy Leopold Kantrowitz

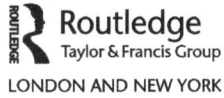

Routledge
Taylor & Francis Group

LONDON AND NEW YORK

First published 2020
by Routledge
2 Park Square, Milton Park, Abingdon, Oxon OX14 4RN

and by Routledge
52 Vanderbilt Avenue, New York, NY 10017

Routledge is an imprint of the Taylor & Francis Group, an
informa business

British Library Cataloguing-in-Publication Data
A catalogue record for this book is available from the British
Library

Library of Congress Cataloging-in-Publication Data
Names: Kantrowitz, Judy Leopold, 1958- author.
Title: The role of the patient-analyst match in the process and
outcome of psychoanalysis / Judy Leopold Kantrowitz.
Identifiers: LCCN 2019059032 (print) | LCCN 2019059033
(ebook) | ISBN 9780367483517 (hardback) |
ISBN 9780367483500 (paperback) | ISBN 9781003039488 (ebook)
Subjects: LCSH: Psychotherapist and patient. | Psychoanalysis.
Classification: LCC RC480.8 .K359 2020 (print) | LCC RC480.8
(ebook) | DDC 616.89/14—dc23
LC record available at https://lccn.loc.gov/2019059032
LC ebook record available at https://lccn.loc.gov/2019059033

ISBN: 978-0-367-48351-7 (hbk)
ISBN: 978-0-367-48350-0 (pbk)
ISBN: 978-1-003-03948-8 (ebk)

Typeset in Times New Roman
by codeMantra

Contents

Foreword

Theodore Jacobs, MD

The history of psychoanalysis in the past half century could be written from the perspective of a growing, and increasingly, sophisticated understanding of the centrally important contribution to the analytic process that is made by the interplay between the minds, characters, and life experiences of patient and analyst.

Prior to the mid-nineteen seventies, the focus of analytic interest and investigation was quite exclusively on the patient.

This was a time in many disciplines when the idea of objectivity held sway. Throughout academia, as well as in the professions, there was general endorsement of the idea that objectivity was both possible and highly desirable.

The task of the historian, for instance, was to discover the truth about the period of history she was studying, that of the literary critic the truth about the meaning of a poem or novel, and that of the analyst the truth about her patient's neurosis and the unconscious forces that produced it.

The analyst's job was to listen for that truth, grasp it, and interpret it to the patient who then would be liberated from its influence. The personality, history, life experiences of the analyst, even her countertransference reactions to the patient and the material of the hour, were believed to exert little influence on the course and outcome of the treatment.

Although it was three quarters of a century old, psychoanalysis was still in a comparatively early phase of its development and it remained strongly under the influence of Freud's followers who were fiercely loyal to the Professor.

Like Freud himself, these analysts, many of whom were emigrés from Austria and Germany, feared the alteration and dilution of the precious gift, depth psychology, that Freud had given the world. As a result, these traditionalists, seeking to preserve Freud's legacy, viewed with anxiety—and not a little contempt—any suggestion that analysis was not only a one-, but a two-person psychology.

In this atmosphere, the idea that one would undertake to investigate the interplay between the psychologies of patient and analyst, or even to explore the psychology of the analyst at work, was all but unthinkable.

It was a time, too, when the topic of countertransference lay under a dark cloud. Freud viewed countertransference as a problem of the analyst's, one that could block progress in treatment. This was also the position of the Freudians in America who adamantly opposed the idea put forward by the Kleinian, Paula Heimann, that countertransference represented unconscious transmissions from the mind of the patient which registered in the mind of the analyst.

To the Freudians, who, in general, rejected Klein's views, Heimann's contention was a misguided attempt to elevate countertransference to a place of unwarranted importance. In response, with Annie Reich as their spokesperson, they doubled down on the idea that countertransference is a problem of the analyst's that must be overcome through self-analytic work or additional treatment.

This view, coming as it did from an eminent colleague and echoing Freud's own position, had a powerful effect on analytic practice and education.

Countertransference became a matter not to be talked about, or even acknowledged, except, perhaps, to a few trusted colleagues in a private setting. Students and practitioners alike were afraid to speak of their countertransference experiences for fear that doing so would mark them as troubled individuals and/or insufficiently analyzed and would damage their reputations.

As a consequence of this situation, which had a smothering effect on analysts interested in exploring the phenomena of countertransference and the psychology of the analyst at work, for some fifteen years little or no progress was made in America in advancing our understanding of these two integral, and profoundly influential, aspects of the analytic process.

Judy Kantrowitz grew up analytically in this conservative climate. In her training, the focus was on understanding and interpreting the patient's material. The analyst's job was to listen with evenly hovering attention, grasp the unconscious conflicts and compromise formations that lay behind the patient's difficulties, and interpret them to the patient. The psychology of the analyst was not a factor unless her pathology intervened to disrupt the analytic process. It was generally assumed, however, that the well-analyzed analyst was sufficiently in control of her own issues so that they would not impact negatively on the analytic work.

There was little interest in, or curiosity about, the impact that the psychologies of patient and analyst had on one another.

To Judy Kantrowitz, this omission constituted a significant scotoma in the traditional understanding of the analytic process. Appreciative and respectful of the Classical tradition which she has valued throughout her career, Dr. Kantrowitz nevertheless realized that the way of thinking about the analytic situation that she was being taught did not do justice to the fact that two people are continually interacting in treatment: two individuals who bring their own psychologies, histories, belief systems, values, biases, defenses, and reactions to one another into the consulting room.

Judy Kantrowitz knew from her prior work with children, as well as from her observations of how people in close, ongoing relationships, inevitably influence, and often affect change in one another, how important a factor the interplay between patient and analyst is in all that happens in the analytic situation.

She was not alone in recognizing this neglected aspect of analytic theory and practice. The 1980s saw a gradual awakening among traditional analysts to the importance of the interactive and interpsychic dimension of analytic work, and, increasingly, the pages of our journals were filled with articles on the phenomena of enactments as well as papers that dealt with the interplay between transference and countertransference and its impact on the analytic process. The time had come when the idea of analysis as a one-person psychology had given way to the recognition that analysis inevitably involves two psychologies in continual interaction with one another.

Judy Kantrowitz's contribution to this shift in our conceptualization of the analytic process and to the consequent growth and development of the entire field of psychoanalysis has been immeasurable. Arguably her body of work, as amply demonstrated in this truly wonderful collection of her papers, constitutes the single most important influence in bringing psychoanalysis into the 21st century.

Unlike other clinicians who have made notable contributions to our understanding of the interactive aspect of analytic work, Judy Kantrowitz is not only a superb clinician, but an outstanding researcher.

Her publication in the late 1980s of her research on the subject of the match between patient and analyst established without question that the extent to which the personalities, styles, conflicts, and defenses of the two participants in analytic treatment either meshed in a favorable way or failed to mesh was a major determinant of the outcome of the analytic work.

This study put an end once and for all to the long-standing belief of the traditionalists that in a well-conducted analysis, the personal qualities of the analyst played little role in affecting the course and outcome of treatment.

This was of monumental importance because Kantrowitz's study made clear, not only that the traditional understanding of the analytic process was incomplete and limited, but that analysts needed to revise their ideas concerning the therapeutic action of psychoanalysis. No longer was it possible to maintain that it is solely the uncovering and working through of unconscious conflicts and compromise formations that is responsible for therapeutic change. By demonstrating that the person of the analyst, her way of working, and the way she interacts with the patient unquestionably contributes to the therapeutic action of analysis, Kantrowitz's work changed our understanding of how analysis operates.

Judy Kantrowitz's research also acted as a stimulus and encouragement for others to undertake studies of the patient-analyst relationship and, especially, the unconscious transmissions that regularly take place between them. These studies, in turn, greatly increased our understanding of the role played by unconscious communications in analytic treatment.

Judy Kantrowitz's work is unique in another respect. Not only does she open up new areas for study, but in many of her papers she portrays the interplay between patient and analyst with such vividness and richness of detail that the word pictures she creates bring to mind the exquisitely rendered character studies of the 17th-century Dutch master painters.

Originality is a hallmark of Kantrowitz's work, a quality clearly and engagingly illustrated in this invaluable collection of her papers. One such unique contribution is the paper in which, with rare self-reflection, she discusses how her usual and accustomed style of working, one that she took for granted and that, heretofore, had presented no problems, evoked an intensely negative reaction in one patient and very nearly upended the treatment. Because her style of working was so integral a part of her analytic identity and because it had not created difficulties of any kind, for some time she failed to recognize it as the source of her patient's negative reactions.

To write such a paper, an analyst has to have a well-honed capacity for self-reflection as well as uncompromising honesty and a willingness to share her errors—what Jim McLaughlin called our hard spots and dumb spots—with her colleagues. Judy Kantrowitz has an abundance of these qualities, and in this paper, the result of her ability to observe and reflect on herself in the immediacy of the analytic situation is a contribution that is original, insightful, and that, in alerting us to a common and most important scotoma in clinical practice, extremely useful.

Another remarkable contribution that Judy Kantrowitz offers us, one that stands out as unique in our literature, is her account of her son's death from brain cancer and the impact it had, both on her functioning as an analyst and on the several patients who knew about this tragedy.

Nowhere will you find a paper as sensitively written, as moving, and as valuable in recounting the struggle that an analyst undergoes when she attempts to carry on her analytic work during a time of emotional upheaval due to a personal loss or other painful trauma.

This seminal paper will long stand as a model for the way that thoughtful and disciplined self-reflection, along with keen observation of a patient's verbal and non-verbal behavior, allows an analyst, despite her coping with grief or other powerful, potentially disruptive emotions, to stay on course, carry on the work in a productive manner, and as exemplified in this splendid paper, make an invaluable contribution to our literature, a contribution that is unique in providing a resource for those colleagues, not a few in number, who choose to carry on with their analytic work while contending with severe emotional trauma.

This remarkable paper, however, is not alone among Judy Kantrowitz's work in focusing on aspects of analysis that have been little explored. Another original chapter in this book is given over to an examination of the preconscious and its role both in mental life and in treatment.

The term, preconscious, is, of course, well known, but its place in normal psychology and our patients' everyday mental operations has not been well described in the writings on clinical process.

Judy Kantrowitz illuminates the function of the preconscious and demonstrates that it exists as the link between the relational world and that of the unconscious. It is from the preconscious, she points out, that patients' associations emerge and it is to the preconscious that the analyst's interpretations are directed. It is the area of patients' minds that does business with the analyst and the world of objects. As such, we need to better understand it and its role in mental life.

In her discussion of this subject and her clinical examples, Judy Kantrowitz takes us a long way on this path of understanding.

Extremely useful, too, is the chapter in which Kantrowitz demonstrates how valuable it is for a third party to comment on our understanding of our cases and the thinking that goes into our formulations of them. This is not supervision, per se, but rather the creative sharing of our clinical work.

It is particularly useful, Kantrowitz points out, for a third party to listen for the kind of match that has taken place between patient and analyst. Because she may be invested in seeing the match in a particular way, the analyst may not be aware of problems in this aspect of the relationship that are affecting the treatment. Another pair of eyes viewing the way patient and analyst interact from outside the transference-countertransference matrix may offer a clearer view of the kind of match that actually exists.

As a researcher, Judy Kantrowitz is, of course, best known for her seminal work on just this issue: The match between patient and analyst, but her studies of other aspects of analytic work are also important.

In this respect, her paper on the question of how and in what way doing analytic work changes the analyst is a fascinating one.

In typical fashion, Kantrowitz tackles this problem head on. She eschews generalities and chooses instead to undertake an interview of one colleague, in which he describes the process of change that took place in him as he worked with a challenging patient. The unique value in this paper, as is true of many of Judy Kantrowitz's articles, is her ability to give the reader a detailed account of an emotional and psychological process. This greatly enhances our understanding of what actually took place in the therapist's psyche as he worked with his patient, and provides the kind of evidence that can be utilized in future studies. This paper opens up an important frontier in analytic work.

The question of how analysts are changed by their work and by different kinds of patients is a relatively unexplored area. It is one, however, as Judy Kantrowitz points out, that we need to learn a great deal more about as changes in the analyst inevitably affect the patient and the analytic work.

As is evident, Judy Kantrowitz likes to tackle difficult and important topics, one of which is a question that analytic authors regularly face and that plays a central role in advancing our field: writing about patients.

In her typically direct way, Judy Kantrowitz has investigated this issue by eliciting the experiences and views of authors who have published clinical material and have had to contend with this thorny question. Kantrowitz's work has clarified the many dimensions of this problem and the variety of ways analysts seek to deal with the difficulties inherent in each approach, thus providing valuable information for those who wish to publish clinical material.

Readers of this wonderful book are not only in for a great treat—Judy Kantrowitz's papers are most enjoyable to read—but a rich educational experience. For among her many valuable contributions, one that I believe is among her most enduring is her role as a superb teacher.

There is not one paper in this collection that does not enlarge and enhance our understanding of some aspect of the relationship between patient and analyst and hence of the analytic process itself.

What Judy Kantrowitz has given us, then, in this book, is a rare gift, one to be read, re-read, and treasured. It contains some of the most important thinking and writing in the field of psychoanalysis to appear in the past half century.

Reading Judy Kantrowitz, in short, is for all of us, no matter our age, background, theoretical orientation, or our years in the field, a growth experience. She teaches us to think, to explore, to expand our curiosity about ourselves as well as our patients, and to be adventurous. By lending us her knowledge, her wisdom, and her courage, she enlarges our vision, enhances our sensitivities, and, like all great teachers, makes us better at what we do. There can be no greater gift.

Foreword

Donnel B. Stern

Judy Kantrowitz tells us in her introduction about the history of this book. Even though she was a candidate in good standing at her institute, she was required, because she is a psychologist and not a psychiatrist, to create a research project to satisfy the demands of the CORST waiver she needed in order to take on the clinical part of the training. In those days, nonpsychiatrists, who could only be trained as "research candidates" (that is, people who were trained in order to do research, not clinical work), were required by the American Psychoanalytic Association, the professional organization Dr. Kantrowitz hoped eventually to join, to demonstrate their capacity to do research, and their commitment to it. That must have been maddening for someone who, like Dr. Kantrowitz, knew she wanted to be a clinician. (She tells me she was told by her institute that she would be free to be a clinical psychoanalyst if her CORST research addressed a clinical topic, but of course her psychiatrist colleagues faced no such requirement.) Not too many years later, in response to the famous lawsuit mounted by a group of psychologists, the policy of restricting clinical training to psychiatrists was declared illegal, a restraint of trade. No one mourns it.

But Dr. Kantrowitz made a silk purse from a sow's ear. In fact, she did the best job I know of transforming the one into the other. She already felt that it made little sense to claim, as most mainstream analysts of the day did, that the analyst's character and conflicts were not relevant to the process and outcome of treatment. And so she embarked on a project that must have been at least as much a rebellious gesture as an obedient one. She rooted her CORST-qualifying research in her belief that *both* participants' character and conflicts were crucial, and she ended up creating a piece of research that was widely read when it was published and retains landmark significance today. That research on "the match" between the patient and the analyst is presented in this volume, the remainder of which is devoted to the many papers Dr. Kantrowitz has written since then on the clinical implications of the match.

As surely as any research outcome can be, the main finding of this research, and the clinical phenomenon these findings describe, is unassailable: the match between the analyst and the patient is highly significant in predicting the success of psychoanalytic treatment—more significant, as a matter of fact, than the factors, centering on ego strength, that analysts of that time believed were the best predictors. This finding demonstrated not only that the analyst's character and conflicts were important to outcome, though. By implication, it also made it impossible to ignore the effect of the analyst's character on the ongoing psychoanalytic process. In other words, because the match predicted outcome, it could not be ignored that both analyst and patient were part of the process all the way along.

It was a different time in psychoanalysis. Interpersonal psychoanalysts had been creating since the 1930s a theory of psychoanalysis in which Dr. Kantrowitz's work would have been right at home; but their work was vilified in most mainstream quarters as superficial, too present-oriented, and too little focused on the internal world and the unconscious. The interpersonal principle that the analyst's personality was crucial to the nature of clinical process and outcome was simply seen by most mainstream analysts as one more evidence of the same superficial emphasis of the external world. Today those old canards have been abandoned, and interpersonal psychoanalysis (and relational psychoanalysis, which came along a little later) is no longer sidelined; but when she began her work, these were the attitudes Dr. Kantrowitz ran into in bringing her thinking to an audience of classical analysts.

Most mainstream or classical analysts of that day, whose ego psychological theory dominated North American psychoanalysis, believed that psychoanalysis was a technique that, when mastered by a capable practitioner, should lead to a successful outcome in any case in which the patient was properly selected. "Proper selection" was constituted by an assessment of a set of characteristics of the patient, the aspects of ego strength I have already mentioned (Dr. Kantrowitz goes into this matter in detail in the text.) The judgments of these characteristics, together, made up the criterion referred to as "analyzability." (The determination of analyzability, especially its use in selecting training cases, was maintained in some psychoanalytic institutes until recently, and may still exist in some.) From this perspective, when "standard psychoanalytic technique" is properly applied to a properly selected patient, the analyst's character and conflicts should be irrelevant to the outcome.

Dr. Kantrowitz faced closed-mindedness and arrogance in her attempt to write about the match. When she submitted a paper to one of the mainstream journals, one of the editors wrote that she had "a strange idea about psychoanalysis." She seemed to believe, he said, that psychoanalysis involves making the unconscious conscious and also something about the relationship. "You have to choose," he said. The editor's reaction brought those days vividly back to me: there was continuous argumentation in the mainstream, classical journals about the validity of "relational effects," which were often portrayed (when they were considered at all) as inferior to "structural change" brought about by interpretation. About the editor's reaction, Dr. Kantrowitz comments pithily (and wryly, if I read her tone correctly) that, "I felt very well understood, but strongly disagreed with the editor's conclusion."

But eventually, even those who held the most conservative views of psychoanalysis were hard-pressed, in the face of all the evidences to the contrary, Dr. Kantrowitz's writing prominent among them, to maintain their certainty that relational effects were somehow insubstantial and that the nature of the analyst's character and conflicts were irrelevant to the outcome of a capable analyst's work. Over the years, Dr. Kantrowitz refined and expanded her work, until it attained the classic status it now enjoys.

In closing, let me attempt an overview of what Dr. Kantrowitz believes is most clinically significant about the concept of the match. Any time one side of an issue gains prominence, the other side tends to be ignored. Dr. Kantrowitz applies this principle to the relationship of the intrapsychic and the interpersonal/relational. That is, as much as she felt, and still feels, that structure, continuity, and the internal world used to be over-emphasized, she now feels that the pendulum has swung too far in the other direction, so that process and context, discontinuity, and the psychic significance of the external world are now given more prominence than they should be. Dr. Kantrowitz's work, which began as a corrective to the old bias (and still has that meaning for her), has now become, in addition, in her own eyes, a contribution to the correction of the new imbalance. To attend to the match is to attend to structural characteristics of the analytic situation: the character and lifelong conflicts of both the analyst and the patient. Dr. Kantrowitz hopes that analysts will be encouraged by her work to ask themselves hard questions about who they are, and what the effect of their character is on the patient. She accepts the importance of context, of paying close attention to the conscious and unconscious, moment-to-moment events of clinical process, but she also wants us to recognize the effects of the larger, more stable, structural considerations—basically, as she says, internal object relations.

The match, says Dr. Kantrowitz, is important not only in treatment, but also as a lens through which to understand and use supervision. Just as the match in the clinical setting is usually investigated privately by the analyst, the match in supervision is not a joint project, but an activity carried out by the analyst within their own mind. The "triadic match"—the match between patient, analyst, and supervisor—is part of what determines the degree of success of the supervisory work and the kind of growth that can take place through it, for all three participants in it. As is true of the treating analyst in the treatment setting, the supervisor, too, may grow as a result of their investigation of the supervisory match, both dyadic (i.e., the match between supervisor and supervisee) and triadic.

In the end, what is most important to Dr. Kantrowitz about the concept of the match is its encouragement to us to do whatever we can to investigate the effects on the analytic situation of who each of us has come to be. Dr. Kantrowitz hopes that her work will encourage psychoanalysts to learn something about themselves—and then to do it again and again. Attending to the match, that is, can contribute not only to the patient's growth, but also to the analyst's. The significance of the analyst's character to the ongoing clinical encounter changes as the treatment itself changes, but it never ceases to be a crucial consideration. The match is always important and never stands still.

Acknowledgments

There are so many people I wish to thank since this is a compilation of work over my professional lifetime. To begin with the present: I am extremely grateful to Donnel Stern for inviting me to publish in his series. Throughout the process, he has been informative and extremely helpful—wonderful to work with. I also wish to thank Kate Hawes, Hannah Wright and the Routledge staff for the help in making this publication happen. I am grateful to Kim Bernstein for her conceptual editing of the introductory chapter and to Kris Springer for his copy editing the last chapter and the references. Were it not for the encouragement of Ellen Pinsky and Phil Blumberg, I might not have pursued this project. An added thanks to Phil for reading the entire book and offering very helpful edits and suggestions. Some colleagues, like these, also become close friends and enrich my life in a multitude of ways. I do not take this for granted. I am deeply appreciative.

I am grateful to Don Stern and Ted Jacobs for their introductions. Both have been sensitive to my experiences and intent in writing this book. Having both an Interpersonal and a classically trained analyst explicating aspects of my work unites my own thinking—though I would add that Ted and I have both always thought in this fashion. Happily, the psychoanalytic world in North America now has mostly joined this view. Ted's detailed understanding and appreciation of my work moves me deeply. An added benefit of writing, in addition to what we ourselves learn as we do it, is that it enables us to find similarly minded colleagues who enlarge our own personal and professional worlds.

My thanks to Jonathan Palmer for again letting me use one of his beautiful paintings as a cover for my book, as well as for a friendship and colleagueship that nurtures my life.

I am enormously grateful to Olga Umansky for her patience and help facilitating me in contacting publication houses to enable me to get permission to reprint my papers. Olga, our BPSI librarian, has also been a friend and supporter of me, and my work, over the years and so my thanks is far more than just specifically for her latest help.

I wish to thank my colleagues who contributed to the earliest part of my study of the match as research assistants: Judy Singer, Frank Paolitto, Leonard Soloman, Ann Katz, Humphrey Morris, and Deborah Greenman.

Over the years, so many colleagues and friends have contributed their perspectives and editorial ideas about my papers. My writing group—Steve Bernstein, Dan Jacobs, Malkah Notman, and Judy Yanof—has worked together for over 25 years. I have learned a lot from each of them. Many others have read and critiqued some of my writing: Natalie Bluestone, Phil Blumberg, Nancy Chodorow, Bernard Edelstein, Bob Gardner, Fran Givelber, Ellen Golding, Bill Grossman, Tony Kris, Shelley Orgel, Jonathan Palmer, Edith Perlman, Ellen Pinsky, Evy Schwaber, Austin Silber, and Anna Wolff.

My psychoanalytic teachers contributed to my growth as an analyst. I am especially grateful to Bob Gardner who supported attention to my countertransference at a time this was not a fashionable idea in the Boston psychoanalytic community—a time, fortunately, long past.

I have continued to learn about myself, and my work, through on-going peer supervision. For 10–15 years, I worked in peer supervision with both Bill Grossman and Austin Silber. In their very different ways, they both stretched my capacities. I am very grateful. I miss both of them a lot. In subsequent years, I have continued very helpful peer supervision with Gerry Fogel, Brian Robertson, and Judy Chused—each has helped me expand my analytic self. I am also grateful to my peer supervision group: Nancy Chodorow, Alex Harrison, Dan Jacobs, and Jonathan Palmer for the opportunity to continue to learn together about our work. My New York study group—Rosemary Balsam, Phil Blumberg, Dennis Haseley, Ted Jacobs, and Nancy Kulish, which previously included Jay Greenberg, Henry Nunberg, and Shelley Orgel—have also contributed to my growth and pleasure. Steve Goldberg has been my valued intellectual companion in learning about impasses in our study groups about treatment and supervision.

And, of course, I am grateful to all my patients over the years from whom I have learned so much about the human psyche, theirs, mine, and ours together—the topic of this book.

My children, Steve and Amy, have also been my teachers. I love and admire them for their values, and contributions to the world—and just for who they are. They are both creative and generous with themselves. I continue to miss our youngest son Jeff, who died of a brain tumor at 31, but I am grateful for the time we had. My grandchildren—Sophie and Elliot—-inspire me with their warmth, curiosity, fun-loving ways. To see them grow is something for which to be very grateful. And I am grateful to my parents. My father's life was difficult, losing his own father when he was six, helping his mother and siblings to survive, but never losing his warmth, sense of fun and common sense. My mother grew up with more economic privilege, but had to face limiting ideas about what a woman's role should be in the 1950s and 1960s. She was a serious and gifted artist who pursued her work despite these strictures, but never allowed herself to display the fullness of her talent. Both my parents were models to me about how to persevere, as well as enjoy life.

When I was appointed a training and supervising analyst in 1989, I had a dream: I was in my childhood living room. A staircase opened and I descended to my professional office. I said out loud, "How did I get from there to here?" Perhaps what I have just written explains part of it. I was an English major in college, wanting to write short stories as a career, but I soon recognized I really didn't have the imaginative talent for such a career. I knew my interest was in character, and after some exploration, I decided to go to graduate school in clinical psychology. At the time, it never occurred to me that I could have a career as a psychoanalyst. Going to medical school, I knew suited neither my interest nor skills. I never imagined that I could have the kind of rich and satisfying professional life I have had. I could not have done this without the support of all the people cited above. But most all, it was the support and love of my husband which made this possible for me.

My gratitude to my husband Paul is beyond anything I can express. He has supported and encouraged me in my career since we first met in 1957. His belief in me, his patience, kindness, and love have made it possible for me to work and to write and live the kind of professional life I never imagined I would have. He says "genes and luck in no particular order" determine most of what happens to us. We were both so young when we met and married—mostly luck—but also work; I'd say that made our life come out as it has.

My thanks to Sage, Taylor & Francis, and James Harrison, the editor of *The Annual of Psychoanalysis*, for giving me permission to reprint my previously published papers.

Previously published or part of papers reprinted in this volume:

Kantrowitz, J.L. The role of the patient-analyst "match" in the outcome of psychoanalysis. *Annu. Psychoanal.*, 1986; 14: 273–297.

Kantrowitz, J.L., Katz, A.L., Greenman, D., Morris, H., Paolitto, F., Sashin, J., Solomon, L. The patient-analyst match and the outcome of psychoanalysis: The study of 13 cases. Research in progress. *J. Amer. Psychoanal. Assn.*, 1989; 37:893–920.

Kantrowitz, J.L., Katz, A.L., Paolitto, F. Follow-up of psychoanalysis five-to-ten years after termination: III. The relationship of the transference neurosis to the patient-analyst match. *J. Amer. Psychoanal. Assn.*, 1990; 38: 655–678.

Kantrowitz, J.L. The analyst's style and its impact on the psychoanalytic process: overcoming stalemates. *J. Amer. Psychoanal. Assn.*, 1992; 40: 169–194.

Kantrowitz, J.L. Impasses in psychoanalysis: overcoming resistance in situations of stalemate. *J. Amer. Psychoanal. Assn.*, 1993; 41: 1021–1050.

Kantrowitz, J.L. The uniqueness of the patient-analyst pair: elucidating the role of the analyst. *Int. J. Psychoanal.*, 1993; 74: 893–904.

Kantrowitz, J.L. The beneficial aspects of the patient-analyst match: factors in addition to clinical acumen and therapeutic skill that contribute to psychological change. *Int. J. Psychoanal.*, 1995; 76: 299–313.

Kantrowitz, J.L. The Triadic Match: candidate, patient, and supervisor. *J. Amer. Psychoanal. Assn.*, 2002; 50: 919–968.

Kantrowitz, J.L. The external observer and the patient-analyst match. *Int. J. Psychoanal.*, 2002; 83: 339–350.

Kantrowitz, J. L. A different view of the therapeutic process: the impact of the patient on the analyst. *J. Amer. Psychoanal. Assn.*, 1997; 44: 127–153.

Kantrowitz, J. L. The role of the preconscious in psychoanalysis. *J. Amer. Psychoanal. Assn.*, 1999; 46: 65–89.

Kantrowitz, J.L. Privacy and disclosure in psychoanalysis. *J. Amer. Psychoanal. Assn.*, 2009; 57:787–806.

Kantrowitz, J.L. The effect of post-analytic contact. *J. Amer. Psychoanal. Assn.*, 2013; 61:947–956.

Kantrowitz, J.L. Appreciation of the importance of the patient-analyst "match." *Psychiatry*, 2016; 79(1):23–28.

Kantrowitz, J.L. Reflections on mortality: a patient faces death. *J. Amer. Psychoanal. Assn.*, 2017; 65:673–686.

Introduction

When I began writing about the effect of the patient-analyst match on the process and outcome of psychoanalysis in the early 1970s, my theory and clinical work were in reaction to ideas I was being taught that analysts were, or could be, "blank screens," each interchangeable with another. Our patients' defensive strategies in dealing with their conflicts provided a central focus for our study. It was a one-person view of psychoanalysis, taught as a stringent and limited reading of ego psychology, which asserted that if we adequately evaluated a patient's reality testing, level and quality of object relations, affect availability and tolerance, and motivation, we could then predict who would, and could not, be successfully analyzed. Today I doubt that any psychoanalyst, regardless of specific theoretical identification, would subscribe to such a belief. So why is the concept of the patient-analyst match still relevant?

First, let me clarify what I do and don't mean by "match." I am not referring to identity markers like ethnicity or sexual orientation or other externally observable factors. Such factors may be important to the match between patient and analyst, but if they are, it would be because of their meaning to the particular participants, not merely because these sorts of similarities or differences exist between them.

Just as match cannot be reduced to external sociological factors, it is also not the same as empathy. Empathy facilitates connection; it is about how one listens, but it does not address the range and depth of what one can hear or how one responds. Match is about matters of character and conflict, conscious and unconscious, which mesh or clash between patient and analyst. Match is what drives the therapeutic action of psychoanalysis.

A focus on the match between patient and analyst places attention on the dynamic effect of interactions of character and conflict of both participants on the process that evolves between them—a spectrum of compatibility and incompatibility of patient and analyst that is relevant to the analytic work. Match refers to observable styles, attitudes, and personal characteristics that may be rooted in residual and unanalyzed conflicts, triggered in any patient-analyst pair. It includes individual histories, attitudes, and values that predispose analyst and patient, respectively, to certain transference and countertransference responses. Match is neither a predictive nor static concept. Rather, it refers to the unfolding transaction that itself may shift and change during the course of analytic work. A match that is facilitating at one phase of treatment may become impeding to the process at another stage. The match is in an intentionally capacious concept. Some qualities emphasized in one dyad are irrelevant for another dyad while other qualities are important in that dyad. Match is, and is meant to be, a fuzzy category.

How one makes use of the concept of match will depend on one's particular theoretical orientation. Although it is not linked to any particular school of theory, match is salient with respect to other contemporary psychoanalytic concepts such as unrepresented states (Bion, 1971, 2013; Civitarese, 2005, 2010; Ferro, 2002, 2009; Levine, Reed, & Scarfone, 2013), unformulated experience (Stern, 1983, 2012), and witnessing and trauma (Benjamin, 1993, 2017; Laub, 1992; Stern, 2012). For all of these concepts, it is essential for analyst and patient to have sufficient similarity, an aspect of match, to attain an overlap where unconscious resonance can occur, but be different enough for the patient to expand in range and depth of affect availability and tolerance (Modell, 1990, 2006). This is the crucible, wherein both intrapsychic and interpersonal relationships can be transformed.

Match occurs without conscious representation and is hard to predict at the outset. We do not use the match with our patients so much as the match contributes to the shape of our participation. Match is dynamic, not static. A match that allows one to get into the analytic work could keep one from completing it. Both consciously and unconsciously, a similarity may initially facilitate engagement with an aspect of a patient that is troublesome, helping the patient to find ways of expressing this difficulty; however, over time, too much similarity may interfere with the analyst's capacity to expand her engagement with this same part of a patient, limiting the extent of therapeutic gain. For example, a gentle analyst may facilitate an inhibited analysand beginning analytic work, but later in the process, if the analyst doesn't become more assertive, this same gentle style may fail to address the analysand's defenses sufficiently for the analysand to face and resolve conflicts. Too much difference may make it hard to engage initially, but has the potential to lead to great therapeutic change if the analyst is able to find a resonance with patient's areas of distress.

The importance of the match between patient and analyst seemed unthinkable to most classically trained psychoanalysts in North America from the 1950s through the 1970s, because they maintained a one-person model of treatment. The belief that psychoanalytic work was a two-person enterprise did not become a mainstream idea here until the late 1980s, and not a prominent one until the 1990s. But even then, attention to the specificity of the match between the participants was rare. In putting this volume together, it is my hope that analysts will again consider the particulars of overlap and disjunction between patient and analyst as they so profoundly affect the pair's ability to work together.

***

Psychoanalysts trained in the classical tradition in North America were taught that they could, and should, serve as "blank screens" onto which patients projected their difficulties. The expectation was that analysts' conflicts were to have been resolved in their own analyses. In the event that an analyst had countertransference reactions to a patient, these experiences were viewed as unexpected and problematic, a reason to seek further personal treatment. This idealized view of psychoanalysis was maintained by the vast majority of North American training institutes throughout the 1950s and 1960s.

In the context of a belief that only the qualities of the patient determined the outcome of psychoanalysis, it was also assumed that analysts could predict in advance which patients could and could not be successfully analyzed. Given adequate reality testing, affect availability and tolerance, and level of object relationships, if the person was motivated, it was assumed that any analyst of sufficient experience should be able to analyze such a patient. The definition of all these terms remained abstract.

Perhaps not all Institutes were quite so unrealistic in their assumptions as the Boston Psychoanalytic Society and Institute in 1968, but I know from many of my colleagues in other parts of the North America that such convictions were in no way unique to Boston. Although I was a candidate newly learning about psychoanalysis, the idea that patients alone determined the nature of the analytic interaction stretched my credulity. How could a process in which two people were involved depend on only one of them? How could any person, no matter how well analyzed, not have personal reactions that in some way would be apparent to their patients?

Of course, even in 1968, not all North American psychoanalysts subscribed to these views—Interpersonal psychoanalysts certainly didn't. But we had little exposure to those whose ideas that were in dissent. I remember my appreciation of reading Loewald (1960) and Stone (1962) who remained in the ego psychological point of view while still having views that took into account that two people were involved in the analytic process. One of our teachers did introduce us to different ideas these analysts offered. I thought their more complex, nuanced, and humanistic way of looking at analytic work made sense, but when I tried to discuss ideas raised by their thinking, most of my other analytic teachers showed little interest, and certainly no enthusiasm, in pursuing these questions.

During this era, North American psychoanalysts maintained a conviction that only individuals with medical training should become practicing psychoanalysts; this conviction shaped standards for inclusion/exclusion for acceptance for training at The American Psychoanalytic Institutes (APsaA). It was another rigidity of the time. At that time, the only nonphysicians to be accepted for psychoanalytic training, even to take academic courses as Affiliate Scholars, were fully established academics, who learned the psychoanalytic concepts to be used in their own field of study. The only way to gain permission to learn how to analyze patients was to obtain a waiver from APsaA by undertaking a research project. In 1968, the APsaA established a new category: people who showed "promise" to be contributors to psychoanalytic knowledge could be accepted. It was that year when I applied for training. I had recently completed graduate school and was working in a clinic, supervised by training and supervising analysts who encouraged me to apply for analytic training. I also had contributed to a study on dream deprivation by analyzing the Rorschach data; my name was on the publication. I applied to the Boston Institute (BPSI). I was accepted as an affiliate scholar. Because I was a clinical psychologist and not a physician, as expected, I was not permitted to be trained to analyze patients. The only permissible way to embark on learning to analyze patients was by undertaking a research study requiring a waiver from the APsaA—which could not be applied for until *after* I had completed four years of seminars. The waiver, known as the CORST waiver, gave a nonmedical candidate permission to see psychoanalytic patients under supervision, just as all medical candidates automatically did as part of their training. The research project was to enhance the understanding of some psychoanalytic concept in order to justify the nonmedical candidate learning to treat psychoanalytic patients. If that sounds grossly unfair and complicated, it was, but it was the tenure of the times and I wanted the training.

Except during the Vietnam War, when a few psychologists had been trained at the Menninger Foundation, people without medical degrees who trained as CORST candidates had been required to sign a waiver that they would not practice psychoanalysis. I was very clear in my interviews that I was applying as a clinician, not a researcher. My interviewers were equally clear with me that although they personally had no objection to my entering a full training and eventually practicing as a psychoanalyst, the American Psychoanalytic Association would not entertain my applying to be a CORST candidate until I had completed classes. They encouraged me to begin training as an affiliate scholar and later apply for the waiver. I did so, but every year I wrote to the education committee at the Institute, asking them to consider appealing this restrictive position. I explained that not having cases diminished the value of the didactic education. I was repeatedly told to be patient—not my strongest suit!

As soon as I finished all four years of coursework in 1972, I developed a project and applied for a CORST waiver. I had the support of the Boston Institute in this process, though I continued to be clear with them that I would not be willing to sign an agreement forbidding me from practicing as a psychoanalyst. My mentors assured me that as long as my research project was directly related to a psychoanalytic process, which required me to be immersed in conducting psychoanalysis with patients, it would not be necessary for me to sign such a waiver.

It was apparent to me from the start that a good number of my teachers were not in agreement with the prevailing notions that clinical psychologists were unsuitable for becoming clinical psychoanalysts. Many believed that over time these restrictions would be removed. I doubt that without such support that I could have proceeded, since I was aware that some other teachers were not inclined to accept me as a clinician. In fact, a number of the senior analysts strongly objected even to my doing research on the psychoanalytic process. This was the tenor of the 1970s at the Boston Institute.

All these restrictions were soon to be challenged and overturned in response to a suit initiated by the American Psychological Association (APA) against the American Psychoanalytic Association for restraint of trade. In 1983, the psychologists won the suit, and it was not long after that qualified social workers, followed by other mental health professionals, were also admitted for full psychoanalytic training.

It was during the 1980s that North American psychoanalysis began to relinquish many of its orthodox views. My research project on the effect of patient-analyst match on the process and outcome of psychoanalysis provided support for the growing acknowledgment that psychoanalysis was a two-person process. However, my findings were taken seriously only because our psychoanalytic world was ready for such a different perspective on the analytic process.

The subject I chose to examine for my CORST project was a study of patients' suitability for psychoanalysis and the outcome of analysis. The project then evolved to become a study of the patient-analyst match and its relationship to the outcome of psychoanalysis. For this prospective, longitudinal study of 22 supervised cases, I proposed that after these patients had been approved as suitable cases for candidates but prior to beginning their analyses, I would assess their reality testing, the level and quality of their object relations, their affect availability and tolerance, and their motivation for psychoanalysis. These characteristics were ones cited in psychoanalytic literature as necessary to be a suitable patient for the psychoanalytic method. For this assessment, I employed the Rorschach, Thematic Apperception Test (TAT), Draw-a-Person Test, Cole Animal Test, and some sub-tests from the verbal part of the Webster Intelligence Scale for Adults (WAIS). I was not permitted to do a clinical interview since some analysts at BPSI worried it might interfere with the ensuing analytic process.

My design further proposed that a year after termination these patients would be retested on the same measures; at that time, I was permitted to interview the patients since it could no longer interfere with their analyses. In these interviews, I would ask the analysands about their views about what had and hadn't changed for them on these four variables and their views about the analytic process itself. Although it was not stated in my proposal, when analysands talked about the analytic process, this inevitably involved views of their analysts. I would also interview the treating analysts at the time the patients terminated analysis. In this interview, I would ask their assessment of their patients on these same four variables assessed on the psychological tests. I would also ask how they had seen their patients initially and how they believed they had changed.[1] My proposal was accepted for a CORST waiver, and I began this study in 1975.

While the post-analysis assessments indicated that there was often change in the four variables over the course of treatment (Kantrowitz et al., 1986, 1987a, 1987b), none of these variables alone or in combination predicted outcomes. I did not doubt that a requisite amount of the four patient characteristics assessed would be necessary to withstand what were then very classical analyses where modifications, at the time termed parameters, were not entertained.[2] However, in contrast to a belief that the patient's psychological strengths and organization alone could predict whether or not psychoanalysis would be successful, my hypothesis was that the interface of characteristics and conflicts *of both the patient and the analyst* would also inevitably play a role in the course and outcome of the analysis.

In order to assess whether and how analyst variables played a role, I developed a scale for evaluating aspects of the analyst's characteristics, attitudes, and ways of relating to the patient. The data for these evaluations were derived from analysts' spontaneous comments during the tape-recorded post-termination interviews (Kantrowitz et al., 1989). Based on a deconstruction of those interviews, I created a profile of each analyst, which was independently and reliably validated by sets of different independent raters. Two advanced candidates in psychoanalytic training then independently compared the analysts' profiles and the evaluations of changes on the psychological tests for each patient-analyst pair.[3]

My findings showed that when characteristics of the analyst's difficulties were too similar to those of the patient, these conflicts did not change for the better for the patient during the course of analysis. The results also indicated that too great a dissimilarity could also be problematic, yielding limited change. It was the patient-analyst "match"—in contrast to the four variables assumed necessary for analytic suitability—that turned out to be the most successful predictor of the outcome of psychoanalysis (Kantrowitz et al., 1989; Kantrowitz, Katz, & Paolitto, 1990).

While the research methodology was somewhat primitive, my study was, at that time, more relevant to clinical questions, such as the clinical efficacy of the analytic process than many other more empirical studies with greater statistical rigor. I did recognize that there were many limitations to this study[4] and viewed it, accordingly, as a pilot project. I had hoped that others with more sophisticated research skills in this area would follow up this study in a more systematic rigorous fashion.

The concept of match that my study was designed to explore refers to observable styles, attitudes, and personal characteristics that may be rooted in residual and unanalyzed conflicts triggered in any patient-analyst pair. It includes individual histories, attitudes, and values that predispose analyst and patient, respectively, to certain transference and countertransference responses. Match is neither a predictive nor static concept; rather, it refers to an unfolding transaction that itself shifts and changes during the course of analytic work. The dynamic effect of the interaction of character and conflict of both participants will have influenced what did and did not get attended to in a given analysis.

The pilot study, described above, obviously could not assess all these dimensions based on the limited data available to me, but the fact that the patient-analyst variable showed the strongest relationship to analytic outcome served to support changes in the beliefs of many North American psychoanalysts trained in American Psychoanalytic

Association-affiliated institutes, who had already begun to take serious issue with the idea of a one-person psychology.

***

Psychoanalyses take time; I could not return to my prospective study, begun in 1975, until the participating patients had completed their analyses. In the interim, I wrote a clinical paper illustrating my idea about the patient-analyst match. In 1980, I began submitting this paper—the one that begins the collection of papers contained in this volume—to the mainstream classical psychoanalytic journals: *The Journal of the American Psychoanalytic Association* (JAPA), *The International Journal of Psychoanalysis* (IJP), and *The Psychoanalytic Quarterly* (PQ). All three rejected it. One editor pithily summarized the reason for the paper's rejection, writing that I had a strange idea about psychoanalysis: that it involved making the unconscious conscious as well as something to do with the relationship. In short, he proclaimed, I had to choose. I felt very well understood, but strongly disagreed with the editor's conclusion.

By then I knew that although my ideas about match did not seem to be represented in the mainstream psychoanalytic literature, I was far from alone in my belief that analysts' personal qualities and conflicts played a significant role in what transpired in analyses. Bibring (1936), Berman (1949), Anna Freud (1954), and Greenson (1967) had all cited their awareness of the inevitability of countertransference; they also recognized that each analyst's uniqueness meant that their particular qualities would likely influence their responses to each patient. Nonetheless, these ideas had not been part of my training. I did not discover Racker's influential paper on the analyst's countertransference (1957), for example, until after I had graduated. I also was not aware of North American analysts, such as Kernberg (1965), who elaborated on the uses of countertransference. Analysts in other parts of the world had been exploring the world of object relations; papers such as Sandler's "Countertransference and Role Responsiveness" (1976) indicated an awareness of the two-person process and had illustrated its importance in analytic work. But neither these works nor the work of the Interpersonalists was part of our training, nor were they viewed as significant to an appreciation of what transpired in psychoanalysis by most of our teachers at the Boston Institute in the 1970s.

By the mid- to late 1980s, not only were some of the foundational classical psychoanalytic beliefs of North American psychoanalysts being questioned by many experienced and respected analysts in North America, but ideas about the importance of how the analytic personal qualities influenced the anlaytic process started to appear in the mainstream psychoanalytic journals. In 1981, James McLaughlin, who had the respect and admiration of many classical psychoanalytic adherents, published a paper in *The Psychoanalytic Quarterly* on the analyst's transference to the patient. In the paper, he elaborated on the clinical impact of his "blind spots" based on his own personal history and conflicts, "hard spots" due to his adherence to particular theories, and "dumb spots" as a result of his ignorance. Then in 1983, Irwin Hoffman published his now classic paper "The Patient as the Interpreter of the Analyst's Experience." While Hoffman was not viewed as a classical analyst in the way McLaughlin was, he was a disciple of Merton Gill, whose ideas about transference were influential in most psychoanalytic institutes. A shift in the zeitgeist of North American psychoanalysis had begun.

More attention was being given to analyst factors. Irma Brenman Pick's 1985 paper on countertransference sensitively elaborated the tightrope analysts walked: failure to recognize one's own personal conflicts, stimulated by the patient's conflicts, would lead to enactment rather than interpretation. Neither Pick nor Sandler was referring to the analyst's reactions specifically as "the match" between patient and analyst, but this is, of course, what they were describing.

Finally in 1986, *The Annual of Psychoanalysis*, which often accepted more controversial material, published my paper on the match. The following year, American psychoanalytic journals began to publish the results of my follow-up study.[5]

Prior to attending the Institute, I had read and appreciated works of Harry Stack Sullivan (1953), though my training had not included the Interpersonal perspective being taught at the William Alanson White Institute, or anything about the importance of the clinical relationship—as I previously said, Loewald (1960) and Stone (1962) being notable exception. I'm sure my earlier exposure to Sullivan had influenced my thinking. I knew who Clara Thompson was. I think

I had read some of Thompson's papers outside the Institute curriculum, but I knew nothing of her writing about the match between patient and analyst. It wasn't until 2015, when the editor of *Psychiatry* invited me to write a commentary on it, that I discovered Thompson's "Notes on the Psychoanalytic Significance of the Choice of Analyst" (1938). In it, Thompson proposed that the personality of the analyst played a role in the therapeutic result of a psychoanalysis and observed that this fact was seldom (or ever?) reported. Chapter 6 presents my thoughts and reactions in response to reading her paper.

How could I have not have known about this article? There was so much we were not taught. Like other Interpersonalists of the era, Thompson understood 82 years ago that the character and conflicts of the analyst influence the process of analysis and that the extent to which this was pivotal depended on the amount of overlap with the character and conflicts of the patient. It has taken many more decades for psychoanalysts across the spectrum of rivaling schools of thought to acknowledge that who the analyst is as a person inevitably has an impact on the process. But Thompson, more than anyone before or since, viewed the interactive effect of the character and conflict of patient and analyst as central to the analytic outcome in explicit terms that parallel mine. I regret that I did not know about and cite Thompson's article in my work from the 1970s onward. But I also realize that even if I had, most psychoanalysts trained in American Psychoanalytic Association institutes at the time would not have been ready to receive her ideas as support for undertaking my study, for its findings, or for subsequent clinical application of these ideas.

As the zeitgeist changed, however, psychoanalysts became better able to embrace previously rejected ideas. My work on the patient-analyst match was part of a sea change that was occurring in North America. By the mid- to late 1980s, the concept that two people, not one, influenced, if not determined, what occurred in psychoanalysis became a widely accepted idea. Countertransference, previously viewed as pathology that personal psychoanalysis should have resolved, became a topic for exploration.

By the late 1980s and into the 1990s, more classically trained analysts in North America began to attend to and publish papers about what patients were stirring in them, a factor on which their Interpersonalist colleagues had always focused attention. Abend (1986) noted that when analysts faced stress in their own lives, countertransference reactions would more easily disrupt their analytic functioning. Cooper (1986) addressed problems in analysis that could arise from the analyst's masochistic or narcissistic "burnout." Poland (1988) called attention to how, in the context of a unique dyadic relationship with the analyst, analytic insight develops. Jacobs' *The Use of the Self* (1991) introduced an intersubjective perspective, removing the stigma from countertransference reactions while simultaneously making them a rich source for psychoanalytic inquiry. I tried to provide further support for this point of view by interviewing analysts about their use of countertransference reactions (1996, 1997). In the 1990s, I also published some papers, included in this volume, illustrating the effect of the match in clinical work (Kantrowitz, 1992, 1993a, 1993b, 1995, 2002).

Still, at this time, the majority of analysts trained at the American Psychoanalytic institutes seemed to remain unaware or failed to acknowledge that the analyst's character and personality inevitably lead to countertransference reactions that influence both the process and outcome of psychoanalysis—a fact that both Interpersonal and Relational analysts had always taught. Today, these ideas are so widely accepted that it is now hard to remember just how vigorously the idea of the analyst's presence as co-participant was once resisted. But despite the fact that both research and clinical data have made it clear that who the analyst is as a person, including the analyst's character and conflicts, have a significant effect on his or her patients, it seems noteworthy that a focus on the specificity of the interdigitation of character and conflict between analyst and patient currently remains relatively neglected as a focus of inquiry. Perhaps the topic has been overlooked because so many analysts have illustrated countertransference reactions in the psychoanalytic literature and how they have used them in their work that analysts didn't think about it further. Whatever the reason, the concept of match that I'm talking about is broader and more inclusive than countertransference.

Freud's (1910a, 1915a) original discussions of countertransference restricted it to those responses aroused in the analyst by the patient or the patient's transference that resemble responses experienced in relation to significant people in his or her own past. In contrast, "match" covers a broader field of phenomena in which countertransference is included as one of many factors that constitute match. The individual history, characteristics, attitudes, and values of each analyst and patient predispose them, respectively, to certain countertransference and transference reactions. As stated earlier, match also includes observable styles[6] of engagement, attitudes, and personal characteristics that may be rooted in residual and unanalyzed conflicts, shared or triggered, in any patient-analyst pair. While many of these characteristics may not prove to be problematic in general or with many patients, in some instances, unless they are recognized, they may be a source of disturbance or even impasse in the analytic work.

As Thompson noted, the extent of influence the analyst's character and conflicts have will vary depending on the character and conflicts of the patient. Overlaps may create clashes or blind spots—situations that may also offer opportunities for the analyst's personal growth. If, for example, an analyst can recognize that something is impeding the work with a particular patient, he or she may through consultation, further personal treatment, or effective self-analysis find a way to resolve the impasse. Then, not only the patient, but also the analyst, can grow and change in the process of the work (Kantrowitz, 1992, 1993a, 1993b, 1995, 1999, 2002).

I would add again that the match between patient and analyst can shift over time, and what was particularly facilitating at one point in psychoanalysis may become an impediment at a later time. Repeating an example presented at the beginning of this introduction, which comes from my research project, an inhibited, frightened patient whose analyst's gentle style initially helped the patient to gradually open up later in the analysis proved to be a hindrance when this patient was ready to more directly address her conflicts. Although she had changed, his hesitancy to bring up her conflicts and her defenses against them continued, limiting her from deriving a fuller analytic benefit.

***

It is not my intent to give a comprehensive history of the developments of North American psychoanalysis; however, to the extent that two-person theories became prominent in the late 1980s and dominant in the 1990s, I do want to distinguish the ways in which my ideas about the effect of the match between patients and analysts are similar and different from other dyadic theories, Interpersonal and Relational, that came to dominate psychoanalysis in North America.

A caveat as well: no brief description of a theoretical school of psychoanalysis encompasses all the variations within the group. Like with classical Freudian theory, the analysts who subscribe to the Interpersonal and/or Relational schools vary significantly in both what they believe and what they do in actual practice.

Interpersonal psychoanalysis had always focused on the effect of experiential-based relationships with other people, influences not just from the early years, but throughout development (Sullivan, 1953). The internalizations of these relationships lead to patterns of behavior for adults. Constitutional factors and drives are not in their purview; the inner world is structured by the outer world. Analysts, like patients, are inevitably influenced by their history of interpersonal relationships as well as other broader environmental factors (Levenson, 1972). All Interpersonalists agree that the analyst's subjectivity and its influence on the patient are inevitable; the analyst is a "participant observer" in the process (Sullivan, 1953). In the treatment setting, Interpersonal analysts tend to focus on here-and-now interactions between patient and analyst, both conscious and unconscious, actively addressing what transpires between them.[7] Enactments are viewed as inevitable and necessary, a source of clinical information about both participants; in fact, they form the basis for the analyst's understanding about him/herself and the patient (Bass, 2003; Benjamin, 2017; Bromberg, 2003; Davies, 1996; Stern, 2003). Over time, the relationship is transformed, and a new interactional experience occurs.[8] This transformation in the relationship is what is mutative in the Interpersonal perspective. Like most classical analysts, Interpersonalists adhere to the idea that interpretations of transference experiences enable the patient to perceive previously unrecognized aspects of the self, facilitating a recognition of differences between self and other; the integration of such interpretations constitute the therapeutic action according to this perspective (Mitchell & Aron, 1999). Relational theory developed from the Interpersonal tradition (Greenberg & Mitchell, 1983).[9]

Like the Interpersonalists, Relational analysts tend to focus on the here-and-now relationship between patient and analyst, the irreducibility of the analyst's subjectivity (Renik, 1993), and enactments as inevitable and informative. Some Relationalists view enactments as continuously occurring, as part of the unconscious engagement of ongoing relatedness. Relational analysts view what transpires in the work as cocreated; a shared responsibility for who is introducing what is seen as reducing patients' tendency to feel shame about aspects of themselves which patients' may experience as unacceptable (Bromberg, 2001, 2003; Harris, 2011). Some Relational theory developed out of work with patients' "real" experience and their relatedness in the analytic encounter; negotiation about the meaning of what occurs in the analytic work is vital and ongoing (Bass, 2003; Pizer, 1998). Some Relational analysts specifically developed their ideas from their work with traumatized patients (Grand, 1997; Harris, 2011), for whom dissociation is a primary defense (Bromberg, 2003; Davies, 1996; Howell, 2006; Stern, 1997). But more broadly, Relational theory tends to see the self as decentered and dissociation as a natural function of self-experience that can become pathological under ongoing duress or in response to overwhelming trauma. Relational views of extreme dissociation do not necessarily focus on merging dissociated aspects of their subjectivity, but more often on helping patients to find footing in their own inherent complexity. The idea of merger into a single, essential self does not correspond to the Relational view of self-experience, which is more akin to a large table where every part of the personality has a voice (Bromberg, 1998; Davies, 1996; Howell, 2006; Stern, 1997).

Many Relational and Interpersonal analysts have similar attitudes about use of self-disclosure as well as sharing many other attitudes about their ways of working and the belief that inform their work. They are both open to using self-disclosure in their work (Bass, 2015; Benjamin, 2017; Davies, 1994; and many others), though with somewhat different intentions and ideas about its effect. Relational analysts believe that analysts reveal themselves in so many nonverbal ways that making their contribution explicit by putting it into words seems more an acknowledgment of what in other ways is already apparent; self-disclosure may also serve as an acknowledgment of error, easing impasses (Aron, 1991; Benjamin, 2017; Davies, 1994). Some Relational analysts have been strongly influenced by Ferenczi, 1931 and use a variation of his model of mutual analysis, though at the same time they are almost always careful to critique his practice of mutual analysis, often characterizing it as a failed experiment (Bass, 2015; Harris, 2011; Hirsch, 1996).

For Interpersonal analysts, self-disclosure seems used more in the service of interpreting their patients' transferences; they do so by pointing out the patient's impact on them, to enable a clearer sense of self and other; but this approach is not characteristic of all Interpersonal analysts (Levenson, 1972; Mitchell, 1998).

My focus on the patient-analyst match also emerged from a disagreement with classical psychoanalytic theory about the one-person nature of analytic work. In this respect, I join both Interpersonal and Relational analysts in the belief that we analysts are always part of what transpires in the treatment. Our subjectivity, in tandem with the subjectivity of our patients, is inevitably involved.

I agree with the Relational and Interpersonal cohorts that the character and intrapsychic conflicts of both participants inevitably play out in their interpersonal engagement. In my view, enactments are inevitable—perhaps continuous—and happen without analysts' conscious awareness. It is only when they rise to an intensity that catches one or both participants' attention that they can be examined. My general perspective, however, comes closer to those of Object Relational analysts, who see psychic structures as arising from internalized object relationships and for whom, in the therapeutic setting, the focus is on the difficulties the patient presents. What I learn about myself from our interactions, I hopefully use to inform me about how my conflicts and character have intruded in an unhelpful way, but it is not my practice to examine these recognitions with my patients.

Sometimes we become aware of disruptions within ourselves, not necessarily perceived by our patients. When, for example, patients' views of, or ways of treating, us or others, stir affective reactions of approval/disapproval in us, make us feel good, or make us distressed, the analyst's self-reflection is necessary. In this respect, my ideas are similar not only to Interpersonal and Relational analysts, but also to most mainstream psychoanalysts in North America today. But I do my self-exploration outside of the treatment setting. In my view, the content of this kind of personal work on the part of the analyst is not usually to be shared with patients. While I do see the therapeutic engagement as mutual, in that both patient and analyst inevitably participate in what occurs and learn from it, I do not see it as equal in terms of where attention should be focused when we are engaged in the work. My focus remains on the patient; how he or she perceives me and reacts to me is what I explore with them. Consideration of the ways in which we analysts are similar to and/or different from our patients provides a lens into why our affect is aroused, why our judgments get made. But perceiving a match between a patient and me does not mean that I share the details of this recognition.

In keeping with this view, while after personal exploration I tend to apologize for errors I've made when I recognize them, I would not explore or explain my own dynamics and conflicts with my patients. I would likely clarify factual misperceptions on either of our parts after they are explored and understood, would not negate a perception of anything attributed to me that corresponded to actions or aspects of me which I knew to be true, and would not assume that the patient's view was inaccurate, even if it remained out of my awareness. I also rarely reveal personal information, my reactions to my patients, or their impact on me. What is stirred in me by my patients' character, conflicts, and transferences to me I view as places for my private exploration.[10]

I am describing my personal way of working as an analyst; however, what one learns from a focus on the match could be worked with differently depending on personal proclivities and clinical beliefs. Racker's ideas (1957) about identification and counter-identification with patients, which have also been central in Relational scholarship and clinical work, most closely cohere with my own view. When our countertransference to our patients is, as Racker calls, "concordant," they enable us as analysts to become more empathic with the patient and more tolerant of ourselves. Such reactions lead to feelings of closeness and intimacy; however, when similarities result in the analyst overlooking a mesh of attitudes, values, beliefs, defenses, or character styles—too concordant—important areas of conflict may be overlooked. The edge of growth for the patient may be diminished when asymmetry dissolves and aggression and separateness are minimized in the dyad. In contrast, the kind of countertransference that Racker calls "complementary" can lead to an explicit and/or implicit clash with patients. At these times, the analyst identifies with significant others in the patient's life with whom there has been conflict or disappointment; in the transference, old patterns repeat themselves, usually making use of the analyst's character and conflicts that resemble these important others from the patient's past.[11]

In other words, considering our match with patients is a vehicle for self-exploration. It offers a lens of specificity by suggesting that analysts scrutinize themselves in relation to their patients in conscious areas of overlap or disjunction; these explorations may unearth less conscious aspects—mutually unsymbolized material—of both the analysts' and patients' character and conflicts that may be interfering with the analyst's ability to deepen analytic work, leading to disruptive enactments or creating impasses or other forms of interference. In our work with patients, what they arouse in us (or fail to arouse) we may recognize with them, but in my view, we should explore it on our own time. Such explorations can be undertaken in our personal treatment, supervision, or consultation; more informally with close friend-colleagues; or in private self-scrutiny of our responses. Affective states and reflections stirred by our patients and, of course, our dreams can open a path of new discovery of previously unconscious aspects of ourselves. What is discovered may lead to growth in both participants. It is an extra benefit from our work, one I believe we should be cautious about exploiting with our patients.

Two North American analysts, Warren Poland and Jay Greenberg, in different ways, offered views very parallel to my own. In his paper "The Analyst's Witnessing and Otherness," Poland (2000) presents a theoretical view of analytic work as both one-person and two-person in nature: "the presence of a dyadic viewpoint does not cancel out the critical developmental shift in self–other distinction that can be seen from the one-person and interactive two-person perspectives. Unified field intersubjectivity does not undo individuality" (p. 30). Like Poland, I believe we create a false dichotomy to think of our analytic work, and specifically our engagement in it, in any other fashion. Poland's view, like my own, is that three different perspectives contribute to analytic work: the intrapsychic worlds of both patient and analyst; their interpersonal, interactive engagement with each other; and something new and unique that is created between them.

Greenberg "interactive matrix" (1995) offers a similar perspective on how this plays out in clinical work. His concept of an interactive match is most similar to mine in that its focus is on the specific "beliefs, values, commitments, hopes, needs, fears, wishes and so on that both analyst and patient bring to any particular moment in treatment" (p. 11). Greenberg is clear that he is referring to conscious as well as unconscious dimensions of both the analyst and the patient that each brings to their interaction. Overlaps in personality may keep the analysis going smoothly when concordant, while when discordant, such overlaps can bring problems to the attention of the participants. In these ways our views correspond. While our views on the patient-analyst interface are the same, what we do with them is different. Greenberg's overall focus is more on the appreciation of this phenomenon and how analysts may accommodate their approach based on an awareness of the patient's proclivities in order not to prematurely clash; my focus, in contrast, is more toward how analysts can use awareness of these overlaps to increase their self-awareness, understand enactments and other disruptions, and free the analytic work from impasses.

***

By the 1990s, both the inevitability of analysts' countertransference reactions and the acceptance of analysis as a two-person enterprise had become commonplace psychoanalytic ideas. But another shift was under way. While previously focus had centered on the patient, attention was now turning toward the analyst. The debate over whether psychoanalysis was an intrapsychic or intersubjective process was receding, as many analysts (Levine & Friedman, 2000) had come to view that distinction as creating a false dichotomy arguing that, inevitably, it must be both.

Psychoanalysts were increasingly exploring the two-person nature of the analytic encounter: Enactments gained attention as expressions of transference-countertransference engagements that could be productively examined in analytic work (Bass, 2003; Bromberg, 2001; Chused, 1991; Ehrenberg, 2005; Friedman & Natterson, 1995; Hirsch, 1993; Hoffman, 1983; Jacobs, 1986; Maroda, 1998; McLaughlin, 1991a, b; Stern, 2003). Beebe and Lachmann (1998) specified an interactive self-regulatory process that "flows in both directions," "between both participants" (p. 509). Cooper (1998) advocated using the analyst's disclosure of his subjectivity to facilitate the patient's exploration of a new understanding. Adler and Bachant (1998) asserted that it was the analyst's subjectivity, along with the patient's, that influenced what would become part of the analytic process as well as what would be resisted. Almond (1999) focused on the effect on the analyst's expectations on the analysand. Feinsilver (1999) attended to the effect of the analyst's counteridentification with the patient. Ogden (1994a) described how the analyst's subjectivity was used to process the patient's subjectivity. Renik (1993) stated that the analyst's subjectivity was inevitable and irreducible. Similarly, Stolorow and Atwood (1997) perceived the psychoanalytic situation as an intersubjective system of reciprocal mutual influences to be understood through a process of empathic immersion.

The idea of mutual influence became central for many psychoanalysts (Aron, 1996; Hoffman, 1996; Ogden, 1994). In 1995, at annual winter meetings of the American Psychoanalytic Association, there were had two panels on interaction: Toward a Definition of The Term and Concept of Interaction and Interpretive Perspectives on Interaction. Also in 1995, two edited volumes were published: a 1,000 page compendium of encyclopedic chapters devoted to basic clinical and theoretical topics on Interpersonal psychoanalysis (Lionells, Fiscalini, Mann & Stern, 1995), and a collection of articles written by the first two generations of Interpersonal writers (Stern, Kantor, Mann, & Schlesinger, 1995). The two-person nature of psychoanalysis had become center stage, a dominant psychoanalytic interest in North America. My work was part of what was now a mainstream wave.

While classical psychoanalysts in North America increasingly welcomed ideas about the patient's and the analyst's reciprocal impact on each another, the idea of the effect of the specific patient-analyst match was troubling to some of them. Vaughan and Roose (2000) expressed concern that this shift in emphasis could be "luring analysts into attributing stalemates to a 'real' factor," which could then "serve as an asylum from tenacious exploration of often painful countertransference problems" (p. 898) and the transference meaning to the patient of what they perceived. Vaughan and Roose's critique of the concept of match was primarily based on analysts' accounts of "real" character overlaps—primarily sociological ones. And there were accounts by prominent analysts of all schools, ones not cited by Vaughan and Roose's paper, who did point to the effect of the analyst's "real" character, attitudes, or visible style on the patient's transference (Baudry, 1991; Chused, 1992; Levenson, 1972; Mitchell, 1988a, b, Orgel, 1990; Viederman, 1991). I believe the error in Vaughan and

Roose's critique was the assumption that attention to these "real" characteristics meant forsaking an exploration of unconscious elements related to them. None of the analysts whose work I have cited abandoned such self-scrutiny.

A change in emphasis had occurred. Having contended so long with the view that countertransference was something to be expunged, many analysts—now classical trained analysts as well as Relational and Interpersonal analysts—created a new atmosphere where there was an acknowledgment and appreciation for the struggles that patients stimulated in them; this recognition became a natural part of the clinical process (Bass, 2014; Davies, 1994; Ehrenberg, 1992). But at times, it could seem as though it was the analyst's experience (Aron, 1991, 1992; Renik, 1993), rather than the patient's, that was becoming the focus. Eagle (2000) observed:

> Although an examination of one's emotional reactions may further one's understanding of the patient's unconscious transference, I believe that in the current climate, too much emphasis has been placed on the thoughts and feelings that automatically emerge in oneself as an epistemological tool in trying to know and understand another and too little emphasis has been put on additional means of understanding.
>
> (p. 36)

His perception, like mine, was that the reconceptualization of transference and countertransference was an important corrective to the idea of the analyst as a blank screen, but that the prominence accorded to countertransference (Renik, 1993) could detract attention from the complex nature of the patient-analyst interaction. And while Ogden (1997) illustrated how his reverie, stimulated by the patient's material, related to the patient's process, it is notable that psychoanalytic candidates at the time often seemed far more interested in the reverie than in how it illuminated the patient's concerns. The pendulum had swung.

And it soon became apparent that many analysts, primarily but not exclusively with a Relational perspective, had turned away from thinking about the specificity of either patient's or analyst's individual characteristic as the concept of an analytic third became prominent in

North America (Benjamin, 2004, 2017; Ogden, 1994a, 2004). Gerson (2004) posited a relational unconscious that further broadened ideas about the interactive effect of the patient and analyst's unconscious interaction, in a fashion that seemed to subsume individuality under this merger of unconscious minds. Stern (1983), too, proposed a relational unconscious of "unformulated experience," though he was explicit in maintaining that the individuality of subjects was not subsumed.

In his critique of Relational psychoanalysis, Mills (2005) contended that in their privileging of intersubjectivity over subjectivity, some Relational theorists end up refuting the existence of the individual and a unique, subjective process. Similarly to Eagle, he argued that Relational theorists' embracing of postmodernist thinking was leading them to "one unanimous implication… the demise of the individual subject" (p. 165). Mitchell's beliefs about a cocreated process (1998) led him to reject the idea that the analysand brings dynamics to the process that are "pre-organized in the patient's mind" (p. 18),[12] while Ogden's third (1994a) usurped the individuality of patient and analysand:

> The analytic third is a creation of the analyst and analysand, and at the same time the analyst and analysand (qua analyst and analysand) are created by the analytic third (there is no analyst, no analysand, and no analysis in the absence of the third.)
>
> (p. 17)

Although Ogden (2004) seemed to move away from this position over time, since later he maintained "a successful psychoanalytic process involves superseding of the unconscious and the reappropriation of the (transformed) subjectivities of the participants as separate (and yet interdependent) individuals" (p. 193), this caveat seems like an afterthought (an inadequate response to that critique) to Mills.

And then a revival of interest in Bion, especially developed by the field theorists, primarily outside North America, concentrated in Italy/Europe and South America, brought attention to the unconscious of both patient and analyst (Civitarese, 2010; Ferro, 2002). Like the Interpersonalists, they consider a broader surround—the total world of both participants—as the field for analytic exploration. Field theorists also view what emerges as a kind of third—developed from, but larger than, the conscious and unconscious contributions from both participants. It is a unique construction, developed from their total interaction with each other. Through what the field theorists call reverie—a kind of waking dream in which they associate to their patients' material—they give symbolic representation to what the patient conveys through a combination of unformed thoughts and feelings represented through "characters" in the patient's associations and the effect of the field of the patient's projections. Their intention is to facilitate the patient's capacity to think, to feel, and to symbolize. While they also emphasis that each patient-analyst pair creates their own unique construction, the specificity of character of the patient analyst is not a source of exploration or considered of importance to its creation. The analyst's "dreaming" pulls for heightened scrutiny of their own associations. These associations stem, of course, from their exchanges with their patients, but in a sense, it seems to me that these field theorists have almost returned to a one-person psychology since the field they study is a singular one, a merger of unconscious associations where the participants individuality disappears—though I realize this is contrary to their intention. While analysts use themselves as a vehicle for synthesis and symbolizations, they do not seem to be giving thought to the content stemming uniquely from themselves as part of this meaning making.

Field theorists make note of the uniqueness of the dyad; however, the field they examine seems to be the content of the patient. The analyst functions within the field as the "processor"; the content that emerges from his or her own character and world, though abstractly acknowledged as contributing something, in the specific seems to be viewed as irrelevant to the analyst's reverie within the dyadic engagement. "It is the patient's projective identifications and emotions, and these alone, that must enter into stories" (Ferro, 2002, p. 57). The analyst's attention is directed to enable the analysand to develop, to think, to grow; the specificity of conflict is not the focus of scrutiny.

The process described by the Field theorists often seems very fruitful. However, as I see it, the immersion in one's own unconscious process can sometimes lead to self-deception on the part of the analyst. The literature offers numerous examples of this approach, having expanded patients' experiences and freed them from internal constraints, but like with any theory, it doesn't mean these benefits are always accrued. While insight was overvalued within psychoanalysis in the past, there may be a tilt that overvalues unrepresented phenomena today.

Like with many Relational theorists, attention within field theory often seems centered on more primitive mental processes. As such, what can be constructed over time about the beneficial or detrimental nature of the match seems vague, harder to assess. It would seem that one could do so only once the process ends—for better or worse. And while in some ways this may also be true in any analytic process, historically earlier psychoanalytic construction of what transpires enabled analysts to have a clearer view of how they were, or might have been, getting in the way of analysands' progress when they perceived impediments in their analytic interactions. Knowledge based on an understanding of their own history and character could alert them to meanings of enactments, defensive avoidances rather than an expectation—vague in its form—that eventually a new creation would occur from their engagement.

Since field theorists work with the assumption that the patient's and analyst's unconscious processes are shaping the analytic engagement, an assumption I share, I would think that the character and conflicts, that is, the personality, of the analyst and their overlap with those of the more psychologically troubled patient would be crucial to the effectiveness of the analytic work—perhaps even more so than with patients whose difficulties are in the neurotic spectrum—since sensitivity to affect tolerance along with timing and tact of communication are so important for patients who are less sturdy in their development. While Field theorists note awareness of the impact of their own distraction or personal preoccupation (Ferro, 2002), it would seem that they have no self-reflection about the absence of the effect of their own characters and conflicts built into their theory. Relational analysts (Stern, 2013) similarly note that the field theorists have an absence of attention to "the revelation of transference, affect regulation, mutual recognition, or the expansion of freedom in the relationship between patient and analyst" (p. 636). Once there are no longer two distinct people—an analysand or analyst—ideas of specificity (Bacal, 2010; Kantrowitz, 2014) vanish. A concept such as match then becomes meaningless, because convergence and disjunction of personal characteristics and conflicts no longer seem central to the psychoanalytic enterprise.

Perhaps the lack of further attention to the idea of match between patient and analyst as centrally important in psychoanalysis and its outcome is related to the ascendency of postmodern ideas in contemporary Relational theory and Field theory. The postmodern views of psychoanalysis (Eagle, 2001) have provided a needed corrective in questioning the idea of an analytic authority: who could know the truth of another's mind? But many analysts have swung to the other extreme, writing as if each person were constantly in flux, created anew by each interaction with one another (Atwood, Orange, & Stolorow, 2002).[13] In such beliefs, there would be no relatively stable self. If patient and analyst are both fluid without stable characteristics of their own, the idea of a match, any convergence or divergence between them, would make the idea of "blind spots" due to meshing or clashing meaningless.

Previously, the analytic process seemed too narrowly focused on the patient; currently, the scope of the analytic purview is so wide that the specificity of individual character and conflict and their overlap seems lost. To me, an analytic process requires attention to the particulars in both analysand and analyst and in the way the specifics of their respective histories, temperament, character, and conflicts intersect in the work. Much can also be learned from exploring the broader surround of both. Again, to me, these are not either-or matters.

Yet even in the 21st century, concurrent with the contemporary broadening of the field of inquiry, some attention to the effect of a particular analyst on a particular analysand remains. Ferro and Basile (2004) think of the psychoanalyst as individual: self-analysis and gradient of functioning. Kite (2008) describes the traction developed from a particular patient interaction with the character of a particular analyst. Susan Levine (2007) describes an unarticulated concept, the persona of the analyst, which guides the analyst's decision-making in relation to boundaries in self-disclosure; Smith (2004) also writes about the analyst's fantasy of the ideal patient.

I continue to believe that thinking in terms of the match with our patients provides a lens that can keep us steady in the midst of tilts too far in one direction or another. In this volume, I trace the development and provide illustrations of the concept of match. In the initial chapter in this volume, I present my first paper about match. The research to support these ideas is in the appendix. Chapters 2–6 are illustration of specific issues of match. The next section—Chapters 7–10—offers an educational perspective. They show how the issue of the match can be used in supervision and for self-discovery. The last three chapters—11–13—present factors of match in a more implicit fashion, continuing to demonstrate the interactive effect of self and other on the analytic work in day-to-day interactions. The last two chapters are written in a more personal way, revealing how my out-of-the-office personal life intersects with my work with my patients.

Notes

1   The details of this methodology are published in an article in the *Psychoanalytic Quarterly* (Kantrowitz, Singer, & Knapp, 1975).
2   As I was taught, we were to be relatively silent. To facilitate the development of the transference neurosis we were to be primarily "blank screens." Our interventions were primarily to be interpretations.
3   "Their task was to assess whether or not the match of patient and analyst influenced the success of the patient's analysis. To do this, they listed the central characteristics and issues for the analyst as revealed in the profile developed by the raters from the analysts' interviews, and the central problematic issues or areas for the patient as revealed in the post-analysis test report. They were then asked which, if any, of these issues interdigitated for patient and analyst in a manner that they thought might influence the success of the analysis. They were asked to evaluate the amount of influence, the centrality, the direction (i.e., negative or positive), whether it impeded or facilitated the engagement in the analytic process, the course of the analytic work or the completion of the process, and the degree of certainty they had in their evaluations. The judges also grouped the cases into two broad categories of outcome, based on psychological test results: improved and little or no improvement. Next, they reviewed the actual interview with the analyst to corroborate or modify their impressions. They did not make major shifts in their assessments based on these reviews of the transcripts. Each judge wrote a summary paragraph describing, with documentation, his or her perception of the influence of the patient-analyst match on the outcome of treatment. While this method did not allow for formal tests of reliability, the agreement between the two raters was high. Differences were

only in terms of emphasis (Kantrowitz et al., 1989, pp. 901–902). A full account of the method for evaluating the overlapping characteristics and conflicts of the patient and analyst is contained in the 1989 article.

4   The limitations of the data were cited in the study. These limitations included (1) small sample size, (2) lack of comparable data for the patients and analysts, (3) lack of experience of the treating analysts, (4) inability to take into account the effect of supervision on the analyst, and (5) lack of comparability of the analysts' interviews in terms of openness and completeness.

5   As I have explained, empirical studies of psychoanalysis are not easy to undertake. And research studies at that time required a kind of rigor that did not accord with the complexities of actual analytic clinical work and/or the theories that guided it.

6   Interpersonalists and Relational analysts do take for granted the significance of observable styles, but they do not necessarily consider that the particular styles of the participants may contribute to or interfere with the efficacy of the pair's analytic work.

7   In responding to Jay Frankel's characterization of interpersonal analysts as harsh and confrontational, Hirsch (1998) points out the great variations in therapeutic technique among individual analysts who ascribe to this school of thought and practice.

8   This point is strongly characteristic of the interpersonal literature. Stern, Kantor, Mann, and Schlesinger (1995) have all presented ideas about transformation for many years before they became central in the Interpersonalists' literature.

9   Mitchell wrote that Relational psychoanalysis was anchored in three different sources: Interpersonal psychoanalysis, object relations, and Self-Psychology. The Interpersonal contribution was most basic for him (personal communication from Donnel Stern).

10   One reason for my disinclination toward self-disclosure is that I really cannot be sure that what I understand at any particular moment or even on reflection is the whole story. Self-analysis takes time. What I discover may be modified by what further self-scrutiny illuminates. Another reason I do not offer self-revelations is that I view the time I work with a patient as time that should be focused on the patient. They are free to explore me as part of their work. That I may learn from this is to my benefit, something that in some general way I might acknowledge at some point. But in the context of the work, I am there to be used for their benefit, and they are my focus.

11   I think of countertransference as reactions that are stirred in me by transferences my patients bring to their perception of me in our work. I think of my transference to my patients, what I perceive of as character and conflicts in their personhood, as my reactions to them. In actual

analytic work, the distinction between these two descriptions can become blurred.

12 Mitchell later clarified (2000) that he did not mean to suggest that he thinks of the mind "as pre-existing but not pre-organized"—a distinction that baffled Eagle and baffles me as well.

13 Relational analysts, who believe that the field coexists with the individual self, would dispute this characterization as a misunderstanding of their ideas.

Chapter 1

The role of the patient-analyst "match" in the outcome of psychoanalysis[1]

A focus on the match between patient and analyst places attention on the dynamic effect of the interaction of character and conflict of both participants on the process that evolves between them. Match is neither a predictive nor static concept. Rather, it refers to an unfolding transaction that itself shifts and changes during the course of analytic work. In beginning to examine the element of match, it is important to look at the factors leading to change. In order for change to occur, the analyst must be able to enter the patient's subjective world affectively, communicate an understanding of it, and yet maintain a view of the patient's affective and cognitive experience that is different from the patient's in areas of conflict and discomfort. I contend that the analyst's therapeutic effectiveness, reflected in an ability to understand and effectively communicate with a patient, is shaped not only by training and skill, but also by personal attributes. Even assuming adequate training and skill, when the personal characteristics of the analyst are too similar to those of the patient in his areas of specific conflict and/or disturbance, and especially when the analyst is not aware of this overlap as an issue, then analytic effectiveness may be compromised. Too much difference may sometimes lead to an inability for empathy and failure to be sufficiently responsive to the patient. These characteristics include countertransference reactions, personal limitations, and blind spots, as well as personality traits and styles, and personal values and beliefs that are not rooted in conflict. Similarly there may be particular personal characteristics of the analyst that interface with the patient's character and conflicts in ways that are facilitating to the analytic process.

What transpires between the patient and the analyst is shaped by both the nature of the patient and the patterns of relating and reacting that he/she brings from the past and repeats in analysis and the analyst's characteristic ways of relating and reacting, modified by his analytic training and skill. Psychoanalysis is an interplay between two participants that keeps the patient moving forward, regressing and progressing, continuing to deepen his/her affective and cognitive understanding and broaden a sense of possibility in life.

The personal qualities, strengths, and limitations of the analyst and their effect on the analytic process are not frequently emphasized. While analysts are almost always ready to acknowledge in conversation the effect of their personal limitations, as well as the adverse effects of countertransference, they have not always found it necessary to examine their own contribution as fully as they examine their patients' part. Similarly, the analytic literature, while conceding both abstract and specific manifestations of countertransference, rarely considers the impact that the particular qualities of an analyst may have on the treatment process.

Kernberg (1972) views analysts as relatively interchangeable. He observes that the further one moves from employing analytic technique, the more the "real" personality of the therapist is likely to intrude. While this observation seems indisputable, his statement that "less skilled therapists [make] a better contribution to improvement of their patients if the treatment is expressive" (p. 188) (i.e., if the treatment modality employs a standard technique stemming from psychoanalytic theory in which the therapist maintains a position of abstinence and neutrality) is more open to question. The implications of his conclusions are that in analysis there is a uniform analyzing instrument (Isakower, 1938) and the analyst has actually become a "blank screen" by employing it. He virtually dismisses as nonexistent or unimportant the influence of the particular qualities of the analyst.

Such assumptions in fact underly most studies of analyzability. Bachrach and Leaff (1978) reviewed the clinical and quantitative literature in this area. Although they begin their article with a statement that differences in response to psychoanalysis are traceable to "qualities of the analysand, of the analyst and their interaction" (p. 881), the rest of the paper focuses exclusively on the qualities of the patient. They themselves are aware that their review does not include the role that the analyst plays. Toward the end, they admit that in actual practice, the analyzability of a patient may vary with different analysts. They state, "Some people do well with certain analysts and not with others.... This has a great deal to do with what goes into forming a therapeutic alliance between two particular people" (p. 896).

One reason why Bachrach and Leaff do not include a review of the qualities of the analyst may be that the psychoanalytic literature is virtually devoid of such references. A literature on countertransference does exist, but there is little discussion of the interaction between the analyst's specific countertransference reactions, character, and personality organization and the specific conflicts, character, and personality of the particular patient.

McLaughlin (1981) offers an alternative view. He specifically addresses the importance of the real characteristics of the analyst. McLaughlin believes that the analyst brings to bear his total being as a person in the analytic situation. He reviews the concept of countertransference, citing that at least since the 1920s, there has been some acknowledgment that analysts' reactions, like patients', had their origins in infantile experiences. Nonetheless, there had been a model, particularly advocated by North American analysts, of an objective analyst who would conceal all feelings except the wish to help. His role was to mirror the patient and to remain impartial in his inquiry. His care and humanity were to be expressed only through his position as the physician. Deviations from this ideal were seen as lapses to be rectified.

McLaughlin notes that Fliess in 1942 operationalized the concept of the analyst's empathy as acts of introjection and trial identification with the patient. Fliess warned of the dangers for the analyst of counter-identifications and countertransference, of mood alterations and narcissistic vulnerabilities. He saw these as an inevitable part of the analytic process. McLaughlin observes that analysts who subscribe to object relations theory have always stressed the importance of the analyst's personality and behavior, and the patient's consciousness of them.

Similarly, analysts who view the psychoanalytic situation as analogous to mother-child relationships have kept an awareness of the infantile roots that are awakened in the transference for both patient and analyst. McLaughlin concludes that this leads to a view of the analyst as a participant-observer who in the process of analyzing the patient touches on all issues of past development for both the patient and himself. It is assumed that the analyst's ego "keep[s] intact his experiencing, observing and ordering functions" (p. 647), only sampling the intensity of the patient's experiences and using all that occurs, including his countertransference responses for understanding and formulation.

McLaughlin proposes discarding the term countertransference and replacing it with the broader view of transference. He believes that "there is transference in all our processing of experiences, at all times and in all stages of the life cycle" (p. 656). Thus, like the patient, the analyst experiences a transference in the analytic situation, though its intensity and degree, and his freedom of expression, are notably different from the patient's. Shaped by his own analysis, the analyst's "work ego" is characterized by capabilities that specifically apply to doing analytic work. Olinick, Poland, Grigg, and Granatir (1973) describe this "work ego" as being relatively stable and autonomous in its functioning. The analyst's reaction to the patient may run the gamut from trial identification as a controlled empathic response to counter-identification and overidentification as regressive responses. The extent to which ego discrimination and mastery are involved determines where on the continuum the analyst's reaction falls.

Greta Bibring (1936), aware of the potential difficulties of the impact of her particular character or style on a particular patient, described transferring a patient to another analyst because she felt she was too much like the patient's mother in reality. She believed there could be too little "as if" or "distortion" brought about by the transference.

Berman (1949) noted that the analyst's total personality, his attitudes and reactions as a person, his emotional responses that are appropriate or defensive, just as they are in life, contribute to the way in which the analyst reacts to the patient and may "intrude upon or blur the transference picture" (p. 159). Berman differentiates this from countertransference, a term he restricts solely to describing the analyst's response to the patient as "an important figure in the analyst's past life" (p. 159). These more generalized emotional reactions on the part of the analyst may be reflected in temporary and minor changes of voice quality or changes in the quality and timing of interpretations as when, for example, the analyst is suppressing or repressing aggression or reacting to libidinal feelings stirred by a patient. Assuming the analyst is competent, these responses will be predominantly of an appropriate quality. What I am proposing is that even for the competent analyst, there are reactions at times which remain at least temporarily outside of his awareness, and when this is confluent with a patient's difficulty of which he, too, is unaware, the issue will go undetected and therefore unanalyzed unless one of the two recognizes the problem.

Berman himself pointed out that some analyses are poor matches. The patient may accurately sense that the analyst is unable to feel genuinely warm or dedicated to him. At other times, patients may recognize emotional or defensive reactions in their analysts. In some patients, this may lead to their distancing their own reactions and creating a "pseudotranquil atmosphere" (p. 163), resulting in important areas not being analyzed; in others, this may lead to storms in the analysis and acting out. Analyses may terminate abruptly or by mutual consent after such periods of frustration.

Greenson (1967) similarly emphasized the possibility that analysts, while needing to detect and control personal reactions to patients, may find on occasion that they have selected a patient with whom they cannot work. He acknowledged a personal limitation in his not being able to work effectively with patients who had strongly reactionary political or social viewpoints. In illustrating how analysts' values can affect the treatment process, he cited one patient who, noting that the analyst asked for associations whenever the patient spoke positively about conservative politicians or negatively about liberal ones—as if to demonstrate that there was something distorted or infantile in this view—tried to change his political preferences to please the analyst. The analyst was unaware of both his behavior and its impact on the patient until the analysis became stalemated. This dynamic was revealed when the analyst began to question the patient about the reasons for his disengagement from the analytic process. The patient, who was conscious of both his wish and attempt to please the analyst, then elaborated what had taken place. When Greenson became conscious of his behavior and its impact, he was able to pursue both the meaning to the patient of what he had perceived to be the analyst's values and the reason why he had felt compelled to change his views.

Such revelations and consequent awareness are always possible. When they occur, they lead to a deepening of the analytic material and its meanings. In such an instance, an initially problematic match need not inevitably lead to a poor outcome. It does require, however, that the patient and analyst must both, though not necessarily at the same time, become aware of the nature of the impediment and be able to analyze it in order for it to be overcome.

Anna Freud (1954) states that analysts never react and respond in exactly the same manner to any two of their patients. Humor may be used with one while with another the analyst is only serious. The manner of giving interpretations also varies depending on the particular patient—with some the terms are literal while with others similes or analogies make it easier for the patient to accept interpretations. For each analyst, the extent to which a real relationship is allowed to exist alongside of the transference relationship also varies from one patient to another. "The strictiness of the analytic setting" and the degree of the analyst's and patient's ease are also somewhat different for each patient/analyst pair. None of these variations is intended or planned; rather, they occur, she believes, in reaction to subtle nuances and pressures from the patient's personality. If the analyst attends to these variations in his own behavior and reactions, he will uncover many important and previously undetected aspects of the patient's character. Anna Freud elaborates this point by enumerating a series of characteristics, such as "subtleties of [the patient's] healthy personality, the degree of maturity reached by his ego, his capacity to sublimate" (p. 610), all of which reflect the adaptive non-conflictual aspects of the patient.

This focus on the interactive nature of the patient-analyst response is in accord with my position. While I agree that the patient's strengths may be revealed through these observations, I also believe that many subtleties of dysfunction may be illuminated.

Sandler's concept of "role-responsiveness" (1976) is similar. His idea is that the analyst's behavior and reactions may be subtly shaped in response to covert pressures from the patient. Sandler believes that the patient subtly and unconsciously manipulates and provokes the analyst into reactions and behaviors that repeat experiences and relationships crucial to the patient in the past. The analyst's responsiveness to these "proddings" will vary and is often not based on a conscious awareness of what is occurring. When the analyst becomes aware that he is responding to the patient in some manner that is discrepant with his usual way of working, he will scrutinize himself to discover the source within himself of the problems or blind spots that led him to the "irrational response" to the patient. Sandler suggests that these uncharacteristic responses on the part of the analyst may sometimes be considered compromise formations between the analyst's own personally derived tendencies and his unconscious, unintentional acceptance of the role the patient is trying to get him to assume in the transference. The roles to which the analyst will respond, the extent of the response, and the relative proportion of the contributions from the analyst's own issues and those resulting from the patient's pressure will vary in each patient-analyst pair.

It is Sandler's contention that this "role-responsiveness" that shows itself not only in the analyst's feelings but in his attitudes and behaviors toward his patient may be useful in analytic work. He cites several cases where the analyst unwittingly complies with a role the patient unconsciously seeks to establish. The exploration of that analyst's deviance from his usual behavior, once recognized, either by the analyst through his self-analytic work or by the patient who calls it to his attention, led to revelations of crucial dynamics imbedded in experiences and fantasies around earlier relationships not previously within the patient's awareness.

What Sandler has called "role-responsiveness" and I have called "match" may be a factor that, when it is brought within the awareness of the patient and analyst, leads to crucial analytic work. Greenson's case is an example in which this occurred. However, we know of this example because the analyst and patient became aware of the dynamic. If neither patient nor analyst becomes aware of such a dynamic, we cannot be certain, no less prove, that this is operating to impede their work, but it is a plausible hypothesis that needs to be considered when an analysis does not progress. If the analyst responds to the role assigned to him, as Sandler suggests, and remains unaware of doing so, the treatment will only repeat the patient's past experience.

As the Pfeffer (1961, 1963) outcome studies suggest, the internal representation of the analyst then becomes part of a previously established identification and reinforces the old conflicts and maladaptive modes of coping. In successful analyses, unlike unsuccessful ones, new psychic development arises from the interplay of the patient and the analyst (Norman, Blacker, Oremland, & Barrett, 1976;

Pfeffer, 1961, 1963; Schlessinger & Robbins, 1974, 1975). Their interaction affords the patient not only a recapitulation of the past but also an additional new experience.

The crucial question is: assuming a well-trained analyst and a patient whose pathology is not so severe that he is immune to the analyst's reasonable efforts, can any such pair work together and expect to have a successful outcome? Kernberg's (1972) conclusions from the Menninger study suggest an affirmative answer, whereas Pfeffer, in contrast, implies that it is the factor in the analyst's attitude (though he does not focus on the specific qualities and characteristics of the analyst) that is different from the patient's attitude that leads to a transformation in the patient.

Shapiro (1976), too, in evaluating the outcome of training analyses relates unsuccessful results to the personal qualities of the analyst. He reports that "one fourth of the analysts (32 in total) who responded to a questionnaire about their analyses ascribed one or more severe or major difficulties to their training analysts" (p. 23). One-sixth of this group felt countertransference reactions on the part of their training analyst were responsible for the problem. One-tenth of the group held other factors responsible for their difficulties: for example, "inimical personal attributes," such as the analyst's "depressive character," "rigidity and remoteness," "his desire to adopt me," or "the similarity of the analyst and myself" (p. 23). Shapiro concludes that in situations where the initial pathology of the analysand is not too severe to prevent analytic work from progressing, "the congruence between analysand and analyst may well be the most important element in the process of analysis during training" (p. 26).

Tartakoff (Scharfman & Blacker, 1981) also recognizes the importance of "match" or "misfit" between the analyst and patient. She states that neither transference as a repetition (while central to the analytic situation) nor countertransference were comprehensive enough concepts to account for the "total emotional resonance and cognitive response of the analyst evoked by the patient's productions" (p. 670). In her view, the analyst's personal attributes—in addition to the self-understanding accrued during his own analysis—are critical in determining what the analyst communicates to the patient. Based on her clinical experience, she believed that a successful outcome in psychoanalysis depended on the "patient's internalization of the salient attributes of the affective and cognitive interactions of the analysis" (p. 671) in addition to the rediscovery of unconscious material.

Shapiro (1976) lists a series of characteristics that would ideally create a "good fit" between analyst and candidate. He cites reciprocal role expectations, compatible professional convictions and philosophies, as well as cultural and social values and mutual respect for ethnic or sociocultural differences, "unconscious congruence of reciprocal personality dynamics," and "transference countertransference configurations and personal attributes" (p. 27). These are highly abstract concepts, which are difficult to operationalize. They still seem to fall short of capturing the complexity of the analytic interaction because they are so global.

As illustrated by the papers I have cited, the focus of analysis is beginning to expand. The patient is no longer the only one under scrutiny. No longer seen as interchangeable merely on the basis of training, as many of us trained in the late 1960s were taught, the analyst is now being viewed as a multidimensional person. He is expected by virtue of his training to be able to control, contain, and analyze his personal reactions to his patient. However, there is also a growing realization that the analyst's personal traits and characteristics will inevitably impinge on his patient—for better or for worse.

Although there are clear guidelines to standard analytic procedure and practice to which the well-trained analyst generally adheres, I wish to restate and emphasize my agreement with Anna Freud (1954) that the nuances and subtleties of analytic style may shift, even if ever so slightly, in our personal responses to the particular qualities of the patient. For example, with some patients we are looser, while with others we are tighter. It is not the content or quality of any particular style that is at issue, but the fact that different patients elicit different sets of reactions and responses from us even in the analytic situation. Sometimes these responses can facilitate the analysis and sometimes they may hamper it. We can do better work with some patients than with others because of our own characters.

At times when the analyst's attitudes, views, or stance toward life are similar to those of the patient in areas that are crucial to the patient's core difficulties, there may be little or no change, but this may be more of a factor at some periods of time in the analysis than others. Sometimes explorations of similar problem areas may lead to shifts for both participants, for certainly they will not be exactly the same. While at other times, similarities may lead to a stalemate. When the analyst's set is different from the patient's in critical problem areas, assuming that the analyst is able to grasp and successfully communicate the nature of the patient's experience to him, there may be a new opportunity for the patient to shift and modify his experience of both himself and the world. Through internalizing and identifying with his analyst, as well as gaining insight into and understanding of his own conflicts, the patient may become able to expand his capacities and make a new adaptation.

The particular attitudes, views, stance, and issues that are critical will vary for each analyst-patient pair. Each analyst has his own strengths, assets, and talents as well as foibles, limitations, and even residual conflicts, after his own analysis, and his character and personality will inevitably be felt by the patient and have an impact on the analytic process. Few analysts would assert that their personal treatment resulted in their becoming individuals who respond equally and in exactly the same way to all patients. As Anna Freud (1954), Berman (1949), and McLaughlin (1981) all suggest, this is so not only because of inevitable countertransference reactions, but also because of the constellation of qualities that make the analyst who he or she is as a person.

The personal characteristics of the analyst that impinge upon the patient are likely to fall along a continuum. At one extreme, there are blatant countertransference interferences. Then there are the unresolved issues of the analyst, not troubling enough perhaps to require further treatment, but potentially mobilized under stress and possibly interfering with professional effectiveness. The manifestations of these issues may be related to, but are not identical to, what we generally call personal characteristics. Still further along the continuum are the analyst's particular style, interests, attitudes, and values, which shape his reactions and choices in the world, and of course color how he/she responds, but which are not in themselves therapeutic issues. Like the viewing of ambiguous figures in perceptual studies,[2] where what is figure for one person is seen as ground for another, it is not that one selected focus of attention is preferable to another, but rather that what is selected determines the focus. Both are equally valid but each offers a different view and response to the world. Similarly, there are ranges of tempo and pace, styles of communication that reflect high energy (possibly leading to quick purposeful approaches) compared to low energy (possibly leading to a slow, steady approach). Some of these characteristics may be innate while others may be learned—modeled on important figures from the analyst's past and as such having a specific historical meaning.

If we acknowledge that the real characterological qualities of the analyst are an element in the treatment, the way these qualities intermesh with the crucial areas of disturbance for any given patient are important. The effect of these qualities is perhaps not as dramatic as countertransference interferences, but may be as significant if the analyst remains unaware of their impact on the patient.

Precisely because they do not involve countertransference issues that the analyst's personal treatment has trained him to detect and monitor, the likelihood that the effect of these qualities on the patient will be brought to light and used analytically is small, unless the patient himself raises them as a focus. An analyst whose general stance toward life is pessimistic or fatalistic might not impede the progress of a patient (whatever the nature of his difficulties), in whom this view was not a characterological trait, but might very well be detrimental to a patient whose attitudes tended to be despairing—especially if the analyst was unaware that they shared this attitude.

Material from the following four cases should serve to illustrate the range of effects that might result from "good matches" and the consequences of patient-analyst mismatches.[3] The first case is an example of a match that seemed to facilitate the psychoanalytic process. In the second case, the pairing initially was problematic, but due to the analyst's ability to focus on and analyze the difficulty, the process was ultimately facilitated. The third case exemplifies an initially productive analytic process that may have been impeded by the analyst's failure to recognize and analyze overlapping characteristics of analyst and patient. The fourth case represents a non-facilitating match where the patient was unable to articulate and the analyst was unable to see how their shared characteristics resulted in an analytic stalemate that may have been the result of these shared characteristics. In the first and third cases, I have access to both the patient's and the analyst's perceptions. In the second and fourth, the material is presented only from the patient's point of view.

Case I

A 32-year-old man who himself was a skilled professional in the mental health field sought psychoanalysis because of "difficulties with intimacy." According to the patient, he had several close friends, many superficial relationships, and good working relations with his colleagues. There had been several women with whom he had had long, intense, and intimate relationships. He felt that these had been mutually pleasurable emotionally, sexually, and intellectually. Nonetheless, each of these relationships had ultimately turned out to be unsatisfactory. Either he would end up feeling "used" or the woman would terminate the relationship for reasons that he could not fully understand. When he decided to seek help, he made extensive inquiries of his friends and colleagues about analysts in the community and interviewed several before making his decision. At that time, he could not clearly articulate what he was seeking except to say that he needed to be clear "whose needs were being responded to" and to feel that his needs were being "met." For example, he wanted to have a period of vis-à-vis sessions prior to using the couch. Several analysts with whom he consulted felt that his need for this would be better understood on the couch. While he understood their point of view, he felt that their responses were based on something that had to do with themselves and not with him, and he chose not to see any of them.

The analyst he selected was a middle-aged man who agreed to his request for an initial sitting-up period. This analyst's manner and style were quite different, at least superficially, from those of the patient. While the patient wore stylish attire and was immaculately groomed, the analyst's clothing was designed primarily for comfort, and unshined shoes or slightly tousled hair were characteristic of him. The patient was extremely articulate and used precise figures of speech and literary allusions. Although a wide range of affect was displayed, there was something intellectualized in his manner. The analyst's manner of speaking was more tentative, and he tended to use more affect-laden language. Neither the patient nor the analyst had noted these stylistic differences at the outset of treatment.

After a brief vis-à-vis period, the patient began to use the couch. He talked freely and fluently about his past, his present, and his reactions to the analyst and the analytic situation. He brought in vivid dreams that he worked on and connected to current and past concerns; he cried, laughed, expressed anger and outrage and compassion; he reflected over what he had expressed during the analytic hours and continually expanded his awareness and deepened his understanding of himself. All comments from the analyst were almost immediately responded to and incorporated in his reflections. If he thought they were off the mark, he would state his disagreement and, at times, annoyance at being misunderstood. In short, he seemed to be the ideal analytic patient. Yet his analyst felt that for all the patient's new understanding and strikingly acute perceptions about himself (which he also used to try to behave differently), there was something almost "too good" about the analysis and its progress.

One day after approximately six months of analysis, the analyst noted a pattern in the patient's associations and directed the patient's attention to this by repeating the sequence of the patient's thoughts. The patient, enraged, responded,

> I hate it when you do that—and you rarely do. It feels like you are applying an analytic technique—like a recipe out of a cookbook. The content shows you were listening and heard me, but your way of communicating feels like it is directly out of a course in psychoanalytic technique.

The analyst was struck that the patient's complaint about his manner at this time illuminated what had been nagging at the periphery of his thoughts about the patient. Although rich in both content and affect, it was a bit too much "all the way it should be," like a textbook. Since the analyst was unaware that he had done anything remarkably different on this day, he asked how his usual remarks differed. The patient said that he had never thought about it before, but on reflection he noted that there was a spontaneity and freshness—even a pleasant slight unpredictability—to the analyst's usual interventions. Sometimes the analyst's comments were "short and to the point"; other times they were "a bit long and tentative." There were hours in which the analyst said a fair amount and others in which he hardly spoke at all. The analyst's comments might occur at the beginning of the hour, in the middle, or near the end. As the patient mused over these stylistic variations, he concluded that what he liked was the feeling that whatever the analyst did felt fitted to him at that particular moment and that it lacked the feeling of being a "technique" or coming out of a "theory."

Over the next weeks and months, the patient kept coming back to this hour. Explorations of his reaction led him to realize that one of the factors that had contributed to his selection of this analyst, a factor that he had implicitly continued to appreciate, was what he experienced as his analyst's "genuineness." He felt he was being responded to as an individual. He became increasingly aware that he did not feel himself to be genuine. It was not that his thoughts, feeling, fantasies, or reactions were false, but that he was always trying to please others by trying to be "good" and "living up to their expectations." His life was organized around "trying to master"—a theme that he had extensively explored before but that now took on additional meaning. He was conforming to something outside of himself and had lost a sense of what was "real," "meaningful," or "genuine" to him. When his analyst highlighted his material in a manner he perceived as a learned technique, it "touched a nerve." He now understood that it reminded him of something he despised in himself. If his analyst were to follow "rules of analytic procedure" in this way, he would feel these responses to be "unreal." The sense he had of the analyst's "genuineness" made him hopeful about reaching "genuineness" within himself.

Later in the analysis, this issue manifested itself in the transference. The patient wondered if even though he usually experienced the analyst as "genuinely responding" to him, this might simply be the way the analyst routinely dealt with patients. If the analyst were never to think of him outside of analytic hours and to attend to him only as "a case—a patient," then perhaps what went on between them was still not "real." As the historical material unfolded, the patient came to realize that he had experienced his "seemingly caring and devoted" parents as going through the motions of being "good parents," but often "being preoccupied" and "not really attending" to him. He came to see that though he had viewed himself as "devoted and caring" with his close friends and especially his girlfriends, in fact he was often only going through the motions himself and not really attending to them. He began to see why problems of intimacy arose for him.

While all analysts, I assume, would want to be thought of as genuine, the qualities of "spontaneity" and "slight unpredictability" might be viewed as desirable, undesirable, or neutral in value. They are qualities that, if not excessive, are significant only if they have an impact on the patient. A patient who experienced his early relationships as bordering on the chaotic or painfully inconsistent might find that the mild variability of approach shown by this analyst rekindled the past too traumatically. If this experience could be recognized, acknowledged, and explored, it would not necessarily be an impediment to analytic work; nonetheless, it might increase the patient's difficulty in forming a trusting relationship with the analyst. For such a patient, "steadiness" rather than "spontaneity" would likely lead to a sense of security which would probably be facilitating to the analytic process. On the other hand, the patient whose analysis we have just reviewed, was actively, though initially not consciously, seeking an analytic atmosphere that felt "flexible and responsive" to him. This patient used the stylistic contrast between himself and his analyst both to feel hopeful about the possibility of a future that could be different from his past and to highlight and bring into focus an aspect of himself that he experienced as very troubling.

The aspects of the analyst's style that the patient valued are discernible to most observers but in a much subtler form. His colleagues describe him as having a "casual" and "informal" manner. The patient's sensitivity and responsivity to each manifestation of this quality, no matter how slight, indicates the importance of these characteristics for this patient. It also reveals how he used these characteristics to mean something personal and idiosyncratic. Although objectively there may be nothing more "genuine" about spontaneity than predictability, the personal style of this analyst evidently was experienced by this patient as having an enhancing effect on the analytic process. All one can reasonably claim is that the personality differences between analyst and patient contributed to the fact that this patient's central issue arose so quickly and clearly. Analytic progress might have been made eventually under different circumstances, but there seems little doubt that the "match" facilitated the progress.

Case 2

A woman in her early 20s sought analysis for depression. She had an immediate and intensely negative reaction to her analyst who was an older woman. She perceived her analyst as distant and controlled.

Everything about her was experienced as muted, measured, intellectualized, and impersonal. She could document this in the extreme neatness of the office, the carefully constructed sentences, and the modulated tones in which the analyst spoke. The patient felt deflated and hurt by this neutrality and feeling of distance. For a long time, the patient had no memories that allowed her to root her negative feelings in any historical context, and she continued to rail against the analyst for these traits. The analyst maintained a calm, "neutral" stance while systematically trying to understand the meaning of these traits to the patient. Gradually, over several years, a picture of the patient's mother emerged as a controlled and controlling woman who rigidly adhered to rules and was incapable of spontaneity. It seemed that both the structure of the analytic situation and the personal style of the analyst had instantly recreated feelings for this patient that she had not previously been aware that she had experienced in relation to her mother.

Each analytic hour was experienced as hurtful and demeaning, with rules and the analyst's need to remain neutral more important than the patient's feelings. Over time the patient developed a tolerance for the way the analyst conducted the analysis without taking her style so personally. She increasingly understood the origin of her injury and what in the situation was recreating it. The patient experienced the analyst as very empathic throughout, but this did little to ease her distress. Her hope and relief came from the ever so infrequent moments when the analyst deviated in her procedure. For example, the analyst began the hour following a vacation by asking the patient about how her holiday had been; an act of initiative that the patient experienced as out of character for the analyst and as evidence of a spontaneity and flexibility that she had not felt with her mother. Instances like these were experienced as gestures toward her, giving her the feeling that her request had been heard and responded to, and that she counted as a person. The analysis progressed, and the patient's discomfort within the hours and depression outside both abated. It was only later after her dysphoria was considerably lessened that she also came to study and recognize her own use of projection and externalization.

The analyst's seeming similarity to the patient's mother led to an immediate and intense negative transference reaction, in which the patient was for a long time unable to experience the analyst as separate from the original object. The analyst seems to have continually kept in her awareness the impact that her manner and behavior had on the patient, and this was a central focus in the analysis. The "match," while difficult, did not lead to a stalemate. The question may be raised, however, whether the analyst's awareness of her role and the pursuit of understanding its transference meaning would have been sufficient to facilitate change. Although deviations were rare, it was the patient's feeling that it was the fact of the analyst actually being different from her mother as she experienced her—a fact that was reflected in a different attitude toward rules and spontaneity— that allowed the patient to experience both the analyst and herself in a new way. It does seem, however, that had the analyst not pursued the effect that these characteristics had on the patient, their historical meaning would not have been recovered and the analysis almost inevitably would have failed. Assuming that the patient's perceptions did accurately reflect the analyst's personal style, the analyst did not have a blind spot in this area and was able to undefensively analyze those areas that were so crucial to this patient.

This second example raises another interesting question from the perspective that focuses on the interacting characteristics of analyst and patient. We are introduced to an analyst who not only systematically analyzed the patient's complaints about her but also, at least on occasion, according to the patient's perception, shifted the way she related to the patient precisely in the area that the patient found distressing. How can we understand this? If we assume a well-trained, disciplined analyst, it is unlikely that the analyst had decided that there was analytic benefit in directly gratifying the patient or that out of exhaustion she had given in to the patient's demands.

Let us consider another alternative, again maintaining the point of view, for the sake of our hypothesis, that the patient had accurately perceived something about the analyst's style. If the patient had persistently focused on some external behavior of the analyst that not only was determined by an analytic stance and/or her own transference reaction, but also reflected the analyst's internal conflict, attitude, or characterological stance, then it is possible that the analyst may have gained a new or increased awareness about some aspect of herself. The analyst's self-recognition might then have spontaneously led to some shift in the way in which she related to the patient.

Such a change in behavior would not be a calculated one but would emerge from the analyst's own openness and willingness to continue self-exploration stimulated by the patient's observations. This might result in some internal transformation for the analyst that could then manifest itself in some subtle, or on occasion not so subtle, shift in the analyst's response or style.

In this second example, the patient certainly felt and expressed a greatly increased tolerance over time for what she perceived as the analyst's inflexibility, and also recognized her own initial hypersensitivity and externalizations around this issue. She also felt, however, that there were changes in the way in which the analyst related to her in the latter phases of analysis, for example, the vacation comment as well as occasional direct answers to a question. We cannot, of course, know what actually occurred. We do not have access to the analyst's view of what changed and why. It may be that if the analyst did actually behave differently in the latter phase of the analysis that she did so intentionally. Her approach may have been designed to dilute and facilitate the final resolution of the transference neurosis after the patient had already largely worked through these issues. The patient's perception would contradict this speculation since she firmly believed that it was the shift in the analyst that facilitated the shift within herself. If the patient were correct in her assessment, this "match," while initially problematic, may have been ultimately growth-promoting for both analyst and patient.

Case 3

The patient was an intelligent 26-year-old woman who had repeatedly shifted her occupational choice. She had married early, and while ostensibly satisfied with her marital relationship insisted on trying to control all her husband's activities, just as she felt her mother had tried to control hers. She had sought analysis because she had abdominal pains and had been "told to go" by her internist. As the analysis unfolded, the patient developed a transference in which she experienced the analyst as imposing things on her and not being "warm" enough. The patient was extremely self-critical and externalized most issues. She experienced almost all interactions within and outside of the analytic hour as criticism and blamed the analyst for her discomfort because he was insufficiently warm. The analyst was understanding and accepting of the patient, and he made a systematic attempt to analyze the origin of her sensitivity to criticism and her feelings of being controlled and deprived. He and the patient were in agreement about what was troubling her, and to some extent they came to understand its historical antecedents. He seemed to have successfully entered and understood her world. Objectively there was a considerable measure of success. The patient's abdominal pains became less intense and less frequent, and she was able to give her husband more space to be himself. However, neither the patient nor the analyst was very satisfied with the results. The patient did not blame the analyst for this—an indication of change in itself—but took the responsibility on herself saying that she withheld from and resisted her analyst's interventions just as she had her mother's. She refused to become really involved with him and did not believe that anything really significant for her could change. There was a striking absence of genetic reconstruction; some references to younger siblings seemed important but were never developed. The analyst believed that though some real shifts had occurred, the patient had never really become fully engaged in the analytic process and had always held him at a distance. He felt that all attempts at analyzing her withholding and distancing had been unproductive. Ultimately the patient's seeming lack of interest had sufficiently discouraged him so that he, too, lost interest and felt no hope for change. The analysis ended with both of them feeling that they had reached a stalemate.

The analyst described his style as "very formal and very distant." This is not to suggest that it was only the actual amount of warmth that was the impediment, but that its absence, together with the analyst's inability to persist in reaching out to her to explore her feelings about him, led the analyst into a "mirroring" position—turning away from her, just as she was turning away from him.

Termination of the case at this stage in the analysis may well have reflected an accurate appraisal by the analyst that the patient had accomplished as much as possible. However, it is important to note that this analyst felt and reacted very differently with other patients. He characterized his analytic work with these patients as going "swimmingly." They were described as "wonderfully responsive" and as having "developed transference neuroses that were worked through." He experienced them as "interesting and lively." Terminations with these patients were satisfactory and were arrived at mutually. While it is possible that the patient described here was more difficult, the analyst's affective response of "tedium" and "boredom" in reaction to the patient's "steady demanding of more warmth, more responsiveness—expectations to do something for her—making it difficult to tell one hour from the next" is strikingly different from his appreciative stance toward his other cases. The "responsive," "lively," "interesting" qualities he perceived in these patients evoked a more colorful, lively, positive, and affect-full response from him in describing these cases.

Even if he did not vary his analytic technique in treating these patients, it does not seem implausible to assume that some manifestation, however subtle, of his affective response entered the analytic situation itself. His description of himself in relation to this patient as "very formal and very distant" as opposed to just formal and distant suggests such a possibility.

It could be, of course, that this patient's dynamics may have interacted with the analyst's character in a manner that impeded the completion of the analytic work. Reflecting on this case, the analyst was unaware of any clear countertransference issues or residual conflicts evoked by the patient. While he had "not enjoyed" the work, he felt he had worked hard. His ultimate conclusion was that the patient was not analyzable. The analyst may have been right; or it may be that the patient touched something within him that resulted in the analyst being unable to see further, to step outside the stalemate, and to reopen the analytic work. From this latter point of view, it would seem that by the end of the analysis, the analyst had ultimately joined the patient too fully in her distancing stance and sense of despair.

This situation could be thought of in the developmental terms suggested by Sander (1962) as a repetition from the stage of self-assertion. The child, now patient, pulls away from the mother, now analyst, to whom she was earlier closely attached—an attachment and subsequent loss and disappointment she fears reexperiencing in her analysis. She asserts her need for independence and fights against feeling controlled and criticized, but she also continues to express her longing for "more warmth," which is recapitulated in the transference. The hunger for the return to the earlier stage of attachment is poignantly present in the midst of her embattled struggle. The analyst, through his skill and empathic capacities, was able to help her analyze her sense of being blamed, and her need to control as she felt controlled, without becoming caught in the struggle himself. The experience must have been meaningful and effective for she emerges after analysis as a person less needing to blame and control others. This would seem to be an identification with her analyst's attitude (see Pfeffer, 1963) as well as a resolution of unconscious conflict. However, there remained for the patient an inability to turn back to her mother-analyst, a stubbornly maintained holding at a distance, and an insistence that "warmth" be given to her or nothing could change. It is here that the analyst-patient pair seems to be badly matched.

The question may be raised whether the analyst's failure to persevere represents a residual conflict for him, despite his disclaimer, or whether this is his characterological stance. We might take the position that warmth and a willingness to go 98 percent of the way should characterize everyone's treatment of patients; yet in any professional who is well trained, who cares about his patients' well-being, and who wants to be of service, formality and distance do not necessarily stem from internal conflict and are not invariably impediments to treatment. We could argue that some patients might respond adversely to perceiving the analyst as "too warm." It is the impact of these perceptions on the patient that needs to be analyzed in the treatment. Again, it is the analyst's failure to recognize that something in his behavior may have been disturbing to the patient that seemed to prevent him from exploring the meaning and origin or her responses.

If the analyst does in reality share characteristics with a significant person from the patient's past who had been troublesome to the patient (or characteristics of the patient which are unacceptable or disowned by the patient), this does not necessarily make an analysis impossible. It may, however, make it more difficult since it will be harder for the patient to see the analyst as separate from the original object and experience what he relives in analysis as transference. This increased difficulty may be overcome if the analyst keeps his focus on how and why the patient experiences him as he does. Case 2 illustrated this point.

Case 4

A 33-year-old man, who entered analysis moderately depressed and highly volatile in mood, had previously undergone eight years of analysis with a well-trained and very experienced analyst before beginning analysis with me. He felt that he had gained from his treatment and that it had enabled him to complete his schooling. However, he had sought more analysis because he was again suffering from his inability to commit himself to his work and establish a permanent relationship with a woman. In his first year of analysis, he would often repeat comments that his former analyst had made; almost all of them seemed accurate to him.

Yet there was something about the way he reported what he had learned about himself from his previous analysis that had both an intellectualized and self-flagellating quality to it. This became particularly evident in an hour toward the end of the first year of analysis with me. The patient had been describing his dissatisfaction with himself for staying in a dull job and continuing in a stalemated relationship. In both situations, he was marking time but he could not decide what to do next. His parents told him he was "too good" for both the job and the girl, and though he would argue with them, he felt this too. "This," he said:

> is what my former analyst described as my aristocratic attitude—
> feeling I'm entitled to do better and not doing anything to make
> it better. And he's right. Once again I feel stuck, cowardly, repul-
> sively pursuing a relationship where it's not working and staying
> in a dead-end job. My father's attitude is 'you've got to move on,'
> and I feel that's really right, but I stay around unable to let go. I
> don't like the repulsive quality of it, but I hang on.

I said that since his sense of revulsion was so strong something that pulled him to this must be even stronger and that I wondered what he gained from hanging on. His first thought was that the feeling of holding on to something even if it was repulsive to him was familiar, but he then added that he was enraged that someone wasn't there attending to him, and that he didn't get the job or the person he wanted right away, and that he had to work for them.

The next hour he reported that he was thinking of sitting up—something he had done occasionally during his first analysis. When I wondered what had led to this thought, he said he was feeling confused, angry, out of control, and wanting to regain a sense of control.

He wanted my perspective. I should tell him what I thought. My not doing so made him feel humiliated. I wondered what this was about. In a voice filled with rage, he informed me that he felt analysis was humiliating and demeaning, and that he felt unequal to me and hated this, and that lying down just reinforced this feeling. I recalled to him that these feelings were not new and had come up before, but wondered what was currently setting them off. After a prolonged silence, and with visible bodily tension, he said:

> Yesterday you asked what I gained from staying stuck. I feel both that you know why and won't tell me but make me work to find out, and that you're saying I shouldn't be that way—that I should give it up.

I said, "You felt I both withheld from you and criticized you." He responded, "Yes, like father saying 'move on.' You're all the same: father, Dr. X [former analyst], you—you don't really help and just blame and criticize." I wondered about this blaming and criticizing.

> Well, that's the way it feels, as if you're saying it's all my fault. Dr. X calling me aristocratic, your questioning what I gain from not moving—I felt that what Dr. X described about me was correct and so there was nothing more to say or explore. I'd get so angry and attack him. He was patient and accepting like my mother, never getting angry back. I'd scream for a few days and stop. It was all so familiar and it would happen again and again... he'd point out how I was raging as I had at home.... It was too humiliating to admit that I'd felt humiliated by being criticized. I felt that I should be above being angry about that; that at least would make me more of an equal and if I couldn't be one I could point out his faults... show him he wasn't perfect either.

Both his former analyst's comments and mine seemed to join and reinforce his own self-criticism, against which he would then rebel in explosive rage, verbal assaults, and accusations against others. Previous attempts to understand his rage and what stimulated it had led nowhere until we understood that he had experienced my words as criticism. One question was why had his former analyst not recognized the patient's self-criticism. Even though the patient quickly moved from self-flagellation to attacks on others, there was ample evidence of his self-devaluation. It would seem unlikely that his former analyst had continually failed to perceive how the patient viewed himself. What seemed more likely was that the analyst had not recognized how the patient experienced both his self-criticism and what he perceived as criticism from the analyst, that is, that these were humiliating to him. As the patient continued to explore the issue of his self-criticism, he increasingly became aware of how central it was in his character and how it had kept him from being able to own and explore many of his difficulties and conflicts. He realized that it was not that his self-criticism or his sense of humiliation had been unavailable in his first analysis, but that they had not been focused on. Not having worked through the feelings of shame and humiliation associated with the experience of criticism by self and others, it seems that many of the insights he achieved later remained only intellectual.

Over the next months, he calmed down dramatically, was more productive at work, and began seriously to consider marrying his girl-friend. Flare-ups continued to occur periodically. But each time, as he understood how something I had said or done made him feel bad about himself—misunderstood or blamed, and what it revived in his history—he settled down again. At one point, he said:

> Everything Dr. X said about me was right in its way, but what nei-ther of us seemed to understand was that, at root, the real prob-lem was how bad and unlovable I felt I was. All I really heard him saying was 'this is why you are bad and unlovable.' The accuracy of his observations didn't matter. It just confirmed my worst feel-ings about myself.

The question, then, is why the patient's first analyst did not focus on, explore, and analyze the patient's self-criticism. It is possible, of course, that the analyst did raise these issues but that the patient was not ready to deal with them at that time. Let us for the moment, however, assume that the patient's perception reflects the reality of their interaction and that his experience of self-criticism and humil-iation was insufficiently emphasized. If a well-trained, experienced analyst is not hearing or focusing on the other side of the patient's rage—that is, the patient's self-denigration—then a question may be asked whether there continued to be some unresolved personal issues around self-criticism for this analyst. All would agree that a well-trained analyst should not be judgmental. In this case, Freud's (1910a) statement that no psychoanalyst "goes further than his own complexes and internal resistances permit" (p. 145) would apply. Or did the former analyst's interventions reflect a lack of understanding of the operation of punitive, unconscious self-criticism (unconscious guilt)? Another strong possibility is that the analyst's manner of communicating reflected an authoritative style that would be reacted to adversely by persons who had active or residual issues around self-blame. For such patients, a gentle, more tentative manner might facilitate their ability to hear, respond to, and integrate interpretations.

The analyst's seeming failure to recognize that his patient was responding to his comments as criticisms might suggest a psychological blind spot. He appears to have been unaware of his impact on the patient. It is this failure to see the effect on the patient—whether because of the analyst's own unresolved issues, his failure to understand about unconscious guilt, or crucial aspects of his characterological style—that suggests a seemingly poor "match." If the analyst's limitation was due to unresolved issues or a lack of understanding about unconscious guilt, it is possible that a wide range of patients would be affected; the analyst's need for further analytic or pedagogical work would be at issue. But it is also possible that with patients who were not particularly troubled in this area, his work might be effective.

From the material available, it is not possible to determine which, if any, of these factors determined this analyst's lack of awareness. In this particular case, the omission may seem glaring; regardless of which particular factor led to the analyst's psychological blind spot, a patient who could not persist in saying how criticized he felt and an analyst who did not recognize that he sounded critical to the patient were an unfortunate match. Other kinds of blind spots are harder to detect and are not as easily seen as a personal limitation of the analyst.

Even the ideally trained and well-functioning analyst cannot be expected to be equally effective with all patients. We can find a parallel with the analyst-patient relationship in Sander's (1962) description of mother-infant interactions. Of course the parallel is not exact since these patients, being fully grown adults, bring already formed characters into analysis. Nonetheless, these infant observations show how the particular character of the mother influences both the extent to which she resonates with her child's emotional state and the manner in which she conveys her attunement to her child. These two aspects, the understanding of the experiential state and the manner of communicating this understanding, also have their parallels in the analytic process. The mesh of the particular character of mother-infant pairs also has its parallel in the analyst-patient interaction. The way an analyst understands what his patient expresses and the manner in which he communicates his understanding are elements that are shared by all well-trained analysts and yet vary from analyst to analyst.

The analyst, like the mother with her child, tries to stay attuned to the multidimensional aspects of his patient's experiences. Unlike the mother whose resonance with her child is mostly intuitive, the analyst's attunement with his patient is conscious and disciplined. It is governed by a logical, theoretical construction of a therapeutic process that he believes facilitates change in the patient.

The perspective from "inside" the patient is one the analyst may have difficulty maintaining. What makes it difficult may vary according to the analyst's specific character, his life experiences, and the degree to which his self-analytic function is developed. That is, the similarities and differences between analyst and patient have an impact on whether the analyst can or cannot resonate with the patient, just as the similarities and differences between parent and child affect the synchrony between them. Schwaber (1981) has suggested that one's capacity to enter the patient's world may be impeded by a difference in background or gender. She proposes that there are areas in which "essential human alikeness" is not sufficient to bridge the experiential gap that exists, for example, in a female analyst's possible inability to comprehend the nature of a male patient's sexual experience in all its depth and complexity. Gill (1981) offers the other side of this dialectic by suggesting that when the analyst and patient are actually very different, the analyst may be more likely to keep himself actively attending to the nature of the patient's subjective experience. Being aware that the patient's experience is likely to be so different from his own, the analyst must make a greater effort to comprehend it.

These double dangers of being "too alike" or "too different" threaten both mother-and-child and analyst-and-patient attunement. For the mother, the danger is that her character and style may be so different that she cannot effectively empathize with her child; or that she is so intensely identified with her child that she fails to recognize his separateness. For the analyst, the danger is that his discrepancies in experience and perception are great enough to allow for little or no resonance with his patient; or that their similarities in experience and perception cause the analyst to miss the way in which the patient is unique and different from him. These are some of the issues, attitudes, reactions, and behaviors that may strain or dislodge empathic listening. The disruption of empathic listening is likely to lead to a loss of attunement that may ultimately impede the analytic work.

In conclusion and summary, analysis derives some of its power from the revival of emotional attachment to the analyst in the transference. The transference meanings of this attachment are then themselves the focus of analysis. To the extent that the analytic situation repeats the past in these significant ways, old patterns will be reinforced. To the extent that the past is revived, analyzed, and not repeated, emotional growth is likely to occur. An analyst, because he or she is a person like everyone else—human and therefore imperfect—inevitably will have, along with particular strengths and talents, quirks, blind spots, and residual neurotic conflicts that can be activated under stress. These are not necessarily crucial, unless they intermesh in a significant way with the difficulties of the patient.

This, then, is the issue of patient-analyst "match." Unfortunately, the quality and nature of this match are often unknowable before beginning analysis. Matches with mutual "blind spots" will not become apparent. In other instances, the effect of the match may not become clear until the analytic work is far along, since it is precisely the nature of the transference that makes it both inevitable and desirable for the patient to perceive the analyst "as if" he is like significant others in his past. To quote Freud (1895): "If the perceptual image is not absolutely new, it will now recall and revive a mnemic perceptual image with which it coincides at least partly" (p. 330). The analyst, by keeping in mind his/her role as a participant and focusing attention on what his/her contribution is to making the situation feel "not absolutely new" to the patient, will simultaneously heighten and open for understanding the transference experience. It is the patient's perception of and reaction to the analyst, not the analyst's intention, which needs to be kept in focus in the analytic situation. Undoubtedly, the more the analyst can understand and keep in his awareness what his/her actual contribution to the transference experience is, the less likely it is that his/her personal limitations and the effect of the personality constellation will adversely affect the treatment. However, there are limits for everyone. It is the contention of this paper that even if an analyst is highly skilled and experienced, it should not be assumed that he can analyze everyone. The informal but widespread practice of consultants attempting to match prospective analytic patients with particular analysts acknowledges this reality.

Notes

1 1985 Felix and Helene Deutsch Scientific Paper Award, Boston Psycho-analytic Society and Institute.
2 This concept grows out of research in Gestalt psychology. See Solomon Asch (1952), pp. 53–54.
3 Since difficulties in patient-analyst match are the result of some una-wareness on the part of both participants, I assume that the best ex-amples cannot be drawn completely from my own practice; I cannot, of course, present instances of factors in my own work of which I am unaware. Some of the following anecdotal material was revealed to me in the course of my interviews with analysts and patients as part of my follow-up study of analytic suitability (Kantrowitz, Singer, & Knapp, 1975).

Chapter 2

The analyst's style and its impact on the analytic process

Overcoming a patient-analyst stalemate

Each analyst possesses a characteristic style in conducting analytic work. This style is the result of conscious choices as well as more fundamental, generally unconscious, configurations of character. Of course, each individual style has variations and, depending on the characteristics of the particular patient, some aspects of the analyst's style are more prominent in one analysis than in another. Overall, however, there are identifiable qualities in each analyst's mode of working which are distinctive and certain general tendencies in the analyst's methods that permit broader categorization. One of the possible categories is the analyst's perspective on the patient's experience. Some analysts tend to expand the patient's own point of view, in contrast to offering a perspective emphasizing the differences between the patient's and analyst's views; that is, some tend more often to take an inside perspective, others more often take an outside perspective. While most analysts generally use both modes, and it is unlikely that any analyst employs either of these perspectives exclusively, nonetheless, one mode of perceptual organization often is dominant. The extent to which one mode dominates may be shaped by particular characteristics of the patient as well as the analyst's own proclivities.

A confluence of factors contributes to forming an analyst's style. Many of these factors stem from conflict-free areas; others have their origin in conflict or may be interwoven with areas of unconscious or partially unresolved conflicts. The degree of warmth or coolness, closeness or distance, spontaneity or rigidity, informality or formality, and activity or passivity manifested by the analyst in analytic work may be related to the analyst's ability to modulate and tolerate affect, or to maintain particular self- or object representations, or to the depth and intensity of the analyst's participation in object relations. The function of the analyst's style may be, to varying degrees, adaptive or defensive, and may facilitate or impede analytic progress depending on the particular patient and the phase of analysis. As long as it remains within certain boundaries, the analyst's particular style may be viewed as value-neutral.

In all analyses, features of style, along with other attributes of the analyst, such as skill and areas of partially unresolved conflict or countertransference, will determine, in part, the limits of the analytic work. With certain patients, when there is an overlap in problem areas, when the analyst is either too similar to or too different from the patient, blind spots may make it difficult to work effectively. At times of crisis or stalemate in analysis, these problems of compatibility may necessitate a change in the analyst's stance for the analysis to progress. Such problems undoubtedly emerge most sharply in transference-countertransference enactments, but may also occur in subtler forms more often than we are aware. In this chapter, the aspect of the match that I will describe emphasizes the role of countertransference: my difficulties in working with an extremely self-critical patient where, at a certain phase of the analysis, the treatment had become stalemated until an enactment, influenced by the particular patient-analyst match, occurred. My self-analysis informed me about my countertransference and alteration in my style was facilitated by a consultation; both were necessary for the treatment to progress.

In recent years, analysts have given increasing attention to overlapping experiences and other areas of similarity they share with their patients (Gardner, 1983; Jacobs, 1980, 1983, 1986, 1987; McLaughlin, 1983; Poland, 1988) to supplement the long-standing recognition of the impact of the analyst's countertransference on the treatment. While there has been some attention given to the patient's style (Rosen, 1967), the literature on the effects of the analyst's style on the course of treatment is not extensive. Stein (1981) specifically focused on the different impact of the analyst's taking an empathic or questioning stance in relation to the "unobjectionable parts of the transference," which appear to be rational, collaborative, and seemingly not linked to resistance. He believes that the analyst's choice to accept at face value, rather than question, the patient's "unobjectionable" reactions, while humane, protective, and facilitating to analytic progress in the early phase of analysis, may subtly encourage the perpetuation of infantile patterns, and, in the long run, make a proper termination difficult. An introspective-empathic response may lead to a shared narcissistic regression, which is gratifying for both patient and analyst, but he believes such a response prevents the achievement of understanding of the function and origin of the unobjectionable aspect of the transference as well as other components to which it is linked. According to Stein, analysis requires the analyst's active questioning and interpreting of the unobjectionable elements to reveal their connection to unconscious conflicts.

Other analysts specifically considered the shaping effect of the analyst's character and countertransference on the analyst's style of communication with the patient. Weisman (1973) drew attention to the general role of countertransference in determining the choices therapists make in how they conduct their treatments. He distinguished three sources of countertransference. One source was derived from appetites, aversions, wishes, and fears leading to attractions and repulsions. The second came from the habitual, preferred ways that aid or impede participation in relationships; these responses reflect individual style and the standard ways of responding which limit personal options. The third source of countertransference attitudes arose from the analyst's values, standards, directives, and prohibitions, all of which lead to judgments of right and wrong, good and bad, and successful and unsuccessful. These factors have an impact on the portion of another person's life where they impinge. He delineated several forms of countertransference. In a complementary countertransference, the special strengths of the therapist fit and serve to aid the patient, for example, a steadfast organized therapist with a tumultuous, impulsive patient. In an antagonistic countertransference, the therapist may be disrespectful, belittling, self-righteous to the patient or in his estimation of the patient's way of living. In a parallel countertransference, the patient and therapist share the same problem; and in the tangential countertransference, the therapist's understanding and interventions seem irrelevant, peripheral, or out of focus to the patient. Weisman concluded that how productive or nonproductive such interventions are depends on "how readily and intelligently the therapist can correct his own responses" (p. 115).

The role of countertransference in a therapist's or analyst's decision to confront or refrain from confronting a patient also was given attention. Myerson (1973) underscored that the degree of forcefulness employed in a confrontation is influenced by the therapist's unconscious as well as conscious intentions. Countertransference or counteridentification reactions of irritation to the patient's resistance may be rationalized, and justifications for employing more force offered. Alternatively, countertransference identification with the patient or fear of hurting may lead other therapists to avoid confrontation. In addition to conscious intentions in the manner of conducting treatment, therapists' and analysts' reactions to their patients' reactions to them also influence treatment decisions.

Shapiro (1973) expanded Myerson's focus on the influence of unconscious influences on the therapist's choice in treatment technique to include the character and attitudes of the therapist or analyst. To illustrate his point, he contrasted the treatment of a patient by two analysts. One analyst was unusually giving and kind and unable convincingly to confront the patient's unrealistic expectations. The failure to confront, he believed, offered a temptation to an ego regression to which the patient succumbed. The second analyst, in contrast, while comfortable with exploring primitive fantasies, believed strongly in the patient's need to lean on herself and not on him. The confrontative stance, he claimed, was largely responsible for this patient's mastery of her struggles. The implication of this vignette was that not all therapists or analysts have characters that permit them to be confrontative. He concluded that confrontation must be consistent with the therapist's or analyst's character and attitudes for it to be effective.

Self-critical patients present a particular dilemma for therapists and analysts. No matter how accurately analysts and therapists have understood their patients' dynamics and conflicts or how sensitively and tactfully they have made their clarifications and interpretations, the patients tend to hear these interventions as criticism. For patients suffering from self-criticism, interpretations of defense are experienced as confrontations. Interpretations or clarifications of their thoughts, feelings, fantasies, and actions are experienced as implicit communications that they should not be thinking, feeling, fantasizing, or doing what has been brought into focus. The patients feel humiliated at being exposed, blame themselves, and use this revelation to further confirm their sense of badness or defect. Often, as described by Kris (1977), the pressure of self-criticism mounts too high, and these patients rebel against its demands and blame the outside world. Caught between blaming themselves and blaming others, such patients find no space to make use of observations offered about how they behave. Even techniques like Gray's (1973) analysis of defense, which focuses almost exclusively on shifts within the analytic hour, are still frequently experienced by self-critical patients as meaning that by a shift they have done something wrong.

Kohut's (1971) stance of empathic immersion, a mode of listening and organizing observations, offers a solution to this dilemma. If instead of focusing on the defensive aspect of the patients' behavior, the analyst draws attention to the adaptive function it serves, the patients will feel understood and not criticized. As the self is strengthened through this empathic mirroring, the self-criticism and sense of humiliation lessen, and gradually, previously disavowed aspects of the self are allowed back into consciousness and reintegrated. Sometimes, however, the treatment does not proceed so smoothly, and despite a prolonged period of empathic responding, the patient does not assume ownership for his or her feelings, thoughts, fantasies, or actions.

Modell (1970) believes that patients with acute narcissistic sensitivity need what he calls a "cocoon" period in which they can have the experience of being accepted and understood without facing their defensive operations. Eventually, however, such a confrontation must take place. Unlike Kohut, he does not believe that this will spontaneously occur once the self is strengthened. However, it is only after these patients establish a trust in the therapist or analyst based on the belief that they are accepted and cared about that a confrontation, exposing an area of denial or questioning a belief or a behavior, will have an impact.

The choice of clinical theory is shaped not only by intellectual beliefs, but also by the character of the therapist or analyst. As some of these authors suggest, our preferred techniques are similarly determined by events of the past, our reactions to these occurrences, and all the other factors that contribute to our becoming our adult selves. Weisman's view of countertransference is similar to what I have previously called the match between patient and analyst (Kantrowitz,

1986; Kantrowitz et al., 1989; Kantrowitz, Katz, & Paolitto, 1990c). In choosing the term "match," I mean to emphasize the total interactional nature, the pervasive effect of the interdigitation of the analyst's character, and remaining unresolved conflicts with the character and dynamic struggles of the patient. Countertransference is then one particular facet of the match, an interaction in which the behavior of the patient taps into and stimulates an unconscious aspect of the analyst. Countertransference reactions may result in the analyst enacting some part of a relationship from the past or, possibly, from a current relationship which has a troublesome aspect that is still poorly understood.

Analysts and therapists all do better work with some patients than with others. We are all limited by our characters. Some clinicians have a broader range of patients whom they treat successfully than do others. The extent to which we and our patients are capable of stretching our capacities and modifying our limitations differs for each of us, and there are always limits.

When we have reached these limits is not always clear. We may get caught between two poles. We may be pulled between our striving for perfectionism, where we fail to appreciate our limits, and our intolerance of frustration in persisting in the face of what is difficult. However, in our daily work, we believe, and practice the belief, that people are capable of growth and change well into their adult years. Sometimes the pressure from patients who tap into partially or poorly resolved aspects of our selves may help this growth and change as we struggle to facilitate their development (Kantrowitz, 1986; Sonnenberg, 1991).

Case illustration

This case is presented to illustrate the limitations, at a certain phase of analysis, of the analyst's characteristic style of working, brought into focus by a countertransference enactment. It also aims to show how the analyst's self-analysis allowed a revision of style that produced an expanded mode of response that facilitated the treatment. I shall describe the case of a 30-year-old man who came for analysis because he felt hopelessly stuck in every aspect of his life. He could not commit himself to marriage, complete his doctoral dissertation, or separate himself from a hostile-dependent tie to his parents. He had considerable insight into his conflicts from a previous analysis. He credited that analysis for his ability to enter graduate school and for enabling him to separate from a destructive relationship with a former girlfriend. However, his chronic depression had never abated, and his intense self-criticism and sense of shame and humiliation had remained unmodified. His state of paralysis exacerbated all these painful affects.

We began what was to be a nine-year analysis. During the middle years of analysis, he married his girlfriend and completed his dissertation. However, the painful affective states remained largely unresolved even late into his analysis. What follows is not intended to describe the vicissitudes of the patient's dynamics or of the treatment, but only to illustrate a particular aspect of the patient-analyst interaction. The reader should also be cautioned that external details have been disguised to preserve confidentiality.

The patient was a first, adored child. His father, a well-respected scholar, was the chairman of an academic department. According to my patient, his father was charming, but cool, and demanding in his expectations of his son. While in one sense the patient felt he was intensely valued and special to his father, in another sense, he felt that nothing he ever did was good enough, and that his father viewed him as incompetent and as a disappointment. He described his mother as a warm, empathic person, unsure of herself, and always comparing herself unfavorably with her intellectually achieving husband. She pampered the patient, never requiring that he assume responsibility for himself or be accountable to others. He felt simultaneously gratified and infantilized by her and recalled being demanding and imperious with her. Her seemingly endless patience with him, however, would be unexpectedly interrupted by her abrupt departures, the most affectively memorable occurring at the time of his sister's birth when the patient was seven. He felt betrayed, but also believed he deserved this abandonment as punishment for his objectionable behavior. He dated this time as the beginning of his chronic misery. He claimed that he turned from his parents to his friends and activities.

Until he graduated from college, he was successful both academically and socially. After graduation, he drifted from one activity to another, unable to find direction for himself. It was at this point that he sought his first analysis, which helped him to regain his equilibrium. Despite his proclaimed independence, he had never earned enough money to support himself until midway in his second analysis, in his mid-thirties, when he obtained his doctoral degree and his first teaching position. His insistent denigration of and fury with his family kept him tied to them. While this stance allowed the expression of his aggression, it simultaneously served as a defense against the experience of his positive feelings for his family. Positive feelings for them, he feared, would result in his subjugation to them and cause him to experience the painful longing for his unmet desires. He was intensely defended against mourning his disappointment and disillusionment. To mourn would mean relinquishing power and placing himself at their mercy because he would be acknowledging that he cared. It would also mean accepting both their limits and his own, an acceptance he felt would be humiliating and potentially annihilating to himself. By resisting growing up and avoiding the responsibilities of adult life, he felt he could magically freeze time, keeping his parents young and preventing their death. As long as he needed them in this magical bargain, they could not die. Most of these dynamics emerged only during the course of his second analysis.

His oedipal conflicts had been explored in his first analysis. He understood that he feared displeasing his father. Manifestly, achievement was what his father wanted from him, but he was certain that his father concealed that he viewed his son as a rival whom he did not want to succeed. This left the patient paralyzed, feeling that either way he moved, he would lose. This became the paradigm for all achievement. He would do and undo and procrastinate to maintain a status quo that left him feeling frustrated, inhibited, envious, lonely, and enraged. His barely contained anger due to his feelings of deprivation disrupted his interaction with friends and colleagues and in his daily interchanges.

Over the years of analysis, the various ways the patient had experienced me as failing him were addressed. We had considered these incidents both in terms of the specific ways what I actually did or did not do failed to meet what he wanted, and how these experiences echoed past disappointments. In addition, we had come to see his disappointment with me as a projected disappointment with himself. He felt he had disappointed his parents', his own, and my expectations of him. In this last sense, his berating of me also reflected a projection in which he was beating himself in the displacement. A great deal of work had focused on the severity of his self-criticism, from which he rebelled when it became too severe by blaming others. Often he blamed them for objective failings; nonetheless, this castigation represented an externalization of his virulent self-criticism in which what he criticized in them was an aspect of something he hated in himself. He was caught in an either-or dilemma of finding fault in himself and becoming depressed and passive, or finding fault in the other and becoming enraged and attacking them for these faults. Throughout the analysis, I was rescued from the position of feeling attacked through my understanding that this was both a projection of his own self-criticism and of his lifelong belief that he had been blamed. In the analysis, it was his experience of blame he was trying to relive and master.

In the seventh year of analysis, the patient seemed to be in a different state. His marriage, while far from harmonious, seemed to be a source of pleasure to him much of the time, and he was far more appreciative and accepting of his wife than he had been. He approached his work with new vigor, actively pursuing his own scholarship, writing articles which were accepted for publication, offering support and encouragement to students and colleagues, participating in department committees, and discovering a pleasure in his work which he had not anticipated ever finding. Yet he was reluctant to consider termination. He was still subject to periods of intense disappointment, frustration, and rage. He felt that if he stopped, he would be leaving in anger, as he had in his first analysis, because he still did not take himself seriously or believe in his own capacities. So we continued trying to explore what this meant, but the analytic hours seemed only to repeat what we already had understood.

A turning point in the analysis came when he arrived one hour in acute distress. He had been denied tenure because of a budget freeze in his department. The consequences of his years of procrastination, his denial of the passage of time, and his untested half-belief that once he was ready he could have whatever he wanted, all came crashing down upon him. He attacked himself and raged at the world. I empathized with how disappointed he must feel, how hard he had been working, how painful it was not to get the rewards for his work. He did not feel comforted, but rather attacked me. I could not possibly understand, and it was presumptuous to try. He was sure that my own teaching position was secure since he was certain I would have done everything in a timely and efficient fashion. He raged on and on. He would not accept being refused tenure, and he would not go elsewhere to try again. He would stand his ground and make them give it to him. I interpreted how helpless he felt and how enraged this made him. He continued to rage. I struggled to think what else I might offer as our time was almost over, made some feeble attempt, and ended the hour.

No sooner had I closed the door than I realized I had ended the hour ten minutes early. I went to find my patient who was fuming in the hall fully aware of my error. I apologized, saying I knew how miserable he was feeling, and I was sorry to have added to his pain. He asked angrily if I wanted to talk about it, and returned to the couch. My behavior, he said, just confirmed for him how no one could tolerate his pain. He was an obnoxious, hateful person, and it was no wonder his department did not want to make him a permanent member, and I did not want to spend his allotted time with him. I replied that he was understandably angry at my having cut short his time, and seemed to be turning his anger away from me against himself, something we knew he did frequently. I had done something really hurtful to him, I said, and he was adding his own abuse to this, finding his anger at me at this time unacceptable. "So why did you do it?" he screamed. I told him that was something I would have to try to understand.

As I reflected about what had happened during the analytic hour, I understood my feelings of helplessness at my patient trying to get me to experience actively his feelings of helplessness, and I thought that my self-understanding would allow me to tolerate these feelings. I felt bad for his disappointment. I also knew that I felt rejected and angry that he was pushing away my attempts to be empathic and was continuing to attack me, but it seemed to me that my feelings of frustration were mild in comparison to his and could be withstood. What I was not in touch with was that I had exceeded my own limit for tolerating these affects. My unawareness that I was ending the hour ten minutes early, due to my own intolerance of feeling helpless, brought home to him and to me that I had my limits. In trying to put aside my anger and frustration with him in order to remain empathic, I had gone too far in self-abnegation. I knew this experience of helplessness recreated for me the most painful moments of parenting when I could not find a way to comfort a child in distress. Had these dysphoric affects remained more in the center of my awareness, it is possible I might have felt less helpless and then might not have needed to absent myself from the hour. While ending the hour early was an unconscious expression of the angry feelings I had consciously put aside, I may have also been unconsciously protecting him from the anger I feared I might experience and express were I to remain there in a prolonged state of helplessness. Was I sharing the patient's problem in not appreciating the importance of limits? Did I believe, as he claimed his mother had, that with sufficient patience, tolerance, and care from me over time, he would move on of his own accord, and that it was not necessary to set limits? After careful reflection and self-analysis, I concluded this was true. I saw that, like the patient's mother, I had implicitly given him permission to avoid responsibility for his behavior. I had made something my task that should have been his. By unconsciously trying to contain his painful affects, I saw that in fact I was depriving him of the opportunity to assume the responsibility for himself.

When he returned for the next hour, the patient had reached many of the same conclusions about the meaning of my behavior. He did not press me to confirm his thoughts. Rather, he described poignantly how the experience of my trying to be helpful and patient and then abruptly abandoning him when I could stand it no longer was an exact replay of his experience with his mother. I had been unable to tell him when enough was enough. In addition to expressing his pain and outrage about not getting tenure, he thought he had been sadistic toward me. He had wanted to disrupt my seeming calm self-containment, to pull me into his distress. And he also had wanted me to feel my limits as he was feeling his, wanted me to admit that sometimes there was really nothing one could do. He had not believed that my words about the difficulty in tolerating helplessness and rage were anything more than words. To him, words were cheap. He knew he could talk a good game. So could his mother. So could I. Actions were what counted. As long as I did not by action acknowledge that I had a limit, he could not acknowledge he had one. He would feel humiliated and ashamed of failing to live up to his potential, disappointing me and himself as he felt he had disappointed his father. He would see himself as inferior to me, feeling inadequate, envious, and resentful that he had been deprived of something I had. He also knew that he still hoped what he had seen and was describing was not true, because he did want to give up his belief in the possibilities of my perfection or his own. He was impressed, however, that I had not tried to deny or make him responsible for my failure as he felt his mother had.

Over the next weeks, we reviewed this experience and its meaning to him. We came to see that he had taken my not more actively questioning his reluctance to terminate as a covert promise that he could still attain perfection; it meant neither he nor I was satisfied with him as a reasonably competent, achieving person. He now understood a thought he had had earlier—that he would leave analysis angry as an expression of his belief that I had withheld from him the knowledge of how to be perfect. I wondered with him if he had also felt that my failure to pursue assertively his reluctance to end analysis was a way of holding him back, keeping him dependent. He thought this was correct and added that he believed this was a way I could remain superior. As we reworked what had occurred, how he had experienced it, and his new understanding, we also began to talk about setting a termination date.

Something continued to trouble me. All that we had explored seemed accurate. But was it only anger over my withholding the key to perfection that he had meant when he claimed our work was not done? I understood that in assuming too much responsibility for bearing his affective pain, I had been depriving him of assuming this responsibility for himself and contributing to the delay of a developmental step. But I was not sure that, even having identified the problem, I knew how to treat it. Generally, I was good enough at providing comfort and help as well as letting patients try their wings in their own ways. Also, I was not reluctant to confront patients when I believed they could integrate the issue that was being addressed. But I realized that on this occasion, I had failed to protect myself by too quickly putting aside my anger at being attacked out of fear that I would inflict pain on my patient in his acutely vulnerable state. I was also aware that this was not the only time I had tried to extend myself beyond my limit in trying to meet another's extreme pain, in part unconsciously, to ward off my own sense of helplessness and frustration. There was something I did not understand about the tolerance of frustration and how to help my patient develop it. I had known, and now understood in more depth and complexity, that when I empathized with my patient's distress, in addition to stimulating his regressive wishes, he experienced me as demeaning him, holding him back, treating him as incompetent—in short, expecting too little from him. He knew he was capable of more, but was afraid to even try in his belief that he would lose me. He felt I wanted him to fail, and his unconscious bargain was to try but not to move ahead in order to please me. On the other hand, if I seemed not to accept his stance of incompetence and expect more of him, he experienced me as being like his father, harsh, unfeeling, unable to appreciate difficulties, and intolerant of feelings. This either-or dilemma was old territory, familiar from the early days of the analysis. Both sides had been experienced and explored; the conflict had been interpreted and in many ways seemed lessened. However, when it came to his tolerance for frustration and disappointment, we seemed back in the old bind. I did not know how to do it differently. I tried to think about how I had learned to tolerate my own distress when it arose. My own analysis had been enormously helpful in this regard, but I did not have a cognitive grasp of what had been so effective. I decided to have a consultation with a colleague.

My consultant listened to my quandary and some of the analytic process. His advice was clear and straightforward: watch for the places where the patient abandoned his own constructive efforts and gave up in despair. Observe with him the efforts made and wonder what intervened between his work on his own behalf and his giving up and trying to get others to step in to do the work for him. One watched for the shifts. That is, he suggested that I should communicate to the patient that he could and was doing something constructive that we both could see. The second step was the communication of my observation of his turning away from these efforts. The last piece of the intervention was bringing into focus what was intolerable to the patient that had led him to turn away and hand the control over to others. In essence, this approach was, "You were doing something well yourself. Something made you stop. Let us try to see what you found so intolerable that you threw up your hands and hoped someone else would take over."

As I listened to my patient in subsequent hours, there were abundant opportunities for such interventions. In one hour, the patient was thinking about his lack of motivation. He would like to be more productive, and admired people who were, some of whom he then cited. He had begun to expand his area of work. He wanted to be challenged to grow, but would become nervous, pull back, avoid getting in gear. He needed to work harder, to take on an extra job—maybe tutoring—and make more money. Then: "What do I do with the money my parents give me? I just spend it. That's not earning, or working. I see the issue but I don't do anything!" I observed that he had been talking about generating something for himself and then diverted from what he could do and was considering doing for himself, to what he received from his parents. It was after he had turned away from pursuing his thought about doing his own work and focusing on what he was given that he had become self-blaming. He protested, "I can't... I don't want to." To own his work as his, he had thought he could not do it; it was just too much, and he wanted to give up, to have me take care of him. But he knew I was right. When he gave up, he hated himself; but doing it himself was just too hard. I wondered what had intervened between his thought of doing his own work and thinking of what he got from his parents. He realized the thought had been the same: it is just too hard. I said it was then that he threw his hands up in frustration. "Yes," he said, "because I feel I just can't do it." Following this, he returned to thoughts of what he was doing and what more he could do.

Similarly, in a subsequent session, he explored what he continued to gain by holding himself back. He thought I had been drawing his attention to this conflict. He saw that sabotaging his own progress did not please me as he had believed it would. He knew he had fears of competing, and that his father or I might want him to fail. However, at the moment, this did not seem to be the issue. Right now, he thought what I had been raising with him was his reluctance to test himself. I was trying to get him to test reality, to face his unwillingness to try, so that he might see whether or not he could succeed.

As he thought of it this way, he began to get angry. Why now? Why had I not focused specifically on this issue years ago? He felt livid. It was the right issue, but he was furious that I had waited. He began to berate me. I said that he had started to confront an issue he felt was correct and important and had then turned from it to be angry with me. I told him that while his anger at me might be justified, at this moment he was using it to move away from confronting the issue.

His anger abated, and he became reflective again. He thought about how he had confronted a colleague who was avoiding seeing his own self-destructive behavior. The patient saw that he had been denying that his own behavior was self-damaging. With this acknowledgment, he had felt both afraid and ashamed. It was then that he began to attack me. He had known that he could not stand feeling at fault and at such times often blamed others—though less frequently now. What he had not realized before, because he had never allowed himself to stay with his feelings for long, was that what he could not stand was the feeling of anxiety, the tension about not having an assured outcome about what he could or could not do.

In the following months, over and over again, we examined his intolerance of uncertainty, the difficulty he had bearing frustration, and tolerating ambiguity, and disappointment as they became manifest in the analytic hours. His shame over his aggression and hostility became tempered with an appreciation that he had not known how to act differently. Gradually, his tolerance increased. He began to think he might be able to terminate without being angry. He was able to let go of blaming others and himself as he tried to hold himself accountable in his life both in relation to his work and in relation to other people. A termination date was set. While there was a repetition of much that had been tumultuous in the analysis during this phase, he ended the treatment as planned six months later with a new-found sense of competence and confidence.

Discussion

In the case being considered, the analyst's tendency to work from the perspective of expanding the patient's view was increased by the patient's proclivity to reacting with self-criticism and intense shame and humiliation when interventions were not experienced as empathic. While this approach had been facilitating during most of the analysis, in the latter phase it became an impediment to progress. Two deviations from the analyst's characteristic style of working with this patient occurred. The first was unintentional; it revealed an area of denial and came in the form of an enactment. It was not a conscious decision and reflected a countertransference reaction. My premature ending of the patient's analytic hour forced both the patient and me to see I had a limit to my tolerance, and it was not serving either of us well for me to fail to own up to this directly. The second was a conscious, planned intervention in which I shifted my perspective from empathy with the patient's point of view to confronting him about his avoidance, while simultaneously continuing to acknowledge his positive efforts where they existed. It exposed my patient's evasion of actively assuming responsibility for himself. The intervention was intended to be educational as well as therapeutic. I brought the patient's attention to what he could and was doing for himself and showed him how he abandoned his own efforts in favor of seeking others' help or blaming them for not helping. I then helped him face the affects he was avoiding by these evasions.

It is possible, as Shapiro (1973) stated, that were my character different, I could have confronted my patient directly, and probably sooner, with the necessity of his taking responsibility for himself. It is also possible that had he been in analysis with an analyst whose character was different in this respect, the patient's analysis need not have taken so long. To use Myerson's (1973) construction, my reluctance to confront him directly was, at least in part, due to my countertransference identification with my patient's sensitivity to anything he perceived as criticism.

My attunement to his intense self-criticism had made this problem a central focus in the analysis. That it had not diminished as much as I had hoped or expected by late in the analysis, in retrospect, I think related to the fact that the patient was unable to respect or like himself enough until he was able to assume more responsibility for himself. He had remained self-critical because he appreciated that, although he was conflicted and did not want to relinquish the gratifications that came from being taken care of, he also wanted to be more responsible. He felt guilty about his continual evasion of assuming responsibility for himself. While he was overly harsh with himself and needed to attain a more charitable and forgiving view of his behavior, he feared that empathy from me or himself for his continued reluctance to assume responsibility for himself, for his wishes to indulge his dependency, to react explosively to frustrations, and to blame and attack others when he was no longer able to tolerate his self-abuse, was like condoning sadism and would lessen his motivation to change. Real empathy at that point would have been, and later was, to appreciate that he felt any letting up on himself was permission to be someone he hated. He felt his self-criticism helped keep him in line.

My initial focus on the adaptive aspects of his behavior over time did make him feel relatively safe from attack in the analytic hours, but he could not feel really safe with me until he was sure I would not allow him to take advantage of me as he felt he had his mother. Throughout the analysis, my adherence to 50-minute sessions and prompt focus on when he was late in paying his bill had both surprised and relieved him. He was painfully aware that he had a history of leaving garbage for others to clean up.

In the enactment, however, I came to see how I also was not holding up my end of the work by continuing to offer too much help in the cleanup when it was no longer appropriate to his development in analysis. My enactment showed my rebellion against offering so much help. To continue to do so was not to appreciate his strengths sufficiently. He had interpreted this as confirming his belief in my wish to hold him back.

While I was aware of my increasing impatience with the patient's withholding, avoidance, evasion, and blaming me or others within the hours, I believed that forceful confrontation of these defenses was likely either to increase his resistance or to result in a compliance that reflected a need to please me rather than his taking ownership. However, despite my suppression of rising irritation and my redoubling my efforts to listen and respond from the vantage point of the patient (Schwaber, 1983), my own limits made me at that point fail to understand and retain that perspective. In Sandler's (1976) terms, a role-responsive relationship had developed. The patient's push for me to take over for him had been met by my unconscious pull to be the endlessly supportive and nurturing mother. My failure to more actively question his reluctance to terminate was a broader manifestation of my lack of appreciation of the importance of limits. My enactment of the feelings of having had enough, which I was trying to put aside, led me to rethink and ultimately redefine what constitutes support and nurturance.

Understanding the reasons for and meaning of the enactment did not, however, solve the problem of how to manage intense affects, tension, and frustration, particularly under very stressful circumstances. Just as tolerance and containment of affect were a major part of my patient's struggle, so my prematurely ending the hour was an expression of a similar difficulty, though in muted form. Until this enactment, I would view my patient and me as having a negative complementarity match around the management of tension (Kantrowitz et al., 1989), where a similar problem is expressed by opposite behaviors on the part of the patient and analyst. For my patient and myself, the underlying problem was expressed in behaviors intrinsic to each of our characteristic styles, displaying our habitual modes of tension management that became exaggerated under stress. Although the mode of expression and degree of difficulty in tolerating the tension were different, both reflected a similar struggle. There are, of course, ways in which my patient also suppressed his affective reactions that led to acting them out, but his behavior was generally characterized by volatility rather than inhibition, explosion rather than suppression. In ending the hour ten minutes early, I actively appreciated that under certain extremely stressful circumstances I also did not have the knowledge of how to tolerate this experience of helplessness. My countertransference reaction (the suppression of my affective discomfort in order to maintain a supportive stance, since I believed he could not tolerate a confrontation) to this patient at this phase of the analysis interfered with my ability to integrate knowledge, which had enabled me to treat other severely self-critical patients, or even this patient at other times, without encountering such problems.

While there are undoubtedly dynamic aspects that contribute to difficulties in tension management, I think such difficulties also relate to educational deficits. I had run the gamut of my therapeutic skill in relation to this patient. There was something I needed to learn before I could help my patient learn to tolerate his affect. Having exhausted my own resources, I needed assistance from someone else. I chose to consult a colleague who I knew had an outlook and style that were compatible with my own. While there may have been many other ways of addressing my concern, the consultant provided a kind of intervention that suited my preferred manner of working. It acknowledged and addressed the patient's strengths and opened for inquiry what had led him to feel they were insufficient to the task, leading him to abandon trying. The model was similar to Gray's (1973) technique for analyzing defenses and Schwaber's (1983) attention to the shifts in the clinical moment, in that it focused on the patient's shifts within the analytic hour. However, while Gray interprets a defense against a drive representation and Schwaber emphasizes the change in affect and state, the focus of this intervention is on the relinquishing of self-control.

Anna Freud (1936) states:

> When the ego has taken its defensive measures against an affect for the purpose of avoiding unpleasure, something more besides analysis is required to undo them, if the result is to be permanent. The child must learn to tolerate larger and larger quantities of unpleasure without immediately having recourse to his defense mechanisms... theoretically, it is the business of education rather than of analysis to teach this lesson.
>
> (pp. 64–65)

While in later years, Anna Freud came to believe that she had too greatly emphasized the role of education (1965), focus on the need to learn to tolerate painful affects as a developmental task has continued. In a description of patients suffering from intense self-criticism, Kris (1990a) directs attention to the failure of some narcissistic patients to develop the capacity to tolerate frustration and ambiguity during the latency period. An alliance with an adult to assist with the development of self-control was lacking. For a successful outcome of treatment, he believes that in addition to the analysis of the self-criticism, it is necessary to revive the needed alliance for self-control in the analysis.

My consultation provided me with the educational tools I had failed to integrate. It does not seem likely to me that I would have been able to so easily or rapidly shift my stance had I not first confronted my countertransference difficulties through my self-analysis. Once I had recognized and understood my own limitations and, through the help of a consultant, found a method that allowed me simultaneously to support and to confront my patient, I was no longer in a dilemma about how to work with my patient. My patient responded to this immediately. Years of viewing me as a model of the containment of affect had not helped him identify with this in me. As he explained, he had not been able to understand what allowed me to contain affect. It seemed that I could control myself, whereas he could not control himself. And yet I did not teach him. He had, therefore, interpreted my stance as my wanting him to remain less effective than me, as my way of holding him back by withholding. Attending to, and together elaborating, the step-by-step process of trying to master, becoming frustrated, turning to others, and then blaming others for not providing assistance created what Kris called the alliance necessary for the development of self-control. By assuming this focus, I was providing what the patient needed; therefore, he no longer felt I was withholding and competitive, and he was no longer so angry and accusatory. He began to consider that he might have misinterpreted the intention of my behavior. As he became more confident in his abilities, he also became more tolerant and forgiving of others and himself. Self- and other criticism abated as he experienced he could have things for himself.

For another analyst, undoubtedly, other technical interventions might have worked equally well. With another patient, the difficulties for me in finding a therapeutically effective method might not have been so great. Some difficulties occur with all patients during the course of analysis. The comfortable way each analyst develops in working with a patient at a certain point in the process stops working. I have described this work to illustrate the necessity for self-analysis and for continued education to find methods that suit our characters when such difficulties arise in treatment.

It was necessary for me to face the limits of the effectiveness of my personal style and my failure to realize that I was not correctly using a theoretical model in conducting the treatment of this patient (as well as the limits in some personal beliefs) for me to see that something different was needed. My countertransference response to my state of helplessness was dynamically determined, but I would view my reaching this point as stemming from both an educational deficit as well as from a dynamic and characterological source. If I had known how to work with my patient's difficulty with tension management earlier, we might not have reached the point of confrontation through enactment. However, it would have required my being able to see that this was the source of difficulty sooner. This interdigitation of my patient's and my own character and dynamic struggles illustrates the difficulty that may arise in any treatment as a consequence of the patient-analyst match. We all remain blind to certain aspects of ourselves, and when these overlap with central areas of difficulty for our patients the treatment may be impeded. In the case, I have described that my enactment allowed my failure to confront limits to become a focus of analytic attention and an area for further education for both myself and my patient. Under the circumstances, this aspect of the patient-analyst match that had had an impeding effect on the treatment ultimately proved beneficial to the growth of both the patient and the analyst.

The experienced analyst's style is not usually a focus of attention. Scrutiny of our manner, our ways of communicating, and the content we select for our attention may come about through our patients' responses to us. Otherwise, our style generally remains a relatively unself-conscious aspect of our work. Since analysis takes many years, habitual forms of response develop between the patient and analyst. When an analysis becomes stalled, along with considerations of impediments due to transference/countertransference binds or limitations due to the analyst's understanding or technique, the impact of the particular style, reflected in the mode or manner of approach, also deserves attention. While style is not totally independent of these other factors, consideration of its effect places the focus of inquiry in a slightly different arena. In this paper, one particular aspect of style was considered because of its centrality for this patient-analyst pair; other aspects of the analyst's style may be far more important for other patient-analyst pairs as well as for me with other patients. Our self-scrutiny subjected to self-analysis is always an essential part of our work and becomes critical at times of an impasse. Since so often we tend to remain unaware of our more habitual ways of communicating, we may need an outside perspective to locate the area of difficulty. A consultant's view may expand our knowledge of theory, technique, but also of ourselves, and open the way for further self-analysis facilitating our personal and professional growth.

Chapter 3

Impasses in psychoanalysis

Overcoming resistance in situations of stalemate

In the course analytic work, the analyst inevitably encounters periods of time in which a patient is resistant. When this resistance reaches center stage in analysis, it may be a manifestation of a transference-countertransference reaction that recreates the patient's primary conflict. If acting out does not result in the termination of the treatment, and if the patient continues to associate, such an impasse may represent a crucial juncture in the treatment in which central analytic work can be accomplished. If, however, we fail to understand the reasons for a patient's resistance, we may reach an impasse. The only difference between impasses and other intensely conflicted situations that develop is that in the former, no further analysis is occurring; neither patient nor analyst can see a way out. According to Webster's definition, an impasse is "a predicament from which there is no obvious escape." The predicament usually results from our insufficient knowledge about the patient, limitations in our theory or technique, or countertransference interferences, or as I have defined more broadly, impeding aspect of the patient-analyst match. Patients' intolerance for painful affect stimulated in the treatment can, and often does, result in treatment impasses, but in this chapter wish to concentrate on impasses that arise from the transference-countertransference dynamic.

Most impasses occur when a patient sees the analyst or therapist as having confirmed a preexisting belief that is central to, and possibly the basis of, the patient's primary conflict or primary area of difficulty. I will show that the conviction is bolstered by an unacceptable or frightening self- or object representation. Or the therapist may appear to have confirmed a belief that leads the patient to conclude that there is no hope. An aspect of the patient's self-representation is projected onto the therapist, and the therapist becomes enmeshed in it by an enactment of something complementary, which may or may not be recognized and become a focus for analysis. The patient may then resist experiencing painful affects or painful self-knowledge that likely would be aroused in proceeding with analytic work. The patient has come to fear that the treatment experience will be no different from previously frightening or disappointing interactions. This conclusion may result when the treatment repeats a central conflict or repeats an aspect of the conflict that is crucially connected to the patient's frightening or despairing convictions about himself or others. The extent to which a patient is conscious of interpreting the analyst's behavior as a repetition of a previously painful experience varies from patient to patient. The outcome, however, is that the patient no longer considers it safe or fruitful to proceed, and treatment is stalemated.

Some impasses are brief and some may be permanent. A temporary blocking has the same characteristics as an impasse, except for its duration. We consider brief blockings an expectable part of our work. At the most extreme, impasses that cannot be resolved lead to termination of the treatment. Pfeffer's outcome studies of psychoanalysis (1961, 1963) suggest that in successful analyses, the patient-analyst interaction offers the patient not only a recapitulation of the past, but an additional, new experience. From this interplay, new psychic developments arise. In contrast, in unsuccessful analyses, the internal representation of the analyst becomes part of a previously established identification and reinforces old conflicts and maladaptive modes of coping. Treatments that terminate following an unresolved impasse belong to Pfeffer's classification of unsuccessful outcomes if they solidify central troublesome identifications or beliefs, even when progress has been made in other areas.

How can such an impasse come about when a patient has come to seek help and the analyst or therapist is committed to assisting the patient find freedom from constriction and psychic pain? From the standpoint of the patient, such a situation can occur when the patient no longer sees the analyst as an ally in helping to understand and solve his or her difficulties, but as a perpetrator of this pain. From the standpoint of the analyst, an impasse can occur when he or she is unable to understand what the patient is trying to communicate. Such a failure of understanding may be due to a limitation in theoretical or clinical knowledge of technique. A third possibility is that the failure stems from some psychological difficulty of the analyst that resonates with the patient's problems causing a transference-countertransference bind.

Cooper and Wittenberg (1985) state that treatments become "bogged down" when the analyst has failed to obtain a coherent overview of the patient early in the treatment. While they warn of the necessity of remaining open to new data and of refining previously made assumptions, they believe there is benefit in obtaining this overview of repetitive themes early in order to permit a formulation of the patient's difficulties. While a careful history is undoubtedly helpful in understanding the patient, not all patients are able to give such full accounts, and not all analysts are able to grasp so quickly which aspects are central. In addition, despite their caution to remain open to new material and to allow it to transform previously held conceptions, there remains the danger that too carefully constructed initial formulations may prevent hearing and focusing on other or contradictory material when it appears. Sometimes we cannot understand sufficiently what our patients are struggling with until it becomes a live issue between us.

When impasses occur, transferences and countertransferences have interfered with the mutual commitment to the task of free association, interpretation, and creation of new meaning in treatment. The relative contribution and intensity of these transferences and countertransferences will vary for each patient-analyst pair and in each impasse. While there is a large and increasing literature on countertransference (Blum, 1986; Heimann, 1950; Jacobs, 1983, 1986; Poland, 1984; Racker, 1957; Reich, 1960a, b; Tower, 1956; Tyson, 1986), relatively few authors address the issue in the context of a therapeutic impasse. I shall restrict the literature review to articles directly related to this topic.

Maldonado (1984) contends that patients with a narcissistic need for an illusion of self-sufficiency create a state of impasse in response to an unconscious fantasy in which the patient desires to paralyze the analyst's autonomy and the bond. The aim is to avoid or prevent processes of change in the connection with the analyst. These deadlocked situations are accompanied by verbal material in which there is an absence or marked diminution of visual imagery, concealing unconscious content and creating content devoid of meaning. The analyst may unconsciously contribute to this impasse by trying to analyze and interpret material that is lacking in symbolic value or meaning. In patients who are capable of analytic work, the symbolic capacity is not impaired, but is not being employed because the patient is resistant to change. The analyst may further contribute to the stalemate by accepting a form of compensation from the patient out of a countertransference response.

Herbert J. Schlesinger (1992, unpublished) describes three kinds of therapeutic impasses: one where the patient's emotional intensity intimidates the therapist; second where the patient's anxieties lead to inhibitions that inhibit or frustrate the therapist; and third where the patient's previously active and successful engagement in treatment is replaced by an attempt to continue the contact for the sake of the relationship, and the therapist tacitly complies. The first two forms of impasse involve the patient's regression with which the therapist has actively or passively colluded. In this regressed state, the patient's communication has changed from a verbal mode to an action mode. There has been a mutual blindness on the part of the therapist and patient to some aspect of the transference where a shift has occurred in its nature, intensity, or significance.

Often, it is only in retrospect that we are able to understand why treatment impasses have occurred. James T. McLaughlin (1981, 1991a), in reviewing a failed analytic case, states that preferred theoretical and technical stances, determined by the dynamic forces that shape us and our views, may impede us from seeing what we are contributing to impeding the analytic work. His retrospective view shifts his focus from the impediments created in the treatment due to the patient's character and abilities to the limits created by his own. The analyst's contribution in failed treatments arises from what he calls "dumb spots" based on cognitive or experiential gaps, "blind spots" based on limits of knowledge due to dynamic defensive avoidances, and "hard spots" based on the analyst's insistent maintenance of theoretical beliefs that shape and limit what he or she is able to perceive. I would suggest that these "hard spots" are also shaped by dynamic forces. Our choice of theory is likely to be determined by our character and the degree and extent to which we can and cannot tolerate certain kinds of content and interactions with our patients and ourselves.

As I described in the opening chapter, Sandler's (1976) concept of role responsiveness introduces the idea that the analyst's behavior and reactions may be subtly shaped in response to covert pressure from the patient. I will briefly repeat the central points. The patient's unconscious proddings lead the analyst to respond to varying degrees, often without awareness of what is occurring. Responses that are discrepant for the analyst are compromise formations between the analyst's own personally derived tendencies and his unconscious, unintentional acceptance of the role the patient is trying to get the analyst to assume in the transference. The relative contribution from patient and analyst will vary in each patient-analyst pair. Recognition by the analyst that he or she is reacting to the patient in a manner that is uncharacteristic of his or her usual manner of working may lead to helpful self-scrutiny followed by a discovery of the source of their "blind spots" or problems that led to uncharacteristic responses. When such recognitions do not occur, I think, stalemates are likely to result.

Sandler's concept of role responsiveness is related to what I have discussed in the study of impact of patient-analyst match in psychoanalysis (Kantrowitz, 1986; Kantrowitz et al., 1989; Kantrowitz, Katz, & Paolitto, 1990c). Case studies illustrate problems that arise in treatment when a patient has a central area of difficulty that overlaps with some similar area in the analyst, though this area of difficulty may be much smaller and have minimal impact on the analyst's life and functioning. When the analyst is "blind" to such issues, the treatment is impeded in this area, and stalemates are likely to result (Kantrowitz, 1992).

In the four case studies that follow, I will show how the transference-countertransference dynamic appeared, impeded the treatment leading to an impasse, and came to be understood. Transference and countertransference factors contributed in varying degrees to the relative intransigence and duration of the impasses in these treatments. Self-analysis played a role in enabling an understanding and resolution of the impasse, but it was most central in the first and last examples. The vignettes are relatively brief and are not intended to give a comprehensive picture of the patient or of the treatment process.

Case I

The first case demonstrates how my patient's intense resistance and negative transference were analyzable once my self-analysis led me to confront my countertransference. Our transference-countertransference bind was dealt with openly, and the treatment then proceeded with increased depth.

The patient was an educational administrator in his late 40s who had been referred to me by a colleague who had treated him for many years. The patient had gained a great deal of insight about himself through his therapy, but believed he had reached a stalemate with his therapist. He viewed his therapist as too intellectual and unable to help him come to terms with his emotionally traumatic history. My colleague agreed that the impasse seemed unbridgeable, and thought the patient very likely needed to work with someone else to complete his treatment. The patient had been sexually abused by his mother when he was very young. Memories of this had not been repressed, but their affective significance had been totally denied until his treatment. His therapist had been sensitive and supportive over the years, as the patient revived the affective aspects of his experience. His availability and understanding seemed unquestioned by the patient. It was hard for me to grasp what had become so problematic in the treatment that the patient felt he could not continue. He proclaimed he felt enormous relief in beginning treatment with me.

Over the course of several years, we increased both the frequency of the sessions and the intensity of the work. His terror, helplessness, and distrust were vividly revived in the transference. Once he began to experience his own anger and aggression in identification with his abusing mother, his symptoms abated. This previously inhibited man began to explore in all sorts of ways of being that he had formerly believed forbidden. His sexual functioning improved, and his intellectual curiosity expanded. However, throughout our work, I felt held at an emotional distance. It was in this context that we encountered an impasse.

One day he noticed an unfamiliar car in my driveway and asked directly whose it was. Knowing from past experience that my asking him to explore his thoughts resulted in greater inhibition rather than useful fantasy, and thinking that at this moment a little direct satisfaction of his curiosity might stimulate more, I answered both this question and the two or three questions that followed. My answers, which were about a member of my family, were brief and did not reveal any particularly personal information. The patient dropped his questioning and began talking about material from the end of the previous hour. I wondered about the abrupt shift in topic. He stated that seeing the car had interrupted him from focusing on the material he wanted to consider. When he went back to his thoughts from the last hour, his voice was flat, and he seemed affectively remote. His associations were stilted and did not seem to lead to any new understanding. He did not spontaneously return to our interchange. He continued in this manner over the next several hours.

During this time, I wondered with him what he was feeling, noted that in the past his flat voice had accompanied his being angry, and specifically connected that this state began after he had seen and asked about the car. On each occasion, his response was dismissive, and he remained disengaged. He told me I seemed to be far more interested in the car episode than he was. Later in this hour, in the same flat tone, he described a memory of seeing his mother naked and wanting to touch her genitals but not doing so. I asked what had made him stop. He said he had sensed that she did not want him to touch her, though she had always felt free to touch his genitals and never took into account what this made him feel. I asked how he had known her feelings. He could not explain, but had no doubt about the accuracy of his perceptions. Referring to the car episode, I wondered if he had felt that I did not want him to continue asking me questions. "Well, that was pretty obvious!" he said with intense feeling. I wondered what had led him to that conclusion. He said my answers had been very brief and did not encourage exploration. His questions, he believed, had not been inappropriate or intrusive. Therefore, since I had been so discouraging, he assumed there was something about this person in my family I did not wish to discuss. It made him very angry that I could ask and know everything about him, but he was not permitted to know about me. I asked if his remoteness in the hours had been his response. If I were not going to tell him about me, then he was not going to be available to me. He heartily agreed; this was his mode, tit for tat, but the increased distance remained.

I now wondered if by answering his questions I had unwittingly re-traumatized him by stimulating and then not gratifying him. I offered this interpretation. The atmosphere between us lightened almost immediately. His tone was again animated. He had not been aware that this was what had occurred, but it seemed right to him.

For the first time in several years, he referred to his former therapist who he felt was more comfortable than I was with being self-revealing. His therapist had answered personal questions much more fully and without hesitation, he said. Then the patient fell silent. I asked what he was thinking. He said he did not want to tell me because it would give support to the wisdom of my restrained stance regarding self-revelation. Nonetheless, he continued. In addition to the more innocuous things, similar to the facts he had learned from me, he knew that his therapist had been abandoned by his wife whom he then divorced, and that he had remarried relatively quickly and had moved into a new house. The patient found it hard to understand how the therapist could make a new life so rapidly. It made the patient uncomfortable; he felt critical of the therapist at the same time that he felt empathic toward him. He thought that the therapist was uncomfortable about his own behavior. He believed that every time he approached his feelings about his therapist's new life, the therapist moved away from them because of his own discomfort. He felt a clear message to refrain from going ahead, and he had stopped.

I asked what he thought would have happened if he had gone ahead; the patient became anxious. Going ahead was not an option. His therapist had revealed a vulnerability, and he would not pursue something that would be hurtful to him. I said, "You were afraid that you would hurt him." With intense distress, the patient responded:

Yes… and afraid I would hurt my mother and you. I could not touch my mother because though I didn't understand it then, somehow I did sense that she was frightened of sex. Why else would she be sexually interested in a little boy? And when you were so terse in answering my questions, I felt this must be a vulnerable area for you, and so I stopped asking.

I underscored, as I had in the past, that he knew what it felt like to be hurt, and he did not want to be someone who hurt others. The patient

then realized we had returned to familiar territory. He thought his retreat in his earlier therapy could be dated to the time of his therapist's
remarriage. Once he saw his therapist as vulnerable, he now understood, he had become frightened of his power to hurt him. Although
he knew he was dissatisfied with his therapist's manner of working,
at that time, he had no awareness that he would have the desire to
hurt him. But as he had become less and less able to freely bring his
concerns into treatment for fear he would injure his therapist, he had
become increasingly angry at having to restrain his own needs. So his
anger actually had come through after all. It had been the same with
his mother. This constellation had just repeated itself in miniature
with me.

He had first thought he was holding back because I was holding
back, but he now thought he was actually displaying his anger and
being cruel to me in this passive way because he had felt stimulated
by me, as I had suggested, and then rendered impotent by my display of vulnerability. He had experienced it as an unfair use of both
power and vulnerability—a sadistic act, since it left him powerless
to act unless he was willing to become the abuser. But since I had
not avoided what had occurred, I was clearly not as vulnerable as
he had thought, and this had made it possible for him to continue
to pursue his thoughts and questions about what had transpired between us.

In this case, an intense resistance with temporary cessation of associations had occurred when our transference-countertransference
interaction repeated a central traumatic experience. My answering
the patient's questions was strikingly out of character for me, and illustrates Sandler's point that uncharacteristic behaviors on the part
of analysts suggest they have responded both to a push from the patient and to a pull from something within themselves. It required
self-analytic work for me to understand my wish for personal display,
as minimal as this display was. The patient had complained about
how unseen he had felt by his parents who professed to adore him, but
then never seemed to see who he really was or what he needed. They
used him to serve their own needs while proclaiming they were doing
everything for him. He felt that the worst thing about his mother's
sexual use of him was that she did not take into account how this
made him feel.

In the transference, the patient proclaimed his love for me, but I experienced myself as unseen. Since as an analyst I am used to being seen primarily as others need to perceive me, I did not consciously experience his treatment of me as anything unusual. I was unaware that in this instance, I had come to feel abused and had unconsciously rebelled at remaining so unseen. My behavior represented a countertransference response, stimulated by an identification with my patient as a victim. I should have been alerted, when I thought to stimulate rather than analyze his curiosity, that something in me was disrupting my analytic stance.

This mini enactment of his earlier traumatic experience created a temporary impasse, since the patient no longer felt safe. The danger he experienced was twofold. He felt that I was potentially a dangerous person who might stimulate him and leave him helplessly frustrated and unfulfilled. At the same time, he saw himself as potentially dangerous, as a person who could destroy me because of the vulnerability he believed I had revealed.

Understanding the meaning of this enactment eventually led us to understand why his earlier treatment had been stalemated. The patient's experience of himself as an aggressive, potentially destructive person had not been owned until several years of treatment with me. Previously, he had only known that he feared anger and aggression in others. He had affectively detached himself from his former therapy rather than risk the emergence of a self-representation which he feared and which he believed could not be contained by a therapist whom he had come to perceive as vulnerable.

Since he never told his former therapist his fantasies about him, the patient never had the opportunity to test their validity. He may have correctly perceived that his therapist moved away from material about himself out of discomfort; however, had the therapist possessed the necessary information as to the source of the patient's withdrawal and inhibition in treatment, he might well have been able to address and understand this material.

Case 2

The second case illustrates the emergence of an intense resistance when my patient developed a fearful transference, leading to a brief inhibition in her associations. I was aware of and able to address her contribution to a transference enactment, but the countertransference was not central, and the disruption in the analytic process rapidly resolved.

The patient, a married professional in her forties, had sought treatment for a long-standing depression and general inhibition. Her mother had been cool and controlled, her father hot and impetuous. She had aligned herself with her idealized mother, and looked down on her father, fearing and scorning him for his temper. Her relationship with her father had been filled with anger and also sexually charged. She had reported that her mother had bathed her until she was 12, but her shame around this had been focused on her own dependency. In the transference, I had at times stood for the all-knowing, cool, idealized mother and at other points for the frightening, devalued, and sexualized father. She had come to understand how she used her own sexuality as a source of power. Being "sexy" was the way she drew attention to herself and tried to control men. Until the episode I am about to report, she had not recognized the role of sexuality and power in her experience with women.

While in life she had often had passionate attractions to women, there had been only brief flickers of this in the transference. In the end phase of analysis, having come to a much more comfortable, loving feeling in relation to men, she was exploring the way in which her newly discovered anger toward her mother still remained and felt "hard," like her previous feelings about her father. In one hour, she recalled her adoration of her mother. Her mother had been the center of all her thoughts and attention for years. She wondered why she had never felt in love with me as she had with her mother. I reminded her that in our analytic work she had often expressed a desire to be the center of my thoughts and attention. She quickly agreed, and then recognized that she had wanted me to feel toward her as she had felt toward her mother. She knew she had wanted that power over me, but now considered that behind this must lie other feelings of desiring me.

In the next hour, she remembered her mother when she way young. She thought about her mother's beautiful clothes, her soft lingerie, her silky slips, her white skin. She pictured her mother naked before her. Her mother's body was curvaceous, sensual, undulating; hers was boyish. She pictured the mole near her mother's vagina. She thought of moles as beautiful. They were called beauty marks. Elizabeth

Taylor had one on her cheek. She thought of the Elizabeth Taylor paper dolls she had had and how she used to cut them to accentuate the curves of the body, a memory she had often described in analysis. Elizabeth Taylor accentuated the mole on her cheek. Accentuating the mole was like advertising sexuality. Moles on the face were sexy, sensual. She thought of moles near the lip. I said, "Who has a mole near the lip?" She seemed surprised, unaware she had said near the lip. She felt anxious and slightly aroused. Was I saying I had a mole near my lip? The hour was at its end. As she got up from the couch, she stopped and stared at my face and exclaimed, "Oh my God, you do have a mole near your lip! I didn't know, but I must have known."

The next day she described how exhilarated and excited she had felt. The moment she had stared at my face had felt so intimate to her. She had felt permitted to be close to me, welcomed, even invited. A rush of loving feelings had followed. She had thought about me all day. This quality of experience was something she had described in relation to several women with whom she had felt passionately involved in the past. Suddenly she found she had all sorts of interest and curiosity about me that had been strikingly absent during analysis. She did not expect me to answer her questions, but was delighted to have her gaze firmly focused on me in her mind. She realized she had thought I would reject her love, and was elated to find this was not so. The hour continued in this vein.

She was sleepy and vaguely disengaged during the following hour. She moved from topic to topic, all relevant but with no affective charge. She stopped, recognizing she was blocked. She felt lacking in interest or curiosity about anything. How strange it was to feel this way after she had felt so excited and elated. It was very puzzling. Maybe what she had felt with me had something to do with why she was now so closed off to her feelings. We knew this happened to her when she got frightened. She thought it was ironic that only as she was thinking of terminating had she been able to feel so strongly toward me. She wanted those feelings in her life, but not with me. She was just setting herself up for a loss.

Her voice had become urgent and angry in tone. Why shouldn't she shut off these feelings? It was only self-protective. Besides, why had I waited so long to be responsive to her? Why had I let her come so close now? This gave me power over her; now I could make her do anything because of her feelings for me. She was frightened of her vulnerability and her sense of being at my mercy. This was how it had been with her mother and why she had had to be so good, so worried about doing the correct thing. Sadly, she said:

> I think I seduced you. All these years I've tried one way or another to get you to do what I want, and I finally succeeded. I got you to cross a boundary, something you would never willingly do. Now I feel guilty and ashamed.

I noted that she had begun to feel angry with me for what I had done, but then turned the anger away from me back onto herself; we were very familiar with her doing this. But what was it she thought she had made me do? What boundary had I crossed? She said I had let her look at me, invited her to look at me. I had permitted an intimacy. I said she was experiencing looking at my face as if I had exposed my genitals to her. At first, she was uncomprehending, then she began to take in what I had said. I was right in my understanding of what she felt; what she was having trouble grasping was the discrepancy between her feeling and what had happened. Since she did not look at me in analysis, this she thought explained why she had felt that actually looking at me was forbidden. But she did look at me in her comings and goings. She was very conscious of how I looked, what I wore, of my expression, of the shape of my body. Mostly she avoided talking about this. Although we both knew there were occasions when she commented about my appearance, mostly she did not allow herself to pursue these thoughts, to feel or express curiosity about me and my body. She could see now that I had never forbidden her to follow these thoughts or to look at me. She began to comprehend that it was only her own prohibition she had crossed.

In analysis, we had first seen how she had identified with her mother's passive power in her stance of moral superiority, and then later seen how she had identified with her father as an active aggressor. We now understood her identification with her mother as active seducer. Throughout the analysis, we had understood and explored her feelings of being helpless, dependent, and at times a victim. Her wish for revenge through retaliation in kind had emerged. Over the next days, she expressed relief that she had not been so powerful to get me to transgress. She explored her intense anger over feeling at the mercy of her mother's power because of her intense desire for her. She now understood, with a new force, that sexuality was her weapon with women as well as with men. Originally, it had been a major source of vulnerability, but she had turned it into the source of her power, the weapon for her revenge. She would make others want, desire, feel as out of control and as vulnerable to her power as she had felt. But something had changed. In the last year of analysis, she had finally experienced her love for her husband and realized that she did not want to hurt him and no longer thought he wanted to hurt her. And I had not taken advantage of her or abused her in her vulnerability and need for me.

That night, she had a dream in which her father was intensely involved with his accounting books. The image was of him sitting with his eyes fixed on the pages of numbers. In her associations, she thought about his work as his passion. Then, she recalled how as an adolescent she had noticed his gazing at women's legs, how he bought her underwear. Her mother had not been the object of his attention or of his gaze. She began to feel sorry for her mother. She had left her home and family and moved to a distant city to be with her father. It was understandable that she would have wanted someone's eyes on her, someone to be attentive to her. It was sad that her mother had to turn to her for this gratification instead of getting it from her father. Over the weeks that followed, her "hard" feelings about her mother softened.

The resistance for this patient in the termination phase was brief. It did not result in an impasse because the patient herself was able so easily to work her way free from being blocked. This case clearly and fully illustrates how the meaning a patient gives to an interaction in treatment can lead to the perception of the treatment situation being no longer safe. Shutting down, whether it is for part of a session, as it was in this instance, or for prolonged periods of time, is a way patients try to protect themselves until they can regain trust in the treatment situation. If they cannot do so, often they leave.

For a time, in the hours described, my patient had come to view me first as a seducer who would abuse my power over her, and then as a victim of her seduction where I was and would be at her mercy. In the first instance, she was representing me as dangerous to her.

In the second instance, she was representing herself as dangerous to me. She became frightened by my power and her own; she feared that one of us would abuse the other if either of us allowed ourselves to be affectively available to the other. Previously, she had experienced this constellation of feelings and conflicts in relation to men. But the earlier and deeper origin of her conflicts had not been available to her until this experience in the transference.

When I asked my patient about who had a mole near the lip, I was not certain that she had noticed mine. I phrased it in a way that was intended to allow her to attach the source of her stimulation to me or to some other figure.

In this instance, my contribution to my patient's sense of imminent danger and consequent inhibition was important because of the meaning she attached to my words rather than because of an unconscious collusion on my part. My question was consciously intended to help her become aware of her transference feelings. In this sense, then, she was correct in perceiving my comment as an invitation to look. Her sexualization of looking had led to her inhibition of curiosity. During the course of her analysis, her ability to pursue her thoughts and observations had improved. However, as she herself came to realize, her inhibition of close observation of me, and most particularly of my body, had remained. The reported interaction, which led to a brief impasse in her ability to associate, brought the central features of the patient's conflict into the center of the analytic work. Because of the stage of the treatment, I understood the nature of her conflict well enough to interpret accurately what had occurred, and my patient trusted me enough to push through this temporary blocking.

Case 3

In the third case, a perseverative conviction about a negative self- and object representation led to a transference-countertransference impasse that threatened the continuation of the treatment. This intense transference regression did not yield to either analytic or self-analytic scrutiny. The transference conviction was broken by an accidental occurrence that enabled me to help mutual understanding of the impasse and facilitate movement in the treatment.

The patient was a young married woman in graduate school who was caring for several young children, essentially on her own, while her husband was developing an extremely successful business. She sought treatment because she felt overwhelmed and chronically anxious and depressed. A previous therapy had not been experienced as helpful to her. She felt her therapist had been distant, critical, and judgmental. After a brief period of psychotherapy with me, we began an analysis, meeting four times a week. After about six months of analysis, she requested a fifth hour. Analysis had proven very useful to her. She believed she was gaining a new perspective on her life, but often the intensity of her emotions became frightening to her. At these times, she found the three-day interruption hard to tolerate. In addition, she had a friend, also in analysis, who similarly would feel flooded by intense affect and had found a fifth hour stabilizing.

I was in agreement with my patient that a fifth hour would be of benefit to her, but I did not have more time available. I told her that if she wanted I would tell her when I had an open hour due to a cancelation. And when I had an opening, I would make a regular time for her, but I said I did not anticipate that happening in the near future. The patient said she would welcome the fifth hour any time I could arrange it. I often was able to find her this additional hour, which she usually was able to attend.

The analysis began to deepen, and she seemed to feel less flooded by her affect. However, when six months later I still did not have a regular fifth hour to offer her, she began to press me vigorously for her own additional hour, and became increasingly distressed when I did not offer it.

Soon the analysis became totally focused on my withholding what she wanted. We explored the meaning of this to her. Although she felt humiliated to reveal her thoughts, she described feeling it meant that I did not really want to see her, found her presence burdensome, and did not like her. She wished, if this were so, that I would tell her, since she did not believe it would benefit her to be treated by someone who felt this way about her. The treatment now felt like her previous therapy, and she became increasingly depressed.

Painful memories of feeling devastated when she left her hours with her former therapist were recounted. She wanted me to understand that although in the hours she experienced me as responsive to her feelings and encouraging of their expression, this misery was what she was now feeling again with me. She recognized that she believed her friend who had five analytic hours was valued and cared about by her analyst as she was not by me. She soon realized that she saw her friend as the present-day representation of her older sister whom she believed her parents had favored.

Feeling unvalued by me now, she felt unvaluable as she had in the past. I told her she was very understandably angry at my not providing the time she wanted and was turning that anger away from me and onto herself. I said that I could understand that my not giving her this time could be interpreted as my not wishing to see her, which must be confusing since it was not what she felt when she was with me. She soon began to express her anger about the situation more freely and to tell me how rigid and withholding she found me.

A negative maternal transference became the center of our work. Along with her fury with me, she was able to describe and relive early distress about feeling turned away from by her mother. Her angry and competitive feelings intensified. She felt in a terrible bind; she needed me and my help so much, and at the same time she felt I looked down on her and scorned her and was holding her back due to my competitive feelings toward her as a younger, attractive woman. We were able to explore and expand how her anger and competitive feelings toward me made her feel guilty, and then fearful of my retaliation. I interpreted that she took my not giving her another hour of her own as a punishment about which she had contradictory feelings. She felt she deserved such a punishment for her hostile feelings and wishes toward me. At the same time, she felt my rejection of her as undeserved and unjustified, since she believed she would feel kindly and loving toward me, as she had earlier in the treatment, if only I had positive feelings for her.

Although she readily recognized that these feelings were exact replicas of what she had felt with her mother and her previous therapist, my not finding an additional hour for her made all this understanding only intellectual, and she remained convinced that I wanted her gone. The understanding of her transference did not have sufficient power because my actions, she felt, confirmed her belief that she was unlovable. I felt totally stymied. I was already working more hours than I considered optimal. And while I would have created an hour for any urgent need, I knew I would feel overburdened by a commitment to another regular hour. I had to struggle with and analyze my counter-transference guilt at wanting to spend some time on enjoyable nonprofessional activities since I could have created the fifth hour by cutting into my nonworking time. While I felt for her pain and distress, I believed it was preferable for her to be angry with me than for me to feel resentful of her. If I were to make an extra hour and feel overburdened, I would then actually experience what she already feared I felt. This would make the situation still more difficult to analyze.

The impasse was overcome by a concrete event. The patient's hours were Tuesday through Friday, and I had cancelled a Friday appointment. I was having a tooth pulled, but since it was not my practice to give the reason for absences, I did not tell her why I would not be there. The Thursday prior to this cancellation, she had been so enraged at my upcoming absence and so convinced that it confirmed my wish not to see her that she considered ending the analysis. Nothing I said gave her any perspective or comfort. When she returned the following Tuesday, her mood was totally different. She stated that her fury at my cancelilng the Friday hour had underlying it the fantasy that I was going away for a three-day weekend and had chosen Friday rather than Monday to be gone in order not to see her.

Over the weekend, another friend, who knew she was in analysis with me, reported to her that she saw me at the dentist and overheard that I was having a tooth extracted. This factual information confronted her and led her to recognize that her construction about the meaning of my absence was her fantasy creation and not the reality. She suddenly and powerfully grasped what I had been trying to help her see: I had done something that made her angry and disappointed her, and it was understandable that she would feel that way; however, it did not necessarily mean that what she concluded about the meaning of why I had done that was true. The negative transference dissolved, and she worked productively on what had transpired between us even though it was many months before a fifth regular hour became available. It was not until several years later that we discovered the origin of an unconscious guilt that had substantially contributed to the intensity of her conviction that she was so bad, undesirable, and deserving of punishment.

In this case, the fact of my not providing an additional regular hour was used by the patient to support a conviction about herself. It was similar to how she had previously used her former therapist's style as a confirmation of his similar negative feelings about her. He may not have understood the reason she could not make use of the treatment, since she had not been able to tell him clearly what she felt. She had felt too humiliated to reveal her feelings, being convinced that her perception of his negative feelings about her were accurate. Unconsciously, she believed they were justified. In her treatment with me, I did understand the meaning of my behavior toward her, but not the reason for the depth of her conviction.

While at the time it seemed likely that her conviction that I experienced her as a burden and did not wish to be with her was derived from her relationship with her mother, the tenacity of this conviction seems to have had an unconscious source. When we came to understand the unconscious fantasy from which her intense guilt and self-loathing arose, we could see that her relationship with her mother, while having its troublesome aspects, was being unconsciously laden with meanings from repressed memories and fantasies. Guilt for her hostile and competitive feelings toward her mother concealed a deeper layer of guilt. Therefore, in this instance, the intense negative transference that threatened termination were based on the patient's belief that the analyst was confirming a view of her that was central to her own negative view of herself. This self-representation was a consequence of a core neurotic conflict and the accompanying anxiety and depression for which she sought treatment.

This case illustrates an intense negative transference that repeated only an aspect of the patient's central conflict; it reinforced her conviction that she was bad and undesirable. It did not reveal the unconscious source of her guilt. However, unless it was overcome, she could not explore her conflicts more deeply. The painful work in the negative transference likely contributed to her increased tolerance for dysphoric affects and aggressive impulses, and possibly, over time, she might have been able to recognize affectively as well as intellectually that her conviction was based on a transference. However, as it happened, only when she had the experience of a strongly held belief in a plausible fantasy disconfirmed did she let go of the firmness of her conviction about my negative feelings.

Words were not enough. It should be noted, however, that it did not require her knowing anything about my actual feelings for this change to occur. What was confronted in reality was not what I actually felt, but that the fantasy she had constructed, and was convinced was reality, was proven to be inaccurate. She then was able to entertain the possibility that things she believed so strongly were not necessarily so. It seems likely that the hope that she might find herself less awful than she expected made it possible for her to explore her conflicts in greater depth, producing beneficial results for her mood, her self-representation, and her tolerance of affects.

Case 4

The fourth case illustrates an unresolved impasse where my patient's negative transference results initially in ceasing to associate and ultimately in leaving treatment. The countertransference issue was insufficiently understood during the treatment. Retrospective consideration led me to further self-analysis, and a possible, though by no means certain, understanding of the nature of the transference-countertransference impasse.

The patient sought treatment for difficulties in establishing a committed relationship with a man. A previous therapy had offered both comfort and self-understanding, but had not affected her incapacity to sustain an intimate relationship. She was very fond of her therapist, but had not returned to see him because she believed he was unable to be sufficiently active and confrontational with her. She had addressed this concern with him; in fact, she had pushed the issue so strongly that, according to the patient, her therapist had finally told her that this was who he was and he could not be different.

In treatment with me, the patient explored many of her difficulties with men. While she was perceptive and sensitive, her focus often remained on the qualities of the men rather than exploring herself. We came to understand that her intense self-criticism was too painful for her to sustain a self-focus. She tried to understand and work on her problems in displacement. Her intolerance for her own limitations was, therefore, revealed in what she perceived as others' shortcomings. Her wish for self-perfection then resulted in her intolerance of others' limitations which resembled her own. Having externalized her problem, she would then try to eliminate it by extricating herself from the relationship.

Our work was only intermittently in the transference, until the third year of treatment. At this time, the patient expressed dissatisfaction with my manner of working with her. She wanted me to be self-revealing, to tell her directly about both myself and my feelings about her. While I tried to explore what it was she wished to know, why now, and what various responses and information from me would mean to her, none of these approaches led to anything fruitful.

The patient became increasingly angry and frustrated with me and the treatment. Then, she rather abruptly dropped this pursuit and returned to her usual mode of working. I wondered about the shift, but she shrugged off my questions and continued with the thoughts she brought in. My attempts to reintroduce her abandoned wishes were continually met with seeming disinterest. Not long after, she announced her decision to terminate.

I said that I thought what had happened in her first therapy had happened again with me. She had asked her first therapist to be different and when he had told her he could not, she had felt there was no point in her continuing the treatment and had left. She had asked me to be different, and while I had not told her I would not or could not, I had not done what she wanted. It seemed she had given up hope of getting me to do so.

I suggested that when she found some aspect in another person that she experienced as a limitation, she became enormously disappointed and disillusioned, and the person no longer had value for her. She had had this experience of disappointment and turning away not only in treatment, but in her relationships with the men with whom she tried to become close. She agreed with this formulation, but she showed no interest in exploring or expanding these ideas, or in developing any others. Her material remained rather flat, and she continued her plans to terminate.

In the remaining weeks, I tried to reengage her, specifically addressing how her disappointment in others reflected an intolerance of aspects of herself and her own wish to be perfect, beyond criticism. She was concerned that I was disappointed with the outcome of the treatment and tried to assure me that there were many ways in which it had helped her. She believed she had learned how difficult it was for her to accept others' limits or her own, and agreed that this left her feeling very disappointed and sad. She knew I was trying to help her see that even if she could not have everything she wanted, it did not mean she could not have more than she had. She believed she had gotten what she could from treatment and wanted to stop.

At this point, I too experienced a sense of disappointment, sadness, and feeling of failure that I considered to be a parallel to my patient's. Knowing my own tendency to be perfectionistic and having through self-analysis in relation to another patient (Kantrowitz, 1992) recognized my refusal to accept limits in myself as an analyst, I believed my patient had found in me an area that mirrored her problem. My assessment that she could go further with treatment and that I would be able to help her to do so was probably expecting more than was possible. That is, I was refusing to accept a limit inherent in the situation. The patient perhaps could go further, but probably not with someone who shared a difficulty in accepting limits. It was not that I believed that granting her request for me to change my behavior would have been beneficial; it was, rather, that my not doing so confronted her with a limit of my flexibility.

While I had no trouble accepting that I had such a limit, I was having trouble accepting that there was a lack in my skill to work with this patient. The patient and I had both been humbled, but what I experienced as largely beneficial for my self-understanding, despite the element of disappointment, seemed mainly depressing to my patient, and that was regrettable.

In retrospect, while I think these formulations are correct, I believe they are also partial. I think I became caught in a too-narrow understanding of my patient. I think she needed to see me struggle with and solve the problem she was trying to master—both to find a model of how to do it and in order to believe it was possible (M. Hurwitz, 1991, personal communication).

Limits were a problem for her, but not the problem of the moment. At this point in the treatment, she wanted to be more self-revealing and dared to make it more affectively alive in the transference. I think she worried that I was encouraging her to do something I would not do myself and was testing this out. Had I interpreted that she wanted me to do what she was struggling to do, namely reveal herself and her feelings, this might have released the deadlock. I suspect, however, she still would have required something more than an interpretation.

In McLaughlin's terms, there were both blind spots due to my own dynamic defensive avoidance and hard spots due to my adherence to a theory that was too narrow to reflect the patient's struggle. In Sandler's terms, there was a role responsiveness that was not understood by me at the time. In terms of match, there was an interdigitation of the patient's central difficulty with accepting personal limits with my own difficulty in accepting my limits or the limits of the power of the theory I was employing to be helpful in freeing the patient.

This retrospective construction, of course, may not be accurate. It may be that this patient could not tolerate the intensity of affect in the transference and could not remain in treatment once the work moved out of the displacement. All these theories remain speculative without confirmation from the patient. This case demonstrates an impasse in treatment where I had become stuck in an unproductive way of understanding my patient's resistance and negative transference because of countertransference reasons.

Since I thought I was so clear about my contribution, I had not sought consultation, and I had failed to do sufficient self-analytic work necessary to free myself from this bind. While there is no way to know how it would have evolved had I reached this new construction before my patient terminated, earlier and extended self-reflection would have given the treatment an additional chance.

Conclusion

When impasses have been overcome, it is usually possible to understand the dynamic factors that have contributed to them. Often the work around stalemates is crucial to the discovery of previously unconscious or poorly understood dynamics of the patient. While an overview of the patient's life history is without question an aid in understanding the present difficulty, often we still cannot sufficiently comprehend the reason for the current impasse. Factors relevant to the stalemate are most often already known to us when the impasse occurs, but do not, at that time, attract our attention as being related in meaning. It is only afterwards that these factors stand out and their meaning is newly appreciated. Once we have understood, the reason for a stalemate may seem obvious or even glaring to us. When we report such instances, the reader may wonder how we could have possibly overlooked the construction we eventually came to; however, this is likely to be an artifact of our presentation. We have selected and organized our data in support of our new understanding.

Similarly, events in the treatment, the meaning to the patient of something the therapist or analyst does or does not do, may not be apparent at the time. What to us may seem innocuous or may even bypass our attention, may link with some conscious or unconscious element for the patient that has crucial significance. When patients are aware of this meaning and are able to tell us, as my patient (Case 2) was in the termination phase of her treatment, our work is not so difficult, and reworking of important dynamic material can be facilitated. However, when impasses occur, most often our patients cannot tell us or do not know consciously themselves what has blocked them. It requires that we carefully examine our interventions and ourselves to try to find out how we have contributed to the stalemate.

There is increased awareness by analysts that they play a part when a treatment reaches an impasse. When the impasse is not overcome and the treatment terminates, we can retrospectively review our work and try to learn from it, but our conclusions remain speculative. While our theories may be plausible, we need the confirmation of the patient and the lifting of the impasse to establish their validity. While it is true that the more comprehensively we understand our patients, the better able we are to grasp what has led to the deadlock, some psychological dynamics or crippling unconscious beliefs only become apparent through enactments. Translating nonverbal communications into verbal constructions then becomes our work. When viewed from the perspective of being enacted communications, threatened impasses offer an opportunity for crucial understanding.

Sandler's suggestion that we be alert to any behaviors or reactions that are uncharacteristic on our part is one helpful starting point for self-exploration. Considerations of the ways in which we recognize or can come to perceive the dimensions of our similarities and differences with our patients and their conflicts is another avenue to pursue in self-analysis. Periods of intense negative transference or resistance that threaten an impasse indicate we have come to a place that is emotionally charged for a patient. When we are able to understand what has occurred, we have helped our patient expand his or her intrapsychic world and increased the patient's ability to continue to acquire self-knowledge and trust.

Chapter 4

The uniqueness of the patient-analyst pair

Approaches for elucidating the analyst's role

The role of the analyst's character in psychoanalytic work has received increased attention over the last decade. While there had always been analysts who acknowledged the effects of the analyst's transferences and character on the patient (Freud, 1921; Greenson, 1967 Loewald, 1967; Rycroft, 1956; Schafer, 1959; Stone, 1961; Strachey, 1934; Winnicott, 1969), we had also been taught that the limits of our therapeutic endeavors were primarily determined by the characteristics of our patients. Some psychoanalytic literature presented analysts as "blank screens" (Freud, 1912; Kernberg, 1972) for the patients' conflicts and as relatively interchangeable. Privately, it was understood that skill and talent for therapeutic work would vary as well as the extent to which personal conflicts were resolved. However, in some analytic circles, there was the myth of the perfectly analyzed analyst (Silverman, 1985) and only a limited acknowledgment of the impact of the analyst's character on clinical work (Blatt & Behrends, 1987; Tyson, 1986).

With the decrease in authoritarianism, stemming from the changes in society during the 1960s and 1970s, and the increase in appreciation of the effect of the observer on the observed, from physics the view of therapy as a one-person psychology shifted. With this shift, the impact of the analyst, and even the personal characteristics and conflicts of the analyst, became a generally accepted part of the clinical purview. Once it was accepted that patients' perceptions of the analyst could be based on actual behavior as well as transference (and actual behavior could be put to transference use), it also had to be acknowledged that both factors are in play during the course of every treatment.

It had always been assumed that becoming a skilled clinician required knowledge about oneself, acquired through personal treatment and continued self-analysis. However, historically the purpose of acquiring self-knowledge was to understand and control one's reactions. An analyst's ability to appreciate his or her own dynamic development, conflicts, and vulnerabilities enables him/her to differentiate patients' struggles from his/her own. We learn to detect when our affective reactions stem primarily from our own concerns and when they arise more in resonance with patients' states or conflicts. Such self-awareness also helps us to discern our contribution to our patients' current struggles and distress. Self-scrutiny, then, is not only for the purpose of containing our reactions; it is through this self-other observation that we attain a more complex understanding of our patients and ourselves.

It is the aspects of the analyst's character and characterological qualities that are manifested in the analytic hours through observable characterological traits that impinge on the patient and affect the treatment. Character can be viewed as the central point in a continuum. At one end of the spectrum are countertransference reactions and their behavioral expressions. Under conditions of stress, characterological qualities slip over into conflictual issues and become manifest countertransference difficulties. For example, a characterological tendency toward impatience, characteristically contained as feeling, may be expressed in an unconscious ending of a patient's hour prematurely when the patient frustrates the analyst beyond her tolerance (Kantrowitz, 1992). At the other end of the continuum is habitual, relatively conflict-free, behavioral expression. Generally enduring qualities of style such as tempo, affective tone, and manner of relating, while they are comparatively free of conflict, may also affect the treatment. For example, the same characterological quality of a tendency toward impatience might be manifest in a characteristic of relatively rapid speech. I assume that all patients would have a negative affective reaction to an analyst ending an hour prematurely. However, an analyst's rapid speech might stimulate a variety of different reactions, depending on the patient's transference. For some patients, this might be perceived as energy and involvement; for others, it might be experienced as impatience; another group of patients might have no particular reaction to this characteristic.

Once we are engaged in therapeutic work, the way we respond is not solely dependent on ourselves; we are subtly shaped by our engagement with each of our patients. The individual character of each analyst, as reflected in these traits and behaviors, then influences and, in turn, is influenced by the individual character of each patient, as manifested in the treatment. We respond to differences in our patients with differences in ourselves, though we may not always be aware of these subtle shifts. From the patient-analyst interaction, a new creation evolves in which both participants are recognizable and at the same time, a unique, previously unknown experience occurs. The uniqueness of the interchange is true for both the analyst and the patient.

The limits of the change possible for the patient are dependent on the nature of the particular patient-analyst match and the extent to which the analyst is aware of and responsive to his or her impact on the patient. The analyst, too, may change as a result of the therapeutic interaction, though we generally assume that these changes are more subtle; these shifts in the analyst may also alter and expand the extent of the patient's growth. Once the uniqueness of each treatment situation is recognized, the importance of discerning the impact of the analyst's character on the process becomes apparent.

Elucidating the nature of our impact on our work with patients can be approached in at least three different ways. The first involves being aware of countertransference reactions (Jacobs, 1983, 1986; Mclaughlin, 1981, 1991a, b) Poland, 1983, 1988; Racker, 1968). Countertransference responses provide information about areas of interference in the process and sensitize us to areas for exploration, in ourselves as well as in our patients. The second method stresses the need for attention to patients' perceptions of us (Chused, 1992; Gill, 1982; Hoffman, 1983; Schwaber, 1983). Focusing on these patient reactions enables us to see our contributions to the transference and pave the way to a fuller understanding of patients' perceptions and responses in both the present and the past. A third approach emphasizes the importance of an awareness of areas of similarity and difference with our patients (Kantrowitz, 1986, 1992; Kantrowitz et al., 1989; Kantrowitz, Katz, & Paolitto, 1990c). Heightened awareness of these interfaces serves to warn us of potential blind spots where too much or too little resonance may compromise our work. These three approaches very often overlap, and at times may seem indistinguishable, but each offers a slightly different point of entry for increased sensitivity to our participation and its facilitating and impeding effect on the treatment. On some occasions, or for some particular analysts, one approach may be more illuminating than another.

In all three perspectives, the character of the analyst, as manifested in the treatment, is central to the course of the therapeutic work. In this paper, I will describe these three approaches to discerning the role of the analyst's character in the treatment and offer illustrations of the third method. In addition, I will argue that the quality of each patient-analyst match creates a unique, non-replicable treatment experience.

First, I will discuss countertransference reactions. We are alerted to countertransference interference when we perceive something unusual in our responses: unusually strong affective reactions to patients or situations they present; boredom or disinterest in patients or their hours; lengthening or shortening patients' hours; errors in billing or not informing patients about absences, vacations, or changes in hours; and intrusions of thoughts about the patient in waking or dreaming states. In short, anything that makes our reaction to a particular patient deviate from our usual, expectable responses to our patients. However, just as analysts will differ somewhat in their responses to different patients, so they will also differ in their characteristic reactions to their patients in terms of intensity of affect, level of engagement, frequency of thoughts about patients outside of treatment hours, and so forth. Recognition of deviations in response is always relative to what is normative for oneself. In addition, countertransference reactions are themselves an inevitable part of every treatment. It is not their presence, but the lack of attunement to their presence, which can endanger a treatment. When countertransference reactions are identified, they are a source of information that may facilitate the treatment. As long as our self-understanding enables us to proceed with, and even deepen, the work, countertransference should be considered an expectable part of treatment. It is only when we cannot elucidate and control the expression of countertransference reactions through our self-inquiry that we may need the help of a consultant to understand more fully the nature of the difficulty for and from us in the treatment; if that proves insufficient, a return for further work on our own personal treatment may be in order.

One of the most frequent countertransference reactions occurs when there are similarities of conflicts between patient and analyst. This similarity may result in blind spots that lead to transference-countertransference enactments or stalemates in treatment. In some instances, the analyst experiences the patient as similar to someone emotionally significant from the past; in others, the analyst identifies with the patient or with some important figure in the patient's life. Jacobs (1986), Poland (1988), and McLaughlin (1991) have each given detailed and sensitive accounts of such occurrences. Definitions of countertransference range from viewing all reactions to a patient and the patient's transference under this rubric (Blum, 1986) to the narrower formulation of the analyst's unconscious response to the patient, or the patient's transference, which resonates with his or her own less resolved conflicts (Freud, 1915a). Freud's narrower definition of countertransference seems a more useful delineation for the distinctions I am trying to make and allows us to separate more easily the different aspects of the analyst-patient interaction.

The second method for finding out our impact on our patients is to explore their reactions to and perceptions of us. Hoffman (1983) has emphasized that systematic attention to the patient's associations, to discover ideas related to perceptions of the analyst's countertransference, is crucial to the interpretive work. It also provides the data to keep the analyst from inference based on subjective experience. Increased or decreased affective response; coming early or late for sessions; changes in timing of payment of bills; and change in kind or quality of material, tone, or ability to associate: in short, anything which makes our patient's reactions to us deviant from his or her usual, expectable response alert us to transference reactions.

We need to consider whether these reactions are triggered (Gill, 1982) by something the analyst actually does or does not do. The meaning attributed to analyst's action or nonaction by the patient is what is transferred from the past and may or may not reflect the analyst's actual reactions to the patient. The patient selects the aspect of the analyst that provides material to support his or her earlier view of intimate relationships. The analyst's character, as revealed in the manner of conducting treatment and the particular variations in response to the particular patient, provides the hooks for the patient to play out the transference. When indirect expressions of transference are suggested in changed behavior, we are not always able to perceive that a shift has occurred, and even when we are aware, we are not always able to uncover the stimulus for this change in the patient's reaction to the analyst.

Sometimes we remain blind to such shifts in our patients, if they are too subtle or if they interface with our own need not to see or face something within ourselves with which they resonate. In the situations where we do not detect these shifts, we may not become conscious of the difficulty until transference-countertransference enactments force the patient's experience of distress into the center of our awareness or results in a stalemate in the treatment. Careful attention to the processes and the shifts of defense (Gray, 1973), affect and state of the patient (Schwaber, 1983) in the treatment may be sufficient to help us detect how and when our interventions disrupt or get in the way of the patient's process.

Determining whether the source of disruption comes primarily from the patient's transference or the analyst's behavior is, at times, difficult. Schwaber (1992) calls our attention to the interface between the approach of focusing on data from the patient about ourselves and countertransference. She states that by attending to the subtle shifts of affect and state in our patients, we may be alerted to the impact of our interventions that, due to countertransference interference, have shifted our attention away from the patient's viewpoint. If we are attuned to these subtle shifts, she believes that we may detect our inadvertent participation in reviving the patient's conflicts prior to it becoming a full-blown transference-countertransference enactment.

The patient's and analyst's shared understanding of how a response contributes to the recreation of a previous painful state enables a reorganization of the patient's psychic experiences, which in turn facilitates capacities for self-observation and self-regulation. The particular painful state and the particular quality of the analyst's response or nonresponse, however, will be somewhat different for each patient-analyst pair. Therefore, the reorganization of psychic experiences will take a somewhat different shape depending on the nature of any given pair.

My perspective is that countertransference reactions are sources of information and not simply phenomena to be viewed as interferences and to be disposed of. The amount of relevance to the patient and the analyst differs in each instance, but just as we contribute to the transference evoked for our patients, so they contribute to the countertransference evoked in each of us. Finding the element they contribute may alert us to something in our patients of which they are not yet conscious. For example, on one occasion I thought that a patient had not paid a bill, when in fact it had been submitted to insurance. However, the irritation I felt prior to remembering the insurance alerted me to the fact that I was experiencing the patient as withholding. Listening for this material, I then clearly heard data confirming that the patient was holding back in her relationships with both her husband and me; this perception could then be introduced to the patient. If we are sensitive to patients' readiness and careful about providing data from their material, we can introduce these countertransference perceptions to expand their awareness, deepen their understanding, and broaden their perspective about themselves.

A third source of information about ourselves and our effect on the process can be found through attending to similarities and differences between our patients and ourselves. Transference-countertransference reactions may be the most affectively powerful arena for this recognition, but more subtle resonances and dissonances also occur. These reactions can alert us to areas where we might overlook what may be problematic or overemphasize what may be central to us but not to our patients. The manifestation of the analyst's character in the treatment and the patient's interpretation of his or her perception of the analyst is viewed as critical to the treatment outcome. Both perspectives previously described suggest that no treatment could be free from the analyst's influence; the perspective I am proposing similarly maintains that all treatments are powerfully influenced by the analyst's character, but also by the interdigitation of the analyst's character with the patient's character and conflicts.

In Boston Institute's longitudinal study of analyzability, the interface between the personal characteristics and dynamics of the patient and the analyst emerged as an important factor in the outcome of the treatment. The patient-analyst match was shown to have a facilitating and/or impeding impact, depending on the particular patient-analyst pairs and the particular phase of the treatment (Kantrowitz et al., 1989; Kantrowitz, Katz, & Paolitto, 1990c).[1]

The data suggested that when the analyst had a blind spot about an unresolved conflict, personal style, or characteristic that interdigitated with the patient's problems, these areas were not likely to be recognized, explored, or worked through in the patient's analysis. Similarities in traits, expression of conflict, conflict derivatives, and characterological defense for patient and analyst were one form of impeding match. Negative complementarity was a second kind; here, analyst and patient employed different modes of expression for a similar conflict. The analyst, in these cases, was unconsciously defending against the issue with which the patient was manifestly struggling. The shared problem areas in both kinds of impeding match were always central for the patient, but might or might not represent a major difficulty for the analyst. It was the analyst's "blindness" to the problem because of the overlap that prevented the area from being addressed. A facilitating match, which we called compensatory, existed when the analyst's character or style provided the patient with a quality or dimension with which to identify or modified a previously negative or interfering identification that had impaired the patient's functioning.

While we assume that with well-trained, reasonably skilled analysts, patients who have the capacity for self-observation and self-reflection will analyze areas that are central to their conflicts, the depth and range with which these conflicts and experiences are explored will vary for any given patient-analyst pair. The limits of this exploration, I suggest, are related not only to the limits of each individual, but also to the match between them. Similarly, the possibility for growth is determined by both their individual and interactional characteristics.

When a patient and an analyst have an overlapping blind spot, and when the area of this blind spot is central to the patient's difficulty, the treatment is likely to be stalemated. If this blind spot is not recognized and overcome, the therapeutic work will not progress. I believe that all treatments are affected by the patient-analyst match, but not usually in such a dramatic way. However, all analysts have blind spots and when these interdigitate with a patient's difficulties, enactments rather than a therapeutic process may result. Sometimes these blind spots are due to similarities of conflicts or defenses between the patient and the analyst. In these instances, the analyst's unconscious identification with the patient leads to an unrecognized collusion in which important areas remain insufficiently addressed. On other occasions, these blind spots are due to the analyst's similarities with the characteristics or conflicts of important figures in the patient's life. On still other occasions, the analyst's blind spot may result from a similarity with an aspect of the patient that has been disavowed and externalized in another person. In this latter instance, the analyst has unconsciously identified with a transference representation and is in danger of reconfirming the patient's fears about the nature and outcome of close relationships. If the analyst can recognize the occurrences of these identifications, then they may become a focus for self-analysis and for reevaluation of what is occurring in the treatment process.

It is not only countertransference that creates these blind spots, unless we broaden the term to refer to the total configuration of characteristics and reactions of the analyst—a usage that is too comprehensive to be useful. Countertransference reactions, by the more narrow definition, are in fact the aspects of ourselves that we are the most likely to recognize, since they call forth reactions that are the most deviant from our usual therapeutic responses. We are trained to recognize our conflicts; they catch our attention and make us aware of ourselves in order that we may understand and control ourselves.

In contrast, we are not so attuned to our more general habitual ways of being, thinking, feeling, and reacting. Therefore, their impact and their interface with a patient's character and dynamic conflicts may more easily go undetected. More difficult to detect are those aspects of ourselves that do not pose a source of interference for us in our daily lives or work, but which do overlap positively or negatively with our patients. If this interface occurs in an area of central difficulty for a particular patient and we remain unaware, the potential for interference or avoidance of work in this area is great. Such awareness might help us contain and, one hopes, minimize the aspects of ourselves that may otherwise have an impeding impact on the treatment process.

Blind spots that affect the process of the work in a subtle fashion are often the result of similarities between patient and analyst. There are times when the analyst may not consciously perceive an overlapping area because there is no conscious affective charge connected. I will present two examples where analysts were unaware of any heightened affect in relation to their patients or any difficulty in the treatments until an unconscious identification became apparent. In both cases, the analyst's self-discovery, stimulated in reaction to the patient, led to a more complex understanding and deepening of the treatment.

In the first example, a similarity of situation ultimately revealed an unconscious similarity of conflict. I found that night after night a patient was appearing in my dreams. I was not aware of any particular significance or strong reactions in relation to this patient nor did there seem to be anything troublesome in the therapeutic work; my initial attempts at self-analysis proved unsuccessful in revealing any relevant data. I was sufficiently perplexed and suspicious of the reappearance of this patient in my dream life to consider returning to my former analyst to illuminate the situation. It was in imagining what I would tell my analyst that I understood the meaning of the patient in my dream.

I imagined describing a very painful childhood experience that my patient had been reliving. When he was four years old, he had been left alone with his two-year-old brother. His brother had crawled over to a window and pulled himself up on to the sill. The patient vividly recalled coming into the hall across from the window and seeing his brother fall out; his brother survived but was permanently brain damaged. The patient's mother accused him of pushing his brother out the window. While the patient thought he had not done this, there was always some doubt in his mind, and he had spent his life trying to rescue young boys. I then recalled that when I was four years old, my mother had had a miscarriage. I am an only child and had spent a great deal of time in my analysis bemoaning the absence of siblings. As I recalled an image of my mother from that time and a beach house where we had been staying, I was suddenly flooded with intense feelings of hostility toward this never-to-be-born sibling. Although the memory of my mother's miscarriage was not new, during my analysis I had never got in touch with my wish to be an only child and the benefits accrued from that or with the hostile, rivalrous, hateful feelings I was then experiencing—nor the guilt over my murderous wishes. I was amazed and excited and no longer felt a need to consult my former analyst; I never dreamt of the patient again.

The lifting of my affective repression had an unexpected effect on the therapy. While I had previously been unaware of any particular difficulty in the work, after discovering my own buried hostile wishes and guilt I found myself more actively pursuing my patient's hostile and rivalrous feelings toward his brother. The patient began to express his negative feelings toward his brother in much greater depth and intensity; his compulsive rescuing of young boys began to abate. I recognized that prior to recovering my memory of my own hostile wishes, I had been siding subtly with my patient's protestations of innocence. In order to keep my own destructive wishes toward a potential sibling buried, I had abandoned the position of neutrality in my therapeutic exploration. My subtle siding with the patient's view of himself as a victim of his mother's accusations had prevented a fuller expression of his hostility and feelings of guilt. What is important to note is that prior to the appearance of the patient in my dreams, I had been unaware that I had shifted my stance of neutral listening and had been resonating with his need to claim his innocence and thereby undermining the fuller expression of his resentment, rivalry, and guilt.

I had treated many other patients whose problems centered around feelings of unconscious hostility and guilt without these conflicts being reawakened and without any notable interference in the treatment—though there may, in fact, have been some subtle lack of pursuit of these areas, of which I remained unaware, as was noted in this case. I was neither aware of any major interferences in my own life that stemmed from my repressed hostility and guilt in relation to this unborn sibling, nor that it had played a central role in my dynamics. The similarity of situation with the patient stimulated and revived an unconscious affective memory. Once I was able to more fully inhabit my guilt, the patient's aggressive feelings and fantasies in relation to his brother took on a previously absent vitality and our work deepened. While the patient and I shared an underlying conflict about hostile, rivalrous wishes and guilt over harm coming to a sibling, it was both more central and more conscious for my patient than for me. I had recognized and worked on the conflict with the patient; it was the limited vigor in the work, not the awareness of the conflict, which was the interference. In this example, the issue of match is reflected in the similarity of situation, which became the vehicle for discovering a similarity of conflict and an unconscious identification with the patient that was diminishing the depth of the therapeutic work.

In the second example, a similarity of defensive style served as a collusion against exploring a similar conflict, which was conscious for the patient and unconscious for the analyst. The analyst, a skilled and experienced clinician, was presenting cases to a consultant to further the development of his professional skill. The consultant had been impressed by the analyst's skill, maturity, openness, and non-defensiveness in relation to countertransference issues; he had made very constructive use of consultation and almost always found a way to integrate the ideas in his work. He had presented several other patients before the case about to be described and had no awareness of any particular difficulty in the work with this patient. He liked the patient and looked forward to the hours; he was unaware of any particular intensity in relation to her.

The patient was a schoolteacher who had a warm and playful manner, but was very inhibited in her relationships with men. While previously she had had a few intimate relationships with men, for several years after starting treatment the patient had not dated. She rationalized this social isolation as due to her life circumstances, in which it was relatively difficult to meet men. The analyst, in contrast, believed her social retreat was because she had developed a transference neurosis that focused her affect on the treatment. The treatment, as reported, had an erotic charge in the interchange. The patient would tease and cajole the analyst, barraging him with questions about himself, his thoughts about her, their work, and life in general. While the patient's words by themselves might seem to be aggressive, the tone used by the analyst made it clear that he generally found it pleasing, though sometimes a challenge to deal with. At times, he would respond to her teasing questions with a playful response, and they would engage in a kind of banter, which while never inappropriate, was not furthering the work. This therapeutic style was not usual for this analyst. These interchanges with this patient occurred far more often than he had been aware before presenting the case.

As he reflected on the material he presented, he recognized his manner and tone as characteristic of himself in social settings during his college days, when he enjoyed a reputation for witty repartee, a style that had been toned down over the years. The patient and the analyst, it seemed, shared a playful style that contained more erotic charge than the analyst realized. However, the consultant was struck by the fact that, although this manner of relating was erotically charged, it was also distancing. The playful exchanges served to keep each other at arm's length and prevent a deepening of affect, content, and involvement in the transference. Despite being affectively connected, and in some ways gratified by the treatment, the patient remained enormously frustrated with her life and had made limited progress in understanding the nature of, or reasons for, her inhibitions.

Once the distancing impact of this behavior was pointed out to the analyst, he not only stopped the banter but also considered thoughtfully why it had occurred. Although he had conceptualized the patient's retreat from men as related to her increased involvement in the transference, he now realized that this formulation was intellectual: he had not affectively believed what he had stated. He found it hard to take seriously that the patient was really emotionally or erotically invested in the treatment relationship. He was struck by the fact that the consultant had underscored moments when the patient more directly acknowledged her yearnings for him—for example, she spoke of missing him over the weekend, and of addressing her thoughts to him between hours. He became aware that he had almost not heard, and certainly not registered, these statements. The countertransference, which underlay his distancing and failure really to perceive the transference, was now clear to him.

In his own treatment, he had been unable to take seriously the depth to which he had become affectively engaged in the transference. His style was warm and he easily engaged with other people. It had been very difficult for him to recognize how his affectively charged manner of relating could be employed to create a distance. This distancing had been pointed out to him in his treatment and the impact of its defensive function became increasingly clear to him as he saw how he had inadvertently played this out in the treatment of his patient. He saw that his patient had been less defended against her emerging feelings for him than he had been about his feelings toward his analyst.

Following his insight into the defensive aspect of his style, the analyst not only ceased to join the patient in banter, but he was also able to interpret how her playful questions were a way of holding him at a distance. Simultaneously, he began to address her more direct acknowledgment of feelings in the transference. The patient rapidly began to express previously glossed-over longings and to reveal how vulnerable she felt in acknowledging these feelings. In both present-day and historical material, she elaborated her fear of intimacy. The flirtatious verbal play greatly diminished and, when it appeared, was understood by both analyst and patient as a sign that she had again become anxious about getting close.

The similar defensive style of patient and analyst had served to keep each other at bay and the treatment at a stalemate. Neither seemed aware of the impasse in their work, since there was an affective charge in the hours; however, this affective charge was not of a high enough intensity to alert the analyst to the difficulty in the treatment. The patient was not a countertransference figure for him in the usual sense; that is, she did not represent an important figure from his life nor did her transference resonate with central unresolved issues in his own. She was, however, struggling with an issue that was similar to his own difficulty—a fear of allowing intimacy. The patient's difficulty in this area was deeper and more pervasive than the analyst's. The analyst had a history of intimate heterosexual relationships as well as close friendships with both men and women. But while the patient's difficulties in this area were greater, she was also conscious that she was frightened of intimacy, whereas the analyst was more defended and unaware of his more subtle difficulties in this area.

His own treatment and the consultation worked synergistically for him to gain awareness of this problem. His ability to make use of consultation so quickly to change his treatment approach suggests that his difficulties in this area were not so deeply entrenched, and the consultant had not noted distancing in the other treatments he presented. The patient and the analyst shared a problem: the impediment in the treatment arose from their joint participation. While this patient would undoubtedly have found a forum for bringing this problem into any treatment, since it was her central difficulty, the particular configuration that this treatment took was shaped by the contribution of this particular analyst's conflicts and defensive style.

In both these treatments, the work of analysis had been proceeding without the analyst or patient being aware of a sense of disruption. In the first example, I was alerted to my countertransference by the patient's appearance in my dreams; in the second example, the analyst became aware of a blind spot only after the consultant's observation. In neither instance did this initial intellectual recognition of an interference stir an affective resonance. In the first case, it was my finding the similarity of situation between myself and my patient (i.e., harm coming to a younger sibling when they were four years old) that led to affective awareness and ultimately the similarity of conflict (i.e., the defense against unconscious guilt). In the second case, it was the analyst becoming aware of the similarity of defensive style, which I would view as a characterological similarity that stimulated personal analytic work and led to his affective awareness and recognition that a similar defense was the characterological manifestation of a similarity of conflict about intimacy. For these analysts, the recognition of similarities, one situational, the other characterological, was the pathway to discovering the similar underlying unconscious conflict, which would be defined as a countertransference issue. In other words, once the conflictual area became the surface of the analytic work, the aspect of the match between patient and analyst was in the transference-countertransference arena.

It is possible that careful attention to the process material might have revealed shifts in the patient's affect, state, defense, or transference that might also have alerted these two analysts to pursue areas which their patients were avoiding. However, just as analysts' character traits often lead them to respond differently from one another with their patients, so too may it lead them to gravitate toward different routes for discovery of their impact in the treatment. Our characters determine our differences in many arenas; each analyst's responses inevitably contain aspects of personal style. For each of us, there also are preferred theories of both dynamics and technique; such choices and intellectual predilections are not free from personal developmental influences. Even when we essentially agree on theory, technique, and treatment stance, each of us responds in our own idiosyncratic manner. Our personal histories, including our own treatment experiences and professional training, influence what aspects of patients' material we select for our response.

Thus, there is no single accurate response to a patient's communication; our choice of words and images, our inflection and tone, the timing of our intervention, its length and the extent of interaction, to name just a few areas, will inevitably differ. Orgel (1990) has pointed to the shaping effect that the analyst's particular tone of voice or choice of words has on the patient's affective reality, transference fantasies, and perception of the "real" attitudes and feelings of the analyst in the treatment situation. Each response from us has, in turn, an impact that subtly shapes the subsequent material. Although we remain recognizable in our mode and manner of participation in treatment, patients evoke different aspects of the analyst in response to their particular characteristics. What then emerges has a unique quality: a creation of this particular patient-analyst pair.

To the extent that a patient is open to treatment, the patient is open to a new experience, which means being capable of a new response. To the extent that the patient finds evidence to confirm previously held beliefs about the dangerous or disappointing nature of oneself or others, the treatment will not only fail, but will strengthen the patient's earlier convictions (Pfeffer, 1961, 1963). If, on the other hand, the patient finds evidence that refutes these negative expectations, the treatment will open the possibility for new perceptions about her/himself and others. The analyst's character may contribute to the failure of treatment in differing ways—such as blind spots due to similarities with an aspect of the patient, or an important person in the patient's life, or counteridentifcation with the patient or others significant to him. In contrast, the patient's conclusions when transference fears are confirmed will not show much variation; irrespective of the form of the analyst's enactment, it will be a reinforcement of an old belief about the dangerous or disappointing nature of others or oneself. However, when the analyst's character manifests itself in ways that a patient is able to perceive and respond to as a new experience, then patients may find and develop different aspects of themselves. Such growth depends on the qualities of the particular match. I do not mean that the patient will internalize an aspect of the analyst, though this may, of course, occur. What I am suggesting is that the particular interdigitation of patient and analyst may facilitate the emergence and expansion of certain aspects of the patient—preexisting, but inhibited or unrecognized prior to treatment—and that the nature of each patient-analyst pair will result in some differences about what aspects of the patient develop.

Differences between what emerges in one treatment and what might have emerged from another can never really be tested. Even when there are reports of the impact of a different analyst on a patient (Hurwitz, 1986), the influence of the previous treatment and the patient's different stage of life mean that the treatments are not comparable. We cannot study the impact of the match as if there were laboratory conditions allowing for controls and replication. However, this lack of comparability does not indicate that there are no important differences in approach and character that significantly impact on the patient's capacity to make use of the treatment. I am not suggesting that there is an ideal match. Most patients can work with many different analysts and achieve a successful outcome. Similarly, most analysts can work with many different patients and obtain a successful result. What I am suggesting, however, is that the particular nature of the result will always have some subtle differences—and, sometimes, when there are overlapping blind spots, blatant differences—in range, depth, and even in specific areas of character that are explored, depending on the particular analyst-patient pair.

Unfortunately, we cannot ascertain the exact nature of these differences since we cannot return to an earlier point and redo what has already occurred. Each occurrence has an impact which we make part of ourselves, confirming or disproving previous beliefs and representations of ourselves and others. All we can do is offer examples of cases where we do become aware of a personal impact on treatment. This recognition can alert us to our potential for being caught unwittingly colluding or impeding the process through aspects of ourselves which we have not recognized.

Because we are working with the personal problems of our patients, we are continually engaged in trying to understand intense affective experiences and the defenses against such experiences. Our patients confront us with painful experiential states and conflicts on every developmental level. It is often the defenses by which they manage their distress that we find more difficult than the content of the conflict or state from which they are fleeing. Our shared human experience means that we have all known what it is to be dependent, to feel helpless, to be disappointed, to want autonomy, to be angry, to feel competitive, envious, sexual, to lose and to win, and to face our aloneness and the realization that we will die. Working with patients means that these experiences are never far from our consciousness. The way in which we deal with these experiences, and the extent to which we can tolerate the affects they arouse, will affect our clinical work.

Once our training is complete, and our experience and skill is adequate, our characters as well as our residual conflicts determine the limit of our work with any given patient. Treatment outcomes vary, depending on the nature of the interdigitation of characteristics and conflicts of our patients with ourselves. The three approaches described in this paper offer guidelines for our continued self-exploration. Attention has been drawn to ruptures, dissonances, and disjunctions. The nature of our negative impact—how we interfere or impede treatment—has been illustrated. However, there is little in the literature that focuses on the positive impact of the analyst on the patient; this is certainly an area for future inquiry. Analysts may be disinclined to offer personal examples for fear of seeming boastful or blind to some aspect of the work outside of their awareness that this might expose. However, supervisors and peers could turn their attention beneficially to considerations of the enabling aspects of a particular analyst's character and style in relation to a particular patient, opening up a fruitful area for further investigation of the nature of therapeutic action.

Note

1 A more complete account of this study appears in the Appendix of the book.

Chapter 5

The beneficial aspects of the patient-analyst match

Throughout the history of psychoanalysis there has been a continuous debate about which factors are central to its therapeutic effect. Theorists attempting to identify these factors have tended to polarize between emphasizing the cognitive-affective value of making the unconscious conscious—a focus on content (Bibring, 1936; Bion, 1971; Blatt & Behrends, 1987; Blum, 1979; Freud, 1915a); Glover, 1937; Goldberg, 1979; Gray, 1990; Kernberg, 1992; Kris, 1990a, 1990b; Loewenstein, 1956; Meissner, 1989; Strachey, 1934)—and the primary importance of affective-attachment creating support and promoting growth through a benevolent presence—a focus on the relationship (Blatt & Behrends, 1987; Freud, 1916–17, 1937; Gitelson, 1962; Kohut, 1965; Loewald, 1960; McLaughlin, 1981; Modell, 1976; Nunberg, 1937; Pine, 1993; Reich, 1960a, b); Schwaber, 1990; Spitz, 1956; Stone, 1961).

Outcome studies of psychoanalysis (Kantrowitz, Katz, & Paolitto, 1990a; Wallerstein, 1986) have documented the fact that supportive factors play a greater role in therapeutic benefit than previously had been thought. Pine (1993) specifies the aspects of the analyst's participation in the psychoanalytic process that universally have the effect of support. These mutative factors in the analytic relationship stem from the analyst's reliable presence, neutrality, abstinence, relative anonymity, and focus on the patient. Kris (1993) defines the analyst's activity as support when it counters the patient's self-criticism. Rather than focusing on the general support that the analytic relationship offers, I wish to turn my attention to specific ways the analyst facilitates and enhances psychological growth in the context of the particular dyadic interaction.

Infancy studies provide data for the importance of the constitutional fit between the caretaker and the infant in facilitating or interfering with psychological development. Interactive, nonverbal affective communication shapes the behavior and response of both parties. The aspects of the dyadic interaction that work best for the infant's particular temperament are the ones that persist (Stern, 1985, 1990). While mutual accommodations between caretaker and infant do occur, there are likely to be limits to the extent to which mismatched temperaments are able to shift (Beebe & Lachmann, 1998).

The mutual influence of behavior and response between infant and caretaker is applicable, I believe, in describing what transpires between patient and analyst. Just as the good-enough mother is able to respond to a wide variety of babies and a wide variety of states in one baby, so the good-enough analyst is able to work effectively with a wide range of patients and a wide variety of affects, states, fantasies, and defenses in any one patient. However, the individual characteristics of each analyst determine the particular limitations and strengths that are brought to the analytic work. Previously, I have focused on how blind spots resulting from the interdigitation of the particular characteristics and conflicts of the analyst and the patient impede the analytic process (Kantrowitz, 1992, 1993a, c). In this chapter, I shall focus on the way the interdigitation of the particular characteristics of the analyst and the patient may be beneficial and facilitating to the analytic process. I shall try to show how the positive impact of this interaction often comes from the subtle, nonverbal aspects of the particular patient-analyst pair.

The impact of the real person of the analyst on the outcome of psychoanalytic treatment has not often been a central focus in the psychoanalytic literature. The reason for this neglect is natural. To give theoretical status to the personal attributes and responses of the analyst understandably generates concern that the definition of the analytic process will be clouded and its scientific status compromised (Viederman, 1991, p. 459).

Nevertheless, analysts have recognized that the interests, concerns, values, and attitudes of the analyst inevitably are communicated to the patient (Stone, 1961) and influence the outcome of the analysis, especially in the changes in the patient's self-representation (Dorpat, 1974; Karush, 1967; Viederman, 1976, 1991). What is more, some analysts believe that an analytic process cannot occur if the values of the patient and analyst are too discrepant (Viederman, 1976) and may be seriously impeded if the analyst is "blind" to a problem area because of too great a characterological similarity with the patient (Baudry, 1991; Goldberger, 1993; Kantrowitz, 1993a).

Unconscious attunement to affects and other nonverbal communications are not the usual focus when we try to describe an analytic process. While Jacobs (1973), McLaughlin (1975, 1981), and Schwaber (1981, 1987) have called our attention to the importance of our patients' nonverbal communications, their emphasis is on giving these communications verbal form. Assisting in making conscious what was previously unconscious and giving verbal representation, clarification, and interpretation to patients' verbal and nonverbal communications are our central activity as analysts. I wish to be clear at the outset that by placing my attention on the aspects of our interactions with our patients that often remain outside of consciousness, but which, I believe, nonetheless may have a profound influence on the patient and the analytic work, I am in no way diminishing the importance and centrality of our conscious, active, analytic, interpretive work. My intent is only to draw our attention to the impact that comes from the resonance, often unconscious, of the similarities and differences between our patients and ourselves. This particular aspect of our interactions is a component that contributes to the patient's development. It is not the whole, nor even the major part, of what happens in analysis; it is, however, a factor that has often been neglected when we debate how psychological change occurs.

Analysts have focused on these unconscious attunements to affects and early developmental states when they have tried to apply the findings from infancy studies to the treatment of adult patients. Buie (1993) believes that the therapist's experience of the patient is crucial, since it can be perceived experientially by the patient. The patient's vicarious experience of being securely cared for, seen as real, worthwhile, loved, and having a wholeness of identity through the perception of the therapist's experience of him is the essential interaction for the patient to develop structures that promote an internal restructuring.

Modell (1993) also focuses on the nonverbal communication of feeling and states between patient and analyst. According to his theory, affect in one person automatically induces a similar affect in another person. This contagiousness of affect in one person may occur unconsciously or it may be a conscious experience, but it is always automatic and takes place in an involuntary fashion. Patients who cannot identify, differentiate, or contain their affective responses will unconsciously elicit their analyst's help to provide an affect management retraining. This unconscious attempt to compensate for their deficiency stimulates in the analyst a countertransference experience which he or she uses to give a form and name to the patient's vague and unformed feelings. These responses from the analyst provide the perceptual validation for the patient's experience that previously had been missing. Winnicott's (1965) description of the holding environment provided by the mother for her child and Bion's (1971) view of the breast as the prototype of the container of the infant's emotional states similarly parallel the patient's use of the analyst for the development of self-regulatory functions.

While affective resonance between the patient and analyst is a central dimension in understanding the patient's conflicts and distress, it is not likely to have a one-to-one correspondence with the patient's early life relationship with his or her caretaker. Even if we assume a reemergence of an early unconscious experience, the patient has been influenced by many other people and situations over the ensuing years. These influences result in the patient in the present being different from the earlier self. Even though the specific characteristics of the analyst reverberate with the behavior and response of the patient, similarly to the way the characteristics of the caretaker influences the infant, the extent of the influence is not nearly as great. The analyst's role is not the same as the caretaker's, even though both assist with affect containment and differentiation. In addition, the individual character, style, and residual conflicts of each analyst affects the nature of the interaction with each patient, making it different from the patient's interaction with the original caretaker and somewhat different from the interaction this patient would have with any other analyst.

Once we grant the uniqueness of each analyst, we must begin to consider that the manner in which each individual analyst practices analysis is also, to a certain extent, unique. As Loewald stated,

> timing of interpretations, the context in which they are made, the way they are phrased, the tone of voice, are important elements of therapeutic action... Tact, basic rapport and its fluctuations, the

analyst's breadth of life experience and imagination... are ingredients... without which the most correct interpretations are likely to remain unconvincing and ineffective.

(1979, p. 158)

The behavioral form these dimensions take has infinite variety. The Boston longitudinal study of analyzability provided the first systematic documentation for the impact of the particular analyst's style, character, and conflicts on the particular patient's style, character, and conflict in relation to treatment outcome (Kantrowitz et al., 1989; Kantrowitz, Katz, & Paolitto, 1990b). The patient-analyst match was shown to have a facilitating and/or impeding impact depending on the particular patient-analyst pairs and the particular phase of the treatment. The data suggested that when the analyst had a blind spot in relation to an unresolved conflict, personal style or characteristic that interdigitated with the patient's problems, these areas were not likely to be recognized, explored, or worked through in the patient's analysis. The shared problem areas were always central for the patient, but might or might not represent a major difficulty for the analyst. It was the analyst's "blindness" to the problem, because of the overlap, which prevented the area from being addressed.

It was also found that when an analyst had a characteristic that compensated for some deficit in the patient or which aided in disconfirming some aspect of the patient's transference, the analysis was facilitated. A facilitating match, called compensatory, existed when the analyst's character or style provided the patient with a quality or dimension with which to identify, or when it modified a previously negative or interfering identification that impaired the patient's functioning. In this study, the candidate-analysts did not analyze the facilitating aspect of the match; they seemed to be unaware of its existence. It was only in the retrospective evaluation of the data that it became apparent to the psychoanalytic researchers.

A second kind of facilitating match, not discernible in this study due to the nature of the data, became apparent in clinical material from supervision of analyses. When analysts were able to become aware of blind spots, either through the supervisory process or through the patient's persistent focus on this area, many analysts became motivated to pursue and elaborate these previously closed-off areas. Under these circumstances, both the patients and the analysts changed psychologically as a result of the analytic work. The analysts moved back and forth between elucidating and exploring the patient's material and analyzing their own countertransference and transference responses as a process of joint discovery unfolded.

A third kind of facilitating match is suggested by the infancy studies. Constitutional strengths and positive aspects of early experience may have gone undeveloped or unenhanced in the course of later development. An analyst with similar strengths that are manifested, though not necessarily and probably not usually verbalized, may stimulate the development of these capacities in the patient. Similarly, there may be a characterological match that enables the patient to refind and then expand on early positive experiences which had either not been consciously recalled or which, because they were preverbal, had previously lacked form.

It is in the context of an emotionally important relationship that old conflicts get revived and played out again. This reliving allows the analyst and analysand to examine and understand the constructions that the analysand has formed about the inevitability of the dangerous or disappointing nature of others and/or the self. Through the recreation and analysis of this previously painful state in the context of a new relationship, analysands come to understand how and why they came to feel and believe as they have. If their previous conscious or unconscious fears of danger and disappointment are not confirmed, a modification of self and other representations are likely to occur. Concomitantly, capacities for self-observation and self-regulation will increase, further enhancing self-esteem. But what specific factors are necessary for change to occur?

Clearly, the analysand has to feel safe enough with the analyst to allow the analyst to become emotionally important. Unless the analysand experiences an emotional intensity, the affective reliving will not occur. The analysand must also have the capacity to observe what occurs between them and to tolerate the intense affects that are generated. Analysands must have a sufficient degree of these qualities to be suitable for a form of treatment that facilitates further development of these capacities. When an analysand has a very limited capacity for trust, self-observation, or affect tolerance, it may require an analyst with particular compensatory strengths in the area of the patient's deficit for analytic work to be possible.

In many instances, analyzability is determined by the interactional effect of the particular character and conflict and strengths and limitations of the patient in relation to the particular character and conflict and strengths and limitations of the particular analyst. An analyst whose style is calm and patient may be facilitating for a patient whose tendency is to become emotionally flooded, but possibly less facilitating to a patient who defends by being highly cerebral. An analyst, whose style is more active and affective, might be more facilitating to the more cerebral patient, but overstimulating to the patient who tends toward emotional flooding.

My aim is to define which factors most facilitate change in psychoanalysis and then show how these are manifest in any particular treatment. Often what we describe may seem to be simply good technique or clinical acumen; both of these attributes are, of course, crucial. However, no matter how well trained, experienced, or gifted the clinician, he or she will have blind spots, and all analysts have ways of being with their patients that others could characterize pejoratively in one way or another. Each analyst also has specific strengths; these strengths potentially bring forth or enhance particular strengths of their patients.

While the ideas of what constitutes a psychoanalytic treatment have broadened since the early days when interpretations alone were considered analytic, there was always a recognition that "uncontrollable factors" (Eissler, 1953) such as the match of particular analyst and analysand were an influence in the outcome of the analysis. Alexander and French's idea (1946) that a corrective emotional experience could be attained by the analyst's role-playing a part that counterbalanced the particular patient's expectations in the transference, attests to this awareness. His technique was based on a manipulation, and as such was not only nonanalytic but also likely to fail since transferences are attuned to more subtle manifestations. Playacting is soon likely to be recognized as such and will only reinforce a patient's sense of distrust and disappointment. However, the idea that how the analyst actually behaves in relation to the patient may have a beneficial, corrective impact was well founded.

Although we always know our own patients and ourselves in the most depth and complexity, there are difficulties in using this clinical material to illustrate the beneficial aspects of the match. First, no matter how exacting we are in our self-scrutiny, there are inevitable blind spots when evaluating one's own work. Second, even assuming it were possible to describe objectively a beneficial match of our own, it might well seem self-aggrandizing to do so. In order not to distract the reader from a focus on the impact of match by a temptation to analyze the analyst or the analyst's work, and despite the limitations of secondhand data, it is probably most effective to illustrate this concept through supervisory work.

The first example, disguised to insure confidentiality, illustrates the benefit obtainable from a compensatory match, in which an aspect of the analyst's character makes up for something the patient lacked. This case also illustrates a match of similarity in which the patient employed a less developed aspect of the analyst to support a similar but more specific quality of his own. The patient used his recognition of a shared interest with his analyst to reclaim and develop a previously forsaken gift. In addition, a similar, but developed rather than nascent, strength of the analyst facilitated the burgeoning of a quality in the patient.

The analyst was a youthful-looking man in his late thirties. His manner was warm, open, and direct. A playfulness and gentle vitality were conveyed in his low-keyed humor. He demonstrated considerable skill in his ability both to analyze his patient and to conceptualize the material. His interventions were tactfully phrased and well timed. He was aware of his countertransference experiences and able to explore them productively. These talents made it likely that he would make an excellent analyst for almost any patient. Knowledge of his work with other patients confirmed this impression. I cannot, of course, know how much of this analyst's sensitivity and skill came from constitutional strengths, the security derived from benevolent, loving relationships in his family or later developmental experiences, but his life had been far from free of trauma. His father had died when he was an early adolescent, and a younger male cousin, beloved by the analyst, committed suicide when the analyst was in his late twenties. Although he was now happily married and enjoying his wife and child, his social development had been slow.

The patient was a 25-year-old lawyer who had just graduated from a prestigious law school and joined an equally prestigious law firm. He sought analysis because of his anxiety about being able to perform successfully. It quickly emerged that while his manifest anxieties were about work, he had even more intense anxiety about his relationships with women. Although he had women friends, he had never had a sustained relationship with a woman that was also sexual. His sexual activity was with prostitutes or women he met in bars. The patient's parents had little education and, while they were proud of him, they had a very limited understanding of his world. His brother, three years his junior, had remained closer to them and had established a life more similar to that of the parents. The patient believed that his father had always preferred his brother and that both parents felt more comfortable and closer to his brother. He experienced his father as easily threatened and competitively undermining of him. His mother was warm but insecure; the early closeness he remembered experiencing with her was disrupted with the birth of his brother. The patient had done well in school but felt ostracized socially, though he always had a few friends. He compared himself unfavorably with his contemporaries. He consciously longed for a man to show him how "to be a man."

The analysis began with the patient's dramatic testing of the analyst's capacity to accept and understand him. Not only did the patient appear for less than half of the scheduled appointments, rarely notifying the analyst either before or after, he also increased his sexual promiscuity, placing himself in objectively dangerous situations. He made it abundantly clear to the analyst that he was aware of the risk he was incurring. When he did attend an hour, he was usually late and then actively critical and demanding with his analyst, and finally becoming self-berating. The analyst tried to address his behavior in relation to anxiety stirred by starting psychoanalysis and his difficulty in tolerating the tension, but this did little to abate the patient's actions. Initially, when the patient missed hours, the analyst would call to find out if he was all right. The patient would respond by feeling intruded on or wondering if the analyst thought he had committed suicide. It seemed the patient was challenging the analyst to find him unsuitable for analytic treatment. Indeed, given the patient's behavior, it was more than reasonable to wonder if he had sufficient tolerance for his affects to undergo a psychoanalysis.

For reasons that are hard to make explicit, neither the analyst nor I ever seriously doubted this man's capacity for doing analytic work, though we were both greatly concerned that he might harm himself in his insistence on testing his analyst's capacity to withstand his potentially self-destructive behavior. It was not clear at this point what the patient wished for more specifically from the analyst that was being expressed by this behavior. Although the patient's actions were a source of concern, the analyst described the patient as almost parodying someone who was out of control; the way the patient was able to observe and describe himself made the analyst feel that the patient was not quite in the affective grip of his emotions that his actual behavior suggested. It felt communicative. The analyst both took seriously how desperate the patient felt and, at the same time, held fast to his belief that the patient wanted to and was capable of doing analytic work. His countertransference was to wish to rescue the patient, but he saw that whenever his interventions were of a more supportive nature, the patient would feel undermined and become depressed. Although he found it difficult to tolerate, the analyst gradually came to accept that he could do nothing at this point that would immediately influence his patient's actual behavior. Communicating his understanding of both moment-to-moment affect, state, and defense and the patient's overarching strategy for determining whether his analyst was up to this job, proved to be effective in gradually lowering the patient's anxiety. The patient began to express his underlying sadness, attend more hours, decrease his sexual promiscuity; but then, as he explained later in the analysis, fearing that his analyst would no longer take seriously how troubled he was, he returned to the earlier behavior.

As the supervisor, although I was always somewhat wary of the fact that I was not as worried as the patient's behavior seemed to warrant, I felt a confidence in the analyst's ability accurately to convey and understand the patient's experience. His attunement in the hours and gift in timing and phrasing of inventions made me feel he could handle the situation as well as most of the more experienced colleagues. His sensitivity to his patient's vulnerabilities and tolerance for his patient's enactments made it possible for this very frightened patient to engage in an analytic process. It took over a year of analysis before this patient was able to attend his hours regularly and stop his sexual acting out.

Over the next year, the patient's push toward action greatly diminished, and he began to explore his depression. While at times he pleaded with his analyst to medicate him to relieve his intense anxiety and depression, and threatened to use street drugs to ease his distress and soothe himself, he was able, for the most part, to contain his affect and increasingly able to put his experience into words. He conveyed a picture of a sensitive, talented, lonely boy who felt different from his peers and unable to communicate with his family. He had tried to join the other boys in competitive sports, but being very tall, thin, and nonmuscular, he always felt awkward and ungainly. He hated his body and was certain no woman would ever find him attractive.

At times in the analysis, he would launch into paroxysms of self-hatred, describing the defects he perceived in his body with vivid detail. The patient expressed his despair and self-hatred as intensely as he had previously conveyed his anxiety through action. Although the analyst worried about the extent the patient might regress, he found that employing ego-supportive measures was counterproductive. If the analyst wondered what had set off the patient's attack on himself or tried to put his depression and self-hatred in historical context, the patient would first become enraged at the analyst for not understanding his experience and then increase his self-flagellation. The countertransference anxiety for the analyst was intense, since it reevoked memories of his cousin who had committed suicide. However, rather than being flooded by this anxiety, the analyst was able to contain it and use it to redouble his determination to stay with his patient and try to help him withstand his pain. Instead of trying to shore up the patient's defenses, the analyst then stayed with the patient's affective distress and explored with him in excruciating detail how he saw and experienced his body. The patient reviewed painful and humiliating incidents from his past when he had tried and failed to be competent and manly.

As the patient and analyst explored the patient's fears and anxieties about his body, the patient became less self-deprecating and more at ease with himself. Offhandedly, he began to bring in references to a female colleague in his firm. Gradually, this woman became central in his life as well as in his thoughts. However, when the relationship became sexual, the patient panicked, withdrew from this woman, and reverted to self-deprecation and despair in the analysis. The analyst addressed the patient's retreat in the face of anxiety about a sexual relationship. The patient's associations were to the time of early closeness with his mother and thoughts about the differences between their bodies. His father was never present; he had no sense of his father's body. The analyst wondered whether the patient felt that being with a woman made him feel as if he were a woman. Fears of female genitals then emerged along with the patient's desperate longing to have a man save him and teach him how to be a man.

An idealizing transference with homosexual aspects then dominated the third year of analysis. The patient pleaded with the analyst to teach and guide him. He had fantasies of a ménage à trois in which the analyst would demonstrate how to make love to a woman, whom he would then encourage the patient to seduce. His urgency to have the analyst give to him intensified. He felt humiliated by how important the analyst had become to him and attempted to restore his self-esteem by trying to decrease the analyst's importance through devaluing him and idealizing one of the senior male partners in his firm. The analyst remained patient and steady, reflecting to the patient his understanding of how intense his wishes were, how frustrating and humiliating not to have them gratified, yet simultaneously how reassuring. He also conveyed that he knew that the patient felt he needed his experiences to be understood perfectly. He also explained that this left the patient feeling that what he wished was impossible and fearing that there was not a place for him with his analyst.

The patient experienced intense sadness in relation to what he yearned for and could not have from his analyst. He acknowledged that the limits of the relationship were real to him no matter how much he pushed and tested them. At first, he felt intensely angry with his father, because he felt he could have had what he wanted with him if only his father had been different. Unlike his view of his analyst, whom he saw as steady, emotionally present, and basically benevolent, the patient saw his father as impulsive, unreliable, distant, and undermining of the patient because of his own insecurities.

He felt his father viewed him as a failure, a disappointment, not a real man. He then saw how he had held the same view of his father and his analyst. When he attacked and criticized his analyst, he had chosen the attributes he hated in his father. These qualities, he then saw, were the things he hated and feared in himself and reflected the way he thought his father had seen him. But his analyst seemed to recognize and value his abilities and to have a less stereotyped view of what being manly was. The analyst seemed untroubled by his neediness; his father had pushed him away when he felt and wished to be dependent. As the patient considered what he had got from his analyst and how he felt he had changed, his anger toward his father lessened and he began to consider what he might be able to salvage from the relationship.

Previously unavailable memories of good times with his father began to emerge. He felt enormously sad that in his anger about what his father was not, and in his fear of competing with and outdistancing him, he had deprived himself of knowing what they did and could have together. He had presented and perceived himself as inept, out of control, and unmanly—a parody of his view of his father and of the view he believed his father held of him. He saw how this construction had kept him from having what he could have for himself. Following this analytic work, his interest in women, which had never disappeared, became heightened.

During this time, the patient had begun to paint. Hints of this activity were presaged by the patient's comments about his admiration of the analyst's choice of colors in the office, his appreciation of a lithograph that the analyst recently had hung in the office, and his observation that his analyst must be visually oriented since he chose things with an eye to color and design. He was cautious when he introduced the fact that he had been painting. This activity was the kind he thought his father would mock. In high school, when he had been unable to find pleasure or solace with either male or female peers, in addition to retreating to books, he had taken art lessons. Painting had been a great pleasure for him, and his female instructor had admired his work and encouraged him. But painting had felt like a female activity. Without a man to support this enterprise, to continue to paint endangered his sense of masculinity. He had turned away from the arts to the world of numbers and later torts, which he viewed as shoring up his experience of being male. His father had represented the only kind of maleness he knew, but he could not and did not want to be that kind of man himself. He had often devalued his analyst as too soft-spoken, too tentative, because those qualities seemed like the non-male attributes that he hated in himself. He had tested and baited his analyst, trying to get him out of control like his father or himself, or to crumble and show he could not withstand the attack, like his mother. It was not just cozy between them; there was room for his aggression. With room for his aggression came room for his artistic ability and sensitivity.

Over the next months, another new quality emerged. The patient began to be playful and display a sense of humor. As the consultant who had watched this treatment from the outside, I was unprepared for this new lightness in this previously intensely dysphoric and action-prone man. I wondered if the analyst had had any inkling of this potential in his patient. The analyst himself, while intense and serious, had a playful quality and a gentle, warm humor. The analyst said that while he had never consciously expected his patient to demonstrate a sense of humor, he had sensed his desire to play. Once the first year of crisis in the analysis had passed, he reminded me that he did, at times, gently tease the patient. While he thought this might have more to do with some aspect of his own character, he felt that unconsciously he may have been responding to something in the patient. The patient's humor had a different quality from the analyst's; it was more aggressive and outlandish, but nonetheless good-natured. It had a kind of quirky quality that was reminiscent of something the patient had described about his father. The analyst noted that the patient's playful humor seemed to occur in response to his being playful with the patient. While the analysis continued to be hard work and painful for the patient, the analyst felt that now he and the patient also could enjoy their time together.

The analysis I have described is not complete: it has neither been presented in the full degree of its complexity, nor is it over. What I have presented is a sensitive and skillful piece of work in the early and middle phases of an analysis with a man with whom many analysts would not have felt it wise to work analytically. These early years of the analysis focused on affect management and the establishment of trust; in later material, the conflictual issues moved more to center stage. The analyst is a talented clinician; his tolerance for working with intense affect is considerable; his insight and sense of tact and timing are developed far beyond what is usual for someone at his stage of career. It would be easy to say that his talent for analytic work accounts for the success he had in working with this patient. I would not argue with this construction. What I am proposing, however, is that there are certain specific characterological traits of the analyst, some of which stem from the analyst's dynamics and history and other characteristics, which may be thought of as constitutional or innate, which also facilitated the treatment and may have influenced the development or reemergence of specific qualities for this patient.

The fact that the analyst was so determined to stay with the patient and help him tolerate his pain may possibly be attributable to the analyst's own high tolerance for dysphoric affect. It is certainly true that the analyst's calm temperament, in addition to his technical skill, provided a containment for the patient's impulsive intensity. The alliance to establish self-control (Kris, 1990a) or affect management retraining (Modell, 1993) was aided by this constitutional difference in the analyst. In addition, I would argue that the analyst's own experiences of loss of important male figures increased the analyst's empathy for the patient's yearning for a man. The analyst was conscious of his countertransference feelings of identifying the patient with his beloved cousin whose suicide he had been unable to prevent. The analyst also was acutely aware of his wishes to rescue this patient. Only on occasion did these wishes actively intrude on the process in the form of unneeded supportive measures. I believe that this wish to rescue, the analyst's own unresolved feelings about this traumatic loss of his cousin, and probably about his father as well, entered the treatment situation in the form of the extra energy and intensity that the analyst brought to his work with this patient.

The analyst's heightened energy, affective involvement, and tenacity provided a beneficial balance for a patient whose own father had been experienced as being too little available or engaged with him. The pushing and testing of the analyst by this patient might also have led a less determinedly committed analyst to conclude that this patient could not endure a treatment which required the experience of so much frustration. The analyst's firmly holding to his belief that he would help this man withstand his pain especially because he had been unable to do this for another man was conveyed in nonverbal, as well as verbal, ways, which may loosely have some analogy to the way a mother conveys a sense of safety to an infant. The patient feared he would be too much for anyone, and the analyst made it clear it was not too much for him. In this action-prone patient, it is unlikely that words alone would have been convincing; the patient came to trust that his analyst would not be driven away or give up on believing in the patient's capacities. In a non-role-playing way, the analyst's stance, verbal and nonverbal, provided a corrective emotional experience for the patient. One also could consider the change in the patient as illustrating what Buie (1993) described as the establishment of new structures and connections from the analyst's selective activation and promotion of the patient's preexisting strengths.

I am not arguing that no other analyst could be effective in this respect, nor that an analyst without this analyst's history could not be effective. Many other dynamics and histories might result in an analyst's extra energy, involvement, and tenacity. What I am arguing is that the particular psychology of this analyst, owing to his history and character, was particularly beneficial for this particular patient, given his needs. I refer to this as a compensatory match because the analyst is providing something that the patient was missing and needed in both his ego functioning and his fantasy constructions.

While patients generally wish to feel an investment by their analysts, this patient's need to experience it from the analyst seemed critical to enabling the patient himself to invest in the treatment. For another patient, who had felt affectively smothered, an analyst manifesting such extra intensity might be detrimental to an engagement in the treatment. However, it is also likely that this analyst's benevolent fatherliness might not be so strongly elicited by a patient whose need was for psychological space. The primarily unconscious attunement between patient and analyst had a bi-directionality that resulted in an interactive chain of responses and mutual influencing of behavior and affective response, which bears a loose resemblance to what Stern (1990) describes in the affectively charged interaction patterns between mother and infant.

The second aspect of benefit from this patient-analyst match that I wish to address is based on certain similarities between them. It is clear from the history that the patient had artistic talent that he had ceased to pursue because of conflict. Once the conflict had been modified, however, it was his attunement to his analyst's aesthetic appreciation that facilitated his reopening of an avenue of self-expression he had closed off. The patient was clear that he needed a man to appreciate him and not mock him in order to proceed with his art. The analyst did not actively appreciate or even address the patient's artistic work, except to say that the patient wanted to talk with him about it and feel he would appreciate it. The patient used visually perceivable data about the analyst—the way he furnished his office, the picture he chose to hang—to support his view of the analyst as a man who valued and appreciated aesthetics. The aesthetic aspect of himself was something which he had previously suppressed because he felt it would be scorned.

It is, of course, possible that he would have found other and different evidence to support this gift from some other analyst. I am not arguing that the patient could not have refound his artistic interest and ability in the office of an analyst lacking this analyst's aesthetic sensibilities. Rather, I am proposing that the patient used a real aspect of the analyst (in this instance, the analyst's aesthetic sensibility), which was neither an aspect of the analyst's technique nor generally supportive manner, to increase his sense that a man could be a man while being aesthetically attuned. This specific characteristic of the analyst takes on a particular importance for this patient in the context of the analyst's conveying a certain sense of acceptance of the patient. The flourishing of his artwork illustrates the refinding and expanding on an earlier positive experience suggested by Buie (1993).

Whereas artistic ability was something this patient had demonstrated prior to analysis, a sense of humor was a quality previously unseen. Only later in the analysis were its historical roots understood. The fact that the patient's humor was different in quality from the analyst's suggests that its development was neither imitative nor just an identification. Rather, it suggests that the analyst's playfulness and humor stimulated a nascent quality in this patient that had previously been undeveloped. The outlandish and quirky quality of his humor also captured an aspect of the patient's father. The patient came to experience his mode of expression as a positive rather than negative form of identification with his father. It is not possible to know whether this reflects a previously positive interaction with his father that had been repressed or a more newly developed quality. It seems likely that the patient both rediscovered a positive aspect of his father and incorporated something from his analyst, which he then amalgamated into his own unique brand of humor. We cannot know whether the patient's sense of humor and play would have emerged with an analyst who did not himself have these characteristics. It may be that it would have. We can never return and replay analytic work. Even second analyses never completely satisfy this requirement, since there is the influence of the previous work and a different stage of life to be accounted for (Kantrowitz, 1993c).

The reemergence of a previously undeveloped quality in the presence of an analyst who displays this quality has a loose resonance with infant research that suggests that the aspects of the baby which are stimulated flourish first in imitation and later become developed parts of the self (Stern, 1985). It seems likely that these particular qualities of this particular analyst stimulated a previously underdeveloped aspect of this patient to flourish. With another analyst, another aspect of the patient might have come to the fore in response to some other quality that the patient had in nascent form. In the Boston outcome study (Kantrowitz, Katz, & Paolitto, 1990b), the fit of analyst and patient, which was found to be facilitating at one point in the analysis, sometimes became a handicap at a different point. Since the analysis I have described is still in progress, we can only raise the possibility that impeding aspects of this match may still arise. What I am proposing is that the particular match between patient and analyst influences which aspects of the patient develop.

The construction of this view of the dyad suggests that the patient is to some extent limited by the limits of the analyst. This view is one that Freud took when he stated that no analyst can succeed in analyzing what he has not resolved within himself (1910b). While this proposition has considerable support from clinical work, it is also possible that analysts themselves may grow and change in the course of their work with their patients. In fact, I believe the facilitating effect that analyzing a patient's difficulties may have on the analyst's personal development has been underestimated in our literature and teaching. I would maintain that every analytic patient is potentially an opportunity for the analyst to learn more about himself or herself and to develop. For this to happen, however, it requires the analyst to be vigilant to countertransference reactions, to employ self-analysis, and to seek consultation when one's own efforts do not lead to a deepening understanding.

I will briefly illustrate the way that what was potentially an impeding match between patient and analyst became a facilitating one once the analyst became aware of their overlap. What I am referring to as an impeding match may rightly be considered a countertransference problem. However, the point of the example is that once a characteristic, which initially was embedded in the countertransference, became disentangled from conflict and understood by the analyst, the interfering complementary attitude could be beneficially employed by the patient because of its compensatory quality. Unlike the first analyst, this analyst, being at an earlier stage of her training, was still in analysis; therefore, a multiplicity of factors contributed to her growth.

The analyst was a mature, empathic, sensitive person with considerable experience as a clinician. She was very insightful and sensitive in her interventions. Her most outstanding characteristic, however, was her capacity to make use of her countertransference. She was able to look at herself honestly, with remarkable self-scrutiny and seemingly little narcissistic injury when confronting an aspect of herself of which she felt ashamed or disliked. In part, at least, this lack of vulnerability came from her optimistic view that all things can change. While this undoubtedly had an aspect of grandiosity to it, this analyst believed this capacity for change was equally possible for her patients as for herself. This characteristic, while probably of great benefit in many clinical situations, led her to founder temporarily in her work with the patient while I was her supervisor.

The difficulty the analyst encountered was her initial inability to appreciate her patient's narcissistic vulnerabilities and need for defensive strategies to protect her both from loss of self-esteem and from facing her conflicts. The analyst would direct her attention to the underlying issues of the patient in a tactful and sensitive manner, but she bypassed the analysis of her defenses. As a result, the patient was unable to deepen her work. She was very fond of her analyst, but enormously frustrated and felt as if she were spinning her wheels. In supervision, when I explored with the analyst her ignoring the patient's defenses, she was at first surprised. For all her sophistication, she had failed to understand that her patient could not go directly to her conflicts, since it seemed to her the speediest way to resolve them. What emerged when she began to explore her patient's defenses was that the patient, in contrast to herself, believed that nothing could change; therefore, for the patient to recognize something in herself that she experienced as unacceptable or distasteful felt not only humiliating but sadistic on the part of the analyst.

To the patient, being confronted with her underlying unacceptable wishes or fears felt as if she were having her nose rubbed in something that was as much an immovable fact as the color of her eyes. Once the analyst understood this, she quickly grasped the patient's need to protect herself from seeing her conflicts and was better able to explore at the surface of the patient's awareness. In addition, the analyst also understood that the patient's belief in the immutability of her conflicts was the mirror image of her own belief that all things were changeable. She recognized that these were two sides of the same difficulty. Her capacity to work on her own issues was reflected in her work with the patient, which now deepened and developed.

The analytic work for this patient and analyst had been impeded by a countertransference interference. This match illustrates what I have described as negative complementarity, where a shared difficulty was defended against by antithetical defensive operations. As long as the analyst remained "blind" to the patient's issue, because of her need not to face the reality of limits for herself, the patient could not begin to explore with her analyst her conviction that she could not change, or the dynamics on which this belief was based. Once the analyst was able to focus on her bypassing of the patient's defenses, she was able to explore her dynamic reasons for her stance, face a difficulty in herself, and change how she worked with this patient. A beneficial aspect of this patient-analyst match, which then developed, was that the patient, who tended towards depression and despair, began to experience hope budding when working with this analyst whose outlook was optimistic.

Whereas, in previous papers, I have described how a match between patient and analyst that is facilitating at an early point in the analysis may become an impediment at a later point, in this example, the time of the handicap and benefit of the match was reversed. In other words, after the analyst overcame the countertransference interference, which had been manifested in the negative complementary match, the analyst's characterological style of optimism, initially an impediment, became a benefit; it now served as a compensatory match in which an aspect of the analyst's character made up for something the patient lacked.

While this analyst had the aid of both a supervisor to bring the interference to her awareness and an analyst with whom to work on her conflicts, this kind of shift in awareness and working stance can and does occur long after formal training ends. Usually, however, the difficulties encountered and shifts within ourselves and in our work are all the more subtle in nature. Clearly to be without "blind spots" in relation to an area central to a patient's conflict is desirable. However, we have come to acknowledge that "blind spots" are an inevitable occurrence, though with more experienced clinicians they are usually less blatant. The heightened awareness, vigilant attention, and push toward mastery in an area of previous difficulty for an analyst may bring such an area sharply and beneficially into focus. It may even be that this extra attention to an area of conflict is preferable in certain instances to a more usual evenhanded approach, particularly since absolute evenness of attention and response is probably more an ideal than a reality. Such unconscious tilts in attention may be providing a balance for areas previously neglected or consciously or unconsciously avoided. What is certain is that an initially problematic match may be transformed into a beneficial one when the analyst can focus and work on his or her difficulty.

The beneficial qualities of the patient-analyst match that I am referring to are often subtle. They are conveyed in tone, timing, and responsivity. I am not referring to any particular characteristics or qualities as beneficial; their benefit is specific in the context of the particular patient-analyst pair. Through careful study of the process data, it should be possible to delineate for each patient-analyst pair the central strengths and difficulties in ego function, affect tolerance, and interpersonal connection for patient and analyst and the resultant interplay. From this, we might begin to characterize the subtle manifestation of the analyst's qualities that, at first, may compensate or balance in an area where there is a limitation or difficulty for the patient. Later, if the analytic work is successful in reopening a developmental process, there should be an emergence of some of this quality or characteristic in the patient. On some occasions, this change may reflect an identification with the analyst; on other occasions, it may be more accurate to view it as a previously nascent aspect of the patient which blossomed in response to this quality in the analyst. Most often, it is likely to represent the patient's amalgamation of past and current experience blended in a unique fashion by his/her own particular temperament and style.

The subtle impact of the interaction of the analyst's and the patient's character and residual conflicts on the analytic process is not an aspect of our work that we can teach easily. Only with difficulty can we recognize and monitor it.

Chapter 6

Appreciation of the importance of the patient-analyst "match"

Clara Thompson

In her 1938 paper, "Notes on the Psychoanalytic Significance of the Choice of Analyst," Clara Thompson proposes that the personality of the analyst plays a role in the therapeutic result in a psychoanalysis and observes that this fact was seldom (or ever?) reported. Providing detailed reflections on how particular personal characteristics of the analyst may impede certain patients and benefit others, she concludes that how these characteristics affect the outcome of treatment depends on the nature of the patient's difficulties. Furthermore, sometimes, the nature of what I have called "the match" between patient and analyst while initially detrimental to the analytic work later can be facilitating to the process. Such transformations occur when analysts, through self-analysis or more personal analytic treatment, recognize how their personal difficulties contribute to an impasse and change in their interactions with this patient. To the best of my knowledge, it would be almost 50 years later before any observations of a similar nature appeared in a mainstream psychoanalytic journal (Kantrowitz, 1986).

Thompson focuses her discussion on the factors that influence patients' choosing an analyst. She emphasizes the importance of the analyst's empathy, interest, and understanding to establish a sense of confidence. Although she does not address the ways in which the analyst's personality plays its part in relation to these qualities of engagement, I doubt she would question that personal qualities contribute to conveying them. Rather, she selects gender and age as variables to consider when patients pick an analyst. While not giving short shrift to transference distortions, Thompson wishes to show how perceivable aspects of the analyst contribute to both the selection of analyst and the process and outcome of analysis. For example, choosing an older analyst may be seeking a better parent substitute and someone more mature. Conversely, an older analyst may be preferred to avoid competitive feelings more likely generated by an analyst of a similar age, where resentment might be stirred by the analyst's "superior insight."

While gender and age likely influence a patient's choice of analyst, Thompson states that the analyst's personality is the most complying pivotal factor—"his aggressiveness or passivity, his optimism or pessimism- in other words his personal character structure and problems" (p. 211). A patient's choice of analyst may be based on a familiar feeling of positive attachment or may be a "primarily defensive choice," a pull to repeat previously "unpleasant life problems." She notes however that even such choices may have a favorable outcome if the analyst recognizes the effect of his/her[1] own personality and the aspects on which the patient focuses his/her transference patterns. It is the meaning of the choice to the patient and the analyst's capacity to perceive and work with these meanings that matter, not the facts themselves.

With her characteristic common sense, she observes:

> In this respect, the analytic situation is no exception to the ways of intimacies in general...(personality) is the vaguest, most difficult to evaluate clearly and therefore, an excellent field for errors in objectivity, especially when an error fits into an neurotic pattern of the patient. Also, it is the field in which an analyst himself is most likely to be unaware of some limitation.
>
> (p. 211)

But she continues with a reflection, central to her argument and later to my own, "what can be a limitation in an analyst for one patient can conceivably be an asset with another. Because it may have a different significance in the life pattern" (p. 211). For example, an easygoing analyst may overlook the significance of aggression or delay in addressing it because of his non-reactivity, while an aggressive analyst may be slow in perceiving or in interpreting a patient's masochistic trends. Neither situation necessarily bodes a poor outcome, provided the analyst becomes aware of these trends and addresses the problematic area for the patient. Thompson also notes that the analyst's own residual difficulties, such as "unresolved need for power, desire for admiration... may come out only in the presence of a patient who too completely satisfies an old neurotic pattern of the analyst... and perhaps happen only when the analyst is under some specific stress in his own life" (p. 213), such as physical illness, financial difficulties, or problems in his/her love life.

In considering the importance of analysts' age, gender, and personal characteristics on their patients, Thompson makes the assumption that these analysts are sufficiently well trained and analyzed to work successfully with the difficulties most patients would bring, but refreshingly does not assume that that any individual can be "completely analyzed," "infallible," or totally neutral, as she indicates the psychoanalytic literature of the time might suggest. With delightful common sense, she states, "An individual has some personal reaction to everyone with whom he comes in close contact and an analyst presumably is no exception in this respect" (p. 206).

How sensible and prescient she is. How could psychoanalysts ever have assumed otherwise? As I stated in the preface, for decades and decades, many psychoanalysts did not hold these beliefs. They were taught, and accepted, that analysts, if they were well-enough trained, were, and should be, interchangeable. The method of interpretations, which made the patient's unconscious conscious, was the variable considered the sole agent of change. I will briefly review this history.

While in the current era most American psychoanalysts agree that both patient and analyst contribute to the nature of engagement and outcome of a psychoanalytic process, this point of view was not always the case. As previously stated, for many decades, and most notably in the 1950s and 1960s in North America, many mainstream psychoanalysts believed that they could, and should, be "blank screens" on which patients projected their difficulties. Likely this perspective was more prevalent in North America where the medicalization of psychoanalysis occurred. If analysts could be interchangeable, the process of psychoanalysis appeared more scientific. Analysts' own conflicts were to have been resolved in their own psychoanalytic treatment. If an analyst had countertransference reactions, these experiences were viewed as problematic, a reason to get more personal analytic treatment. It was also assumed that analysts could predict in advance which patients would be successfully analyzed. Given adequate reality testing, affect availability and tolerance, and level of object relationships, if the person was motivated, any analyst of sufficient experience should be able to analyze such a patient.

In 1968, when I began my training at the Boston Psychoanalytic Society and Institute, these ideas are what we were taught. Perhaps not all Institutes were so unrealistic in their assumptions at the time, but I know from many of my colleagues in other parts of the United States that such convictions were in no way unique to Boston. How could a process that two people were involved in be totally dependent on only one? How could any person, no matter how well analyzed, not have personal reactions? I was a CORST[2] candidate. At the time, psychologists were given permission to be trained as analysts only if they engaged in research related to psychoanalysis. Otherwise, if they were admitted, their training was limited to attendance in seminars. For my project, I chose to do a prospective, longitudinal study of the outcome of psychoanalysis. I assessed the patients' reality testing, affect availability and tolerance, level and quality of relationships, and motivation in advance through interviews and projective tests (Kantrowitz, Singer, & Knapp, 1975). A year after termination, I repeated these evaluations and also interviewed their analysts (Kantrowitz et al., 1986, 1987a, 1987b). From a deconstruction of the analysts' interview, I created a profile of the analyst, which was independently and reliably validated.

In parallel with Clara Thompson's observations, my findings showed that when characteristics of the analyst's difficulties were similar to those of the patient, these conflicts did not change for the better during the course of analysis. Too great a dissimilarity could also be problematic. The patient-analyst "match", in contrast to all the variables assumed at the time to be predictive of analyzability, turned out to be the one that predicted the outcome of psychoanalysis (Kantrowitz et al., 1989; Kantrowitz, Katz, & Paolitto, 1990).

How could I have not have known about Clara Thompson's article? Prior to my psychoanalytic training, I had read, and appreciated, works of Harry Stack Sullivan (1953). I knew who Clara Thompson was; I think I had read some papers by her, but I knew nothing of her writing about the match between patient and analyst. The reason I had this gap in my knowledge brings up other parts of the history of psychoanalysis in North America.

North American analysts who were part of the American Psychoanalytic Association were steeped in ego psychology. As I have suggested above, this perspective at the time I was in psychoanalytic training had become very narrow in its focus. In my psychoanalytic training, the commitment to analyze defenses against intrapsychic conflicts consumed all attention; consideration of problems posed by internal, unconscious conflicts was polarized against difficulties stemming from interpersonal conflicts. Many analysts in both camps, but probably more from the mainstream North American group, maintained either-or, reductionistic views about the origin of conflict as well as about how it should be treated; such polarizations characterized frequent battles that occurred in psychoanalysis over the years.

Throughout this time, the William Allison White Institute taught an interpersonal perspective, but American Psychoanalytic Association Institutes, to the best of my knowledge, did not include this viewpoint in their teaching until the late 1980s. Of course, the fact that we weren't taught about the importance of interpersonal relationships didn't mean that we all agreed that they were insignificant.

My research on the patient-analyst match (1993c) was part of a sea change that was occurring. As I noted in the forward, the theoretical/clinical paper I had written on this topic and submitted to major mainstream psychoanalytic journals in the early 1980s had been rejected by all of them. Analysts trained in American Psychoanalytic Association Institutes must have recognized that something was "off" in some of our psychoanalytic literature and what we had been taught in seminars, since by the early 1980s new ideas began to appear. Those of us who published papers on the analyst's role in the process did not know each other at the time. I remember finding James McLaughlin's 1981 article on the analyst's transference (McLaughlin, 1981) and thinking with relief that analysts were beginning to expand their views. Irwin Hoffman's "Patient as the Interpreter of the Analyst Experience" (1983) followed shortly after.

By the mid- to late 1980s, the concept that two people, not one, influenced, if not determined, what occurred in psychoanalysis became a widely accepted idea. Ted Jacobs' intersubjective perspective (1991) not only removed the stigma from countertransference reactions, it made them a rich source for psychoanalytic inquiry. I tried to provide further support for this point of view by interviewing analysts about their use of countertransference reactions in *The Impact of the Patient on the Analyst* (1996, 1997), a study of how analysts changed based on their experiences with patients. In the 1990s, I published papers illustrating the effect of the match in clinical work (Kantrowitz, 1992, 1993a, 1993b, 1995, 2002). Today, all these ideas about the analyst's contribution to the process are commonplace, accepted by almost every analyst.

Both research and clinical data made it clear that who the analyst is as a person, the analyst's character and conflicts, will have an effect on his or her patients. However, it seems noteworthy that a focus on the specificity of the interdigitation of character and conflict between analyst and patient remains relatively neglected as a general phenomenon. Perhaps the topic is overlooked, because nowadays so many analysts illustrate countertransference reactions and how they use them in their work that analysts don't think about it further.

However, as Thompson noted, the extent of influence the analyst's character and conflicts have will vary, of course, depending on the character and conflicts of the patient. Overlaps may create clashes or blind spots. But, as stated before, these situations also offer opportunities for the analyst's personal growth. It bears repeating that if an analyst can recognize that something is impeding the analytic work, and if through consultation, further personal treatment or effective self-analysis, impasses can be resolved, then not only the patient, but also the analyst, can grow and change in the process of the work (Kantrowitz, 1992, 1993a, 1993b, 1995, 1999, 2002).

I would add that a "match" that is particularly facilitating at one point may become an impediment at a later time. An example from my research project was of an inhibited, frightened patient whose analyst's gentle style helped the patient to gradually open up in analysis. However, later in analysis, when this patient was ready to more directly address her conflicts, her analyst's gentleness proved to be a hindrance. Although she had changed, his hesitancy to bring her conflicts and defenses against them to her attention continued, limiting her from deriving a fuller analytic benefit.

In her relatively brief article, Clara Thompson addresses all these points. She knew 77 years ago that the character and conflicts of the analyst influence the process of analysis, and that the extent to which this was pivotal depended on the amount of overlap with the character and conflicts of the patient. It has taken so many decades for psychoanalysts to acknowledge that who the analyst is as a person inevitably has an effect on the process. I regret that I did not know about and cite her article in my work from the 1970s onwards, but I realize that even if I had, most psychoanalysts trained in American Psychoanalytic Association Institutes at the time would not have been ready to view her ideas as support for undertaking my study, its findings, or subsequent clinical application of these ideas.

The zeitgeist changed and with it psychoanalysts became better able to embrace previously rejected ideas. These shifts in ourselves as a profession may parallel changes in the way we view our patients. We now acknowledge what Freud stated early on, both constitution and environment affect who we become. We now view environment in a more comprehensive way. Environment includes our culture in a broad sense, the conditions in the world we live in, our families, and our analysts who help us understand the interplay of these factors while applying self-scrutiny as they engage in a psychoanalytic process.

Notes

1 In Thompson's text, all references to the analyst are as "he." I could not resist making the cultural update by changing these references to he/she.
2 A waiver to be trained as a clinical psychoanalyst was granted by a Committee on Research/Special Training, (CORST) by the American Psychoanalytic Association to nonmedical candidates who were, or would, engage in research related to psychoanalysis.

Chapter 7

The triadic match

The interactive effect of supervisor, candidate, and patient

This chapter examines and illustrates the effect of the triadic match—my term—for the interaction of the characteristics of candidate, supervisor, and patient, and its effects on the candidate's learning and analytic work. A felicitous match can aid professional and personal analytic development. An enmeshment or clash of characteristics, however, may lead to a heightened resistance, which can slow or impede learning and adversely affect the analytic work.

The way character and conflict overlap among these three participants—patient, candidate, and supervisor—influences the direction, nature, and extent of the analytic work in any supervised case.

Furthermore, the impact of the match may change during the course of the work. Each patient presents the candidate with different issues, stirring different countertransference responses. The effect on the candidate of the challenge posed by a specific patient may be exacerbated or ameliorated by particular characteristics or qualities of the supervisor. Therefore, the supervisory experience may impede the candidate's learning, or it may enhance it by balancing or addressing an area of insufficiently resolved conflict or an unrecognized character issue of the candidate that may be especially stimulated by the patient. The effect of the match between candidate and supervisor has some parallels to the patient-analyst match (Kantrowitz, 1986, 1992, 1993a, 1993b, 1995, 1996; Kantrowitz et al., 1989; Kantrowitz, Katz, & Paolitto, 1990). That is, the extent to which the candidate and supervisor are able to become aware of collusions and overcome impasses will be influenced by both participants, their openness to change, and their capacity to act on it.

I focus upon the candidate's capacity to learn from supervised analytic work; the aim is to try to delineate the factors in the match that facilitate or impede this learning. Since it is the meaning of these factors to the candidate that determines their effect upon learning, I present four candidates' evaluations of the impact of triads in which they participated. The supervisors' assessments and my own observations of the matches provide additional perspectives.

I do not assume that there is any ideal match or that there is only one kind of match that can interfere with learning or enhance it for a particular candidate. Rather, I assume that there are as many variations in how the analytic triad affects the candidate's receptivity to learning as there are triadic combinations. The effect of any particular triad may be different at different stages in a candidate's development. The goal of this study is to sensitize both candidates and supervisors to the effect of this three-way interaction.

The data in this paper are based on narratives from candidates and supervisors, gathered from systematic, semi-structrured interviews. Descriptions were collected of interactions between candidate-supervisor pairs as well as of their perceptions and interpretations of each other and of the candidate's experience with his or her patient. As will become clear, in some respects the examples are not comparable. Therefore, somewhat different kinds of exploration were applied in different cases.

In considering the importance of the analytic triad, I am not discounting the effect of individual talent and skill. Some candidates and supervisors are more talented at this work than others. Some patients also bring greater capacities than others for self-observation and tolerance of affect. Talented supervisors are more likely to enhance the skills of a wider range of candidates. Talented candidates are likely to make better use of supervision with more supervisors; they are also more likely to do more thorough psychoanalytic treatments with more patients. Patients with greater capacities for self-scrutiny and tolerance for affects are more likely to achieve self-understanding and therapeutic benefit with candidates of a wider degree of talent, and with less dependence upon the skill of any particular supervisor. The capacity to understand the nature of a patient's difficulties, and the possession of tact and a sense of timing in addressing them, are related to experience as well as to talent.

The role that theory and technique play in this triadic interaction is not independent of clinical skill. Neither are choice of theory and technical approach independent of character and conflict (Aron, 1999; Jacobs, David, & Meyer, 1995; Kantrowitz, 2003). Clinicians who do effective analytic work often seek out theories that help them be self-monitoring in the ways they need. For example, clinicians who themselves have some difficulty in affect regulation are likely to seek theories that address this problem. Similarly, conflicts around aggression, sexuality, or narcissism are likely to lead the analyst to focus on theories that help them stay alert in these areas. The analyst may or may not be conscious of this reason for theory choice. Different patients will stir different aspects of each analyst. The more theories analysts understand, the more affected personal issues may be balanced through compensatory attention to personally relevant theories.

In this chapter, I describe how supervisors helped candidates with patients who challenged them in areas of personal vulnerability. I also discuss the advantage to the beginning candidate of treating patients whose conflicts, at least on a manifest level, are different from those of the candidates themselves. The discussion is limited to the effects upon the candidate of similarities and differences in conflicts and personality traits among candidate, supervisor, and patient in four case illustrations. The chapter does not consider triads that have a negative impact or the working through of candidates' problems in transferences, countertransferences, or enactments that are played out in the supervisory process. While counter-illustrations of this kind are very important, they are material for a different time.

The sample

Method

The four candidate-supervisor pairs are from four geographic areas of the United States. The supervisors are all members of the American Psychoanalytic Association. The candidates have all been trained in APsaA institutes. One of these candidates initiated the idea for this project.

Two advanced candidates who were interested in the project circulated a request for volunteers, both by word of mouth and by e-mail. I then contacted the volunteers. I limited the sample to candidates who were close to graduation, in order to minimize anxiety about evaluation related to progression in training. This seemed likely to allow them to be considerably more open in discussing their experiences of supervision, as well their own analyses. In order to keep the study focused on the interaction within the triad, candidates who were primarily interested in discussing beneficial or detrimental supervisions in ways that did not focus on the triad were not interviewed. I selected two female and two male candidates. All four were older than most trainees. They all had terminated their personal analyses and were close to graduating from their institutes at the time they were interviewed. I interviewed the members of the candidate-supervisor pairs about the nature of their fit with each other in the context of the character and conflicts of the patient. In one instance, since the candidate had changed supervisors, I also interviewed the former supervisor. In the second example also there were two supervisors for the case example; the first supervisor had died approximately a year after the case began.

The interviews

Semi-structured clinical interviews were conducted over the telephone and recorded; each lasted approximately one hour. They were subsequently transcribed. Each interview was preceded by a call from the candidate-volunteer to establish the relevance of his or her particular experience to the research. Thus, the interview began with the candidate's prepared presentation, and I asked for relevant information if the candidate did not offer it. The candidates were first asked to describe briefly the patient's reason for seeking treatment, the patient's history, and the course of the analytic work. The candidate's attention was then directed to her or his perception of overlaps or disjunctions with the patient, in character or in intrapsychic conflict, and to the challenge posed by this enmeshment or clash. The second question concerned the candidate's reason for selecting the particular supervisor, and a description of perceived similarities and/or differences between candidate and supervisor in approach, theory, and character style. The focus was on the characteristics of the supervisor that the candidates believed helped them cope with the patients' issues when these brought up difficulties related to the candidate's character or conflicts. The candidate was asked to assess the concordance or divergence of the supervisor's approach with that of the candidate's training analyst, and also with the viewpoints of any other supervisors. Each candidate gave a brief summary describing his or her other supervisions. All the participating candidates made clear that they had chosen the examples they had specifically because they believed that those particular triadic interactions had had a special influence upon them and upon their capacity to grow and learn psychoanalytically.

Interviews of the supervisors took place after the candidate interviews. Each supervisor was asked for an assessment of the patient, and of the candidate's analytic work, and his or her use of supervision. The supervisors were asked to comment on similarities and differences in theory, technique, and character between themselves and their supervisees. They were also asked about the match between supervisee and patient in terms of character, defensive style, and conflict.

Several limitations of this data should be noted in advance. First, the patient is not interviewed. As a consequence, my knowledge of the patient is entirely secondhand, in contrast to my direct, albeit long-distance, knowledge of candidates and supervisors. Therefore, the representation of the patient is "flattened," and does not come alive to the same extent as that of the candidate and supervisor. This same flattening is encountered in the representation of the candidates' analysts.

Second, the prepared presentations of the analytic and supervisory experiences, while obviously based on the dynamic memory of candidate and supervisor, may have made the relationships appear more static than was actually the case. The nature of analytic work and analytic supervision suggests that there was more complexity than is apparent. The illustrations, being retrospective appraisals, must reflect condensations of evolving relationships and shifting perceptions. Third, in these reports, I consider only the conscious understanding of the candidates and supervisors. Preconscious and unconscious factors influencing their perspectives can be inferred; since these would be speculative, however, they have not been included. Fourth, the effect on the data of my role as interviewer is not assessed. Nonetheless, my participation certainly influenced the material in ways that this study cannot define.

Four examples

For each candidate, the focus of investigation was the impact on the work with only one particular case. In the first two examples, the cases had been supervised by two different supervisors. In the first example, the change had occurred because the supervisor believed there was an impasse in learning. In the second example, the change was necessitated by the supervisor's death. While some of the candidates did briefly discuss their views of their other supervisors in relation to their learning, the triad is examined in the context of only one analytic case each. The first two candidates focused on their development as analysts. The second two candidates also discussed the effect of the triad on the work, but related it more personally to understanding of themselves.

The candidate who wanted her enthusiasm shared

The first case illustrates how a clash in theory, style, and possibly manner of addressing an area of unconscious resistance with one supervisor interfered with growth as a beginning analyst, while a similarity with another supervisor facilitated it. The similarity of style and approach between this candidate and the second supervisor was beneficial to a patient whose style and manifest problems were different from the candidate's.

The candidate, a woman, brought this analytic case, her third, for supervision to a former psychotherapy supervisor, a psychoanalyst who had supported her application for analytic training. The candidate was enthusiastic about her patient, delighted by her psychological mindedness, her "spunkiness," her "naive charm," and her immediate sense of the collaborative aspects of the work

The patient was a woman in her early 20s who was struggling to make independent decisions and become more separate from her parents. She was aware that her anger blocked her from being successful and interfered with her ability to ask for what she needed. Her mother was described as an extremely controlling person who had been profoundly depressed and emotionally absent when the patient was young. Her father was perceived as less "vicious," but also less psychologically minded, than her mother. The patient was much more comfortable with her father.

The candidate and supervisor had worked harmoniously in the earlier psychotherapy supervision, but in this supervision they clashed almost from the beginning. There was disagreement at every level—the supervisor's clinical theory of the patient was that her central problem centered around hostility and guilt; he felt that the candidate was remiss in not addressing these issues. The candidate viewed the patient's central conflict as a separation problem. She believed that the patient lacked confidence in her own beliefs and suffered from low self-esteem. While the candidate saw that the patient did have issues of guilt and hostility, she did not view these as central; instead, she focused on the patient's perceptions of and feelings about herself, her past, and her current relations. The candidate thought the parents' hostility and sadism toward the patient was much more important at that time than the patient's hostility toward them or her. The candidate believed that the patient first had to learn that she did not deserve to be treated the way she had been by parents, friends, and boyfriend before she could begin to address her own aggression and anger.

Candidate and supervisor also differed on questions of technique. Where the supervisor urged interpretation early in sessions, the candidate permitted material to evolve more slowly, intervening only toward the end of sessions. The candidate disagreed with her supervisor on the timing of interventions, both in individual sessions and in the analysis as a whole. She did not think she was afraid to confront anger; rather, she thought it more valuable to follow the patient's material and timing and to build a strong alliance with her. She characterized herself as taking an object relations perspective. The candidate said that she was not troubled by these disagreements; she was, however, disturbed by the difference between herself and her supervisor over her enthusiasm for the patient. She objected to the supervisor's assessment of the patient as ordinary. "Don't be so excited, she's just a patient," was the supervisor's attitude. The candidate, by contrast, thought of her as "a great patient" about whom she gave "glowing reports" to the supervisor at the start of each supervisory session.

After working together for a year on this case, the supervisor suggested that the candidate might feel more secure if she worked with someone who saw the case more as she did.[1] She felt that the supervisor presented this possibility to her in a very respectful way. Initially, she was distressed since she liked and admired her supervisor. However, after discussing the case with another supervisor, she appreciated her first supervisor's reasons for suggesting the change.[2]

Contrasting the two supervisors, she perceived the first as formal, very strongly opinionated, and committed to microscopic analysis of work with patients. She felt that he had been distant and somewhat critical, tending to intervene—"to pounce," as she put it—the moment there was evidence. She described the second supervisor as funny, warm, more casual and comfortable, and taking a more macroscopic view of the analytic material. She perceived him as looser in style, less focused on the particular words used, less apt to be judgmental. She and the second supervisor let the patient take the lead, and worked more "intuitively" than by conscious application of theory. The second supervisor also shared her enthusiasm for the particular patient as "a very good analytic patient."

Both supervisors were men who mentored and affirmed her. She stated that she felt her analyst had also been affirming in manner, similar in her view to the style of both her second supervisor on this case and herself; however, his style was formal as the style of her first supervisor had been. Their support and affirmation were very important to her, since her father had not been "good" to her or helpful.

The candidate felt very maternal toward the patient. She thought her own "gentle" style was helpful to this woman whose parents had been "unstable and unsteady." The first supervisor had advocated a "tough," aggressive approach, while the second supervisor supported her maternal stance and slower approach, viewing it as an asset rather than an interference. The candidate and both supervisors viewed the patient and her difficulties as different from the candidate's; the second supervisor thought that these differences made the candidate's own issues less likely to intrude on the work. The candidate described some of the differences that she admired. The patient told her things "without a lot of embarrassment," something it had taken the candidate a long time to do in her own analysis. The patient had a "naive, fresh way of experiencing things, not jaded by mental health knowledge," while the candidate was steeped in psychological theory.

The first supervisor agreed with the candidate's view that the patient suffered from problems around separation and low self-esteem, although he believed that the patient's avoidance of her aggression was more central than the candidate did. However, he did not concur with her perception of his style. It was not his way to be "nit-picking about theory and technique," he said, but he had "wanted her to not be afraid of the patient's hostility toward her parents... not to shy away from it... to allow it to come into the transference." He did not perceive the candidate's style as "so maternal." Rather, he saw the candidate as "more afraid of helping the patient see and understand how she came to have trouble in relationships."

The second supervisor concurred with the candidate's perception of him, their relationship, and his view of the analytic work. He agreed with the candidate that she and the patient did not replicate each other's conflicts. The patient was compliant; she took from the analyst and gave her a lot of affirmation. The candidate presented herself assertively, but in a way that was very unlike the patient's mother. It was especially facilitating to the analytic work that the candidate was not controlling. While both candidate and patient had doubts about their own abilities, the patient's were conscious and the analyst's were not. The patient "exuded a sense that she didn't think highly of herself." The candidate was manifestly self-assured and freely self-expressive. The patient was quite different—much quieter, less self-centered. The second supervisor stated that his theory and the candidate's were similar; they were both influenced by relational and intersubjective theories. In terms of technique, they were "not way apart." However, the second supervisor tended to be more explorative, eliciting fantasies and affect and interpreting in the here and now. In contrast, the candidate tended to rely more heavily on interpretation within a genetic focus.

In terms of style, they both were outgoing, they both had definite ideas, which they did not hesitate to express, and they both tended to monopolize conversations. They both "wanted people to be happy" with them, but he was less anxious about achieving this, and therefore more attuned. In the interview, the second supervisor said that his mother was a lot like the candidate, "a lot of chutzpah, asking a lot of you, manicky but very nice." The candidate could frustrate him by her need for attention and reassurance, but she did not tend to make him angry.

Both supervisors stated that it was hard for the candidate to "listen, hear, and consider." This difficulty was a central reason for the first supervisor's suggestion that she work with a different supervisor. The second supervisor believed that the candidate became better able to "listen and take in" over time. Both supervisors conveyed that this candidate benefited from having a patient whose manifest conflicts and character were unlike hers and a supervisor whose character, as it was reflected in his approach to analysis and his technical style, was similar to her own. Not being like her patient made the candidate attend more acutely and not assume similarities; her greater similarity to the second supervisor enabled her to feel heard and to hear better. With this basic security, it was easier for her to take in new ideas and approaches, although at this stage primarily ones that extended or modified her own point of view.

In this example, the candidate appeared to treat her patient the way that she wished to be supervised: she affirmed the patient and facilitated the patient's abilities and way of working with a minimum of confrontation. Although she liked and admired the first supervisor, she could not learn his approach; it was too different and too confrontational for her. Perhaps the first supervisor was trying to address what he perceived as the candidate's resistance to dealing with aggression. If so, the candidate's defensiveness was unconscious; consciously she appreciated his input, although she was unable to make use of it. Perhaps she might have been more receptive if she had perceived her supervisor as (or alternatively, if the supervisor had actually been) more tolerant. The difficulty in making use of his approach may also have been due to her identification with her patient as a patient. Her theory of therapeutic action centered on affirmation in the relationship, which she believed had benefited her in her training analysis. The second supervisor's similarity to her in theory and technique made it easier for her gradually to modify her own approach in response to his suggestions. His approach seemed a refinement of her own rather than the imposition of an alien style. It is unclear whether the second supervisor thought the candidate to be resistant to coping with aggression but addressed the resistance in such a way as to avoid raising unconscious defensiveness, or whether he did not consider that the candidate had a difficulty in this area. If candidate and supervisor shared a blind spot about this, the candidate's learning would likely remain restricted in this arena unless subsequent supervision or work with patients brought this limitation to her attention in a form that she could take in.

While differences from the supervisor interfered in the supervision, differences from the patient were beneficial for the analytic work; these differences made it easier for the candidate to be "more objective." Aware of her maternal countertransference, but less defensive about it because of her second supervisor's attitude, she became more alert to her need to be protective of her patient. For this candidate, this particular triadic constellation was favorable to learning. She was grateful to the first supervisor for perceiving a need she had not recognized herself.

The candidate who found a balance of emotional presence and discipline

The second example illustrates a candidate's use of supervisors to expand aspects of himself as they were activated and reflected in his work with his patients. The candidate was a man who had previously had an academic career. Both his analyst and the supervisor of his first case worked from an ego psychological perspective. He felt that this theory was too impersonal and constraining. As a result, he selected a supervisor with a developmental point of view for his second case. He found this to be extremely helpful, especially with regard to affect regulation. For his third case, he wanted for supervision the teacher of one of his seminars, who had impressed him as both flexible and disciplined and at the same time especially attentive to early needs. This supervisor did not have time. The candidate chose another teacher who seemed both kind and open to multiple theoretical perspectives; ten months after they began supervision, this supervisor died. At that time, the supervisor he had originally wanted took over the supervision.

The patient was a young woman who had difficulty sustaining relationships with men. Her father had died during her early adolescence, and her mother quickly got reinvolved with men. The patient felt that she could not compete successfully with her mother, who was a performer. She was very provocative with the candidate, repeatedly threatening to leave analysis. The transference oscillated between what the patient called "a deep feeling of being at home" and devaluation of the candidate as worthless. Although the candidate was more balanced and "self-cohesive" than the patient, he knew his own "propensity to exit relationships when slighted" and that he had his own "oppositional irreverence against [his] dependency wishes," which had been especially apparent in his adolescence.

According to the candidate, the supervisor who died had viewed this case in Oedipal terms. He saw the candidate and patient as having "a passionate marriage of the mind." When the patient dreamed of standing over the candidate "with a sword thrust into his chest," the supervisor saw it as Oedipal aggression as a result of the patient's frustrated sexual desire for the candidate. The supervisor encouraged "erotic repartee," and viewed the analysis as "a creative spinning of the Oedipal myth." For the candidate, the treatment was exciting but also very frustrating. He liked the freedom of expression he had found, but also often felt overpowered by the patient and put in a masochistic position. He regarded the supervisor as accepting and supportive; everything he did was viewed as something to learn from.

When the new supervisor took over supervision of the case, he described the analysis as "chaotic," "lacking a thread that held it together." He thought there was a lack of a primary object identification, and saw the repartee between candidate and patient as a way of maintaining dyadic closeness, but one which the patient eventually found overstimulating and had to back away from. The supervisor's view was that both the patient and the former supervisor had very expressive styles, and that the candidate had joined them. He thought that this had created an overstimulating situation in which the candidate got diverted to side issues and became unfocused. He believed that the banter concealed (and avoided dealing with) the patient's underlying depression and yearnings. The patient had a stimulus hunger, but had trouble staying close with anyone. This new supervisor thought the candidate idealized his (this supervisor's) warmth, and wanted his approval and to be close with him.

At first the candidate felt protective of his work with the initial supervisor, but he knew that there had been an "as if, wheel-spinning quality" to the analytic interactions. The patient's need for admiration and her inability to give much back became clearer to him. The second supervisor was more reserved and neutral. His recommendation was to "step back" and encourage the patient to associate more. The candidate changed his stance. The patient settled down in analysis and life and began to deepen the analytic work.

The candidate observed the shifts in his own style during his training. He believed he was "a bit obsessional, mechanical, and rule-
bound" when he started. He sought ways to integrate more of himself
in his analytic work. He believed that the technical approaches both
of his own analyst and of his first supervisor were too constrictive.
He found greater freedom with the second supervisor, who "dispas-
sionately treated everything as grist for the mill, stayed close to the
material, and was not prescriptive in personal style or theory." The
original supervisor on the third case had a "romantic style, expressive
of a wide range of feelings." This was very freeing to the candidate.
He shifted his stance and became "a more active participant, more
empathic and expressive." But he thought he may have "gone too far"
in this direction. When this supervisor died, the supervisor who took
over for him still gave the candidate "room to move," but in a more
disciplined way; the new supervisor's approach also gave the patient
more room. He took the stance of "an anonymous, neutral analyst, but
one who was also emotionally present." The candidate thought this
supervisor's approach helped him to "rebalance" himself in relation
to his work—that he had "swung too far in the direction of expressiveness" in reaction to his originally having been "too rule-bound."

In this instance, it was the candidate himself who observed and
conceptualized how the various supervisory approaches helped him
grow personally and professionally. His own analyst and his first
case supervisor were experienced as having a style that, although it
dovetailed well with earlier academic work, was too constrictive. The
second supervisor's non-prescriptive style and theoretical eclecticism
helped him become freer in his style and more accepting and analytic
in his approach. The third case supervisor and the patient both had
expansive, affect-laden styles that stimulated and engaged aspects of
the candidate previously held in check. He came to understand how
in the work with patient and supervisor, he had been swept away by
excitement and stimulation while at the same time feeling anxious.
The vivid affective style of this patient as well as her need for containment brought to the fore issues the candidate needed to address
in his analytic work. He was less modulated in his expression of affect
than, in retrospect, he thought desirable. His new supervisor advocated "meeting the patient's psychological needs in the moment and
analyzing them." He had resonated with this approach and with this

supervisor's warmth. He identified with this last supervisor's style as both "emotionally present" and disciplined.

This candidate actively sought out what he felt he needed. He seemed especially responsive to the style of the person with whom he worked. In each experience in supervision, as well as in his personal analysis, he felt reactive and responsive to the limits and scope of his teachers. He believed that he was able to expand his own ways of being when offered a different model.

In the next two examples, the dynamic interplay of the match was related less to training issues than it was to the psychological organization and issues of the candidates. Their self-awareness and self-reflective capacities enabled them to observe the interplay among the participants of their triads and identify the factors that made their particular supervisors especially helpful in these cases, particularly with regard to each candidate's particular character and needs.

The candidate who appreciated affect regulation

The candidate in the third example found that a characterological quality of calm steadiness in her supervisor quieted and balanced her experience of being overstimulated by an exhibitionist patient. She was aware that her own concerns about affect regulation were exacerbated by the patient and eased by the supervisor. This woman was in her mid-50s and already a skilled clinician when she sought analytic training. The supervisor, a man in his early seventies, was one of her admission interviewers. Mutual liking and respect were apparent to both in this first contact, and established a firm ground for their working together. The candidate selected him to supervise her second case before the particular patient was chosen.

The patient was a single man in his early 30s who presented with polymorphous perverse symptoms. He masturbated in front of a window with the idea of a woman looking at him. He also abused drugs and alcohol. His perverse and often outrageous behavior seemed relatively conflict-free, but he wanted to master his perversion, which challenged his sense of masculinity.

The case selection committee considered this man unsuitable for a supervised case. The supervisor, however, viewed the candidate as experienced, mature, and comfortable with overt expressions of sexuality, and thought she would be able to analyze this patient. Since both supervisor and candidate wanted to go ahead, the case was approved. The analysis was filled with action, much of which was highly provocative. The patient presented titillating material, and preferred display to reflection, which he resisted. The candidate at times felt discouraged, worrying that he might in fact prove to be unanalyzable. Her supervisor, however, continued to maintain the belief that the patient could profit from an analytic approach. Although he made suggestions about technique, he believed that his most important role was to convey optimism about this analysis, notwithstanding the discouragement experienced by both candidate and patient.

As the analysis became more focused in the transference, the patient made sexualized intrusions upon the candidate outside the consulting room. He opened the medicine chest in the bathroom, rifled through her things, and peered into her car. He was aggressively derogatory, telling her she smelled bad, imagining menstrual discharge. He feared the candidate would use his florid sexually elaborated fantasies for her own pleasure. The supervisor reported that whatever may have been mobilized in the analyst in response to the patient's sexual, aggressive, or narcissistic fantasies, "she managed it sensitively, interpreting his fears." He also said that "as more of the patient's conflicted life was focused in the analytic process, there was a significant improvement in his work, his relationships with his family, and his attempts at dating a 'real' woman.... Each return to defensive behavior, i.e., withdrawal or florid fantasies... required the candidate's patience, and careful attention to what precipitated them."

The supervisor thought this was a difficult case. While he kept the patient's narcissistic difficulties in mind, his technical approach was to view fantasy as a defense and consider to what extent the patient would be able to see the difference between his fantasies and reality. He thought the analyst was very sensitive to the narcissistic issues. They "saw eye to eye about what was going on in the patient." He did not feel any strain in the supervisory relationship: "We had a friendly alliance." He saw the candidate as experienced, sympathetic to the patient, and liking him, but "a little alienated and overwhelmed by him." Although she could join in the patient's despair, the supervisor believed that she did not avoid the immediacy of engagements with him. "She was very open about her experience,... about her struggling with his derogatory attitude and distancing.... At times she reacted with outrage. So management of her anger and displeasure was a matter of affect regulation. I think I helped by focusing on his changes, keeping his struggle in mind rather than reacting to it. I welcomed her countertransference and understood it as part of the work. I thought she had a pretty firm grasp of that."

The candidate shared the supervisor's view that they had a positive, respectful working relationship. She was not as interested in theory as he. Her supervisor gave her a useful way to think about the patient's aggression. She used theory "to calm me when I'm anxious and not understanding something." During the supervision, she felt liked and respected, but in an impersonal way. She told her supervisor not only about her intense reactions to the patient, but also about important life events, such as illnesses and deaths of loved ones, when they were distracting her from the work. He would respond sympathetically, "of course," but never made further reference to the events. She thought it was in her character to push for a more personal relationship, to seek out more response and reaction, but she also wondered if this patient exacerbated this tendency, wanting as he did to exhibit himself, and to have her exhibit herself to him. She realized in retrospect that she wanted her supervisor both to see her and to show himself to her.

When the candidate talked about her countertransference, her supervisor would listen but not explore it. She assumed that he thought she had understood enough of what was important. He was always respectful of her and of her patient. She "wanted more feedback... maybe more approval." She reported, "I think I'd have welcomed more reaction to what I was doing even if it were critical. I like feedback, but maybe I stopped going for it because he didn't give it. He gave me feedback about the patient, but not about me. Did that give me more freedom to struggle with it myself? Probably."

According to the candidate, she and the supervisor were very different in their personal styles. She sees herself as "right out there.... You can read my affect in my face.... I'm noisier, messier. I have a range of feelings right there.... My style is hysterical." In contrast, she described her supervisor as having "a poker face; you don't know what he is thinking or feeling. He seems more constricted or inhibited."

In reflecting on her experience, what seemed central to the candidate was the "rocklike calm" the supervisor provided. She would feel "frightened... enticed... over-stimulated" by the patient, and the supervisor would absorb the patient's affect and outrageousness. His position was always: "We will talk about it and understand." At first she had not understood how supportive that would be both to her and to the patient. The patient had wanted to be mirrored; she may have wanted something similar in the supervision. Her supervisor kept the focus on the interior of the patient, and helped her learn to do the same.

The candidate wondered: what if the patient had been different, "less colorful"? Would she have found the triad not stimulating enough? Would she have become more outrageous in her efforts to get her supervisor to respond? Did she hide some of her own outrageousness behind her patient's? What she was sure about was that this supervisor was a particularly good match for her with this patient.

The supervisor's focus was on the patient's affect—his experience of it and its expression in the analysis. This had consequences for the candidate's affect experience and expression. The supervisee applied some of the supervisor's comments about the patient's material to her issues, in "muted" form. Thus, she felt that she learned about herself indirectly, by "interpretation in displacement." The supervisor did not consciously intend to interpret the candidate's issues; he believed she was in touch with her countertransference. The effects of his approach, however, enhanced the supervisee's growth in both personal and professional ways.

Her own analyst had been more similar to her in style. He was more "out there." He revealed his own thoughts, opinions, feelings. In fact, he did this much more with patients than she did. The responsiveness and feedback she wanted (and did not get) from this supervisor she had gotten from her analyst and from her first supervisor. Her experience with her second case helped her to tolerate her patient's overstimulating affect without so much personal support from her supervisor. Her supervisor's steady, calm focus on the analytic process enabled her to be less anxious in relation to her patient, and to gain personally in her capacity for greater self- regulation of internal tension. At this point in her training, when she felt more secure and confident, she was better able to benefit from this supervisory stance than she might have been earlier in her analytic career.

The supervisor made it clear, without direct compliments, that he respected and esteemed her. Unlike the candidate in my first example, who experienced her supervisor as not accepting her style and as imposing his, the third candidate experienced the supervisor as accepting, even though he was not responsive in certain ways that she wished. It is interesting that this supervisor was unaware of the effect of his approach and personal style on the candidate. He treated her more as a colleague than a student, and accepted the countertransference reactions she openly presented rather than encouraging self-exploration.

The candidate who wished to feel "speedier"

The fourth example demonstrates again that the particular characteristics of a supervisor may introduce balance into situations where countertransferential responses related to specific character reactions of the candidate are evoked by the patient. This candidate reacted to his patient with feelings of competitiveness and "intellectual slowness." The supervisor's intellectually "quick," confident, and assertive style helped to offset his countertransference reactions. As in the previous example, this candidate, a man in his fifties, was an experienced clinician when he entered analytic training. The supervisor, a woman, had been one of his admission interviewers. Again as in the previous example, there was mutual liking and respect. The candidate selected her as a supervisor for a fifth case for three reasons: the early positive experience, his wish to be supervised by a woman, and her contemporary Kleinian approach, which was different from the ego psychological approach that he shared with his analyst and his other analytic supervisors.

The patient was a young woman graduate student who was bright, quick-witted, verbally facile, and flighty and hypomanic in style. She was a "spiritual seeker." She had experimented with many modes in her quest, including drugs, before entering analysis. She was actively connected with people prominent in the analytic field. Anger was a central problem for her. She was not aware of how alienating she could be.

The analyst's central countertransference to this patient was to feel "slow." He was not into her "grooviness." Her attempts at taking over the analysis, her name-dropping of "analytic stars," and her manic self-interpretations all made him feel superfluous and boring, "like chopped liver." She was very competitive, and stirred his feelings of competitiveness with everyone else who had helped her. At first, it made him feel inferior to them.

He felt that his supervisor's style was also "speedier" than his own. He thought that she was more like the patient, and saw things he didn't see. She helped the candidate be more assertive and confident with the patient. As a result, the patient had greater respect for him. It would have been hard for him to be more assertive without his supervisor, and he thought that the patient would have become anxious. In another respect, however, he saw his supervisor's style as similar to his: both of them were more down-to-earth, straightforward, and tactful than the patient. The supervisor's manner of communicating, which was similar to his own, bolstered his confidence, enabling him to adhere to his own style without being intimidated by the patient's facile, assertive manner and psychological jargon. It helped to dispel his anxiety about "not being swift enough"; in turn, as his supervisor did with him, he was able to help the patient gain stability.

The candidate found the supervisor's theory particularly helpful in relation to this patient. It made it easier for him to recognize the projective aspect of his feeling "slow." With his supervisor's help, he was able to speak to the transference more directly. She encouraged him to be more confrontational, and to interpret the patient's manic defenses and the transference. He would have tended to focus more on other defenses, those related to inhibition rather than expression of affect and impulse; this approach was one he had experienced in his own analysis, and one that had been promulgated by his other supervisors. It fit more easily with his own style and ideas. However, he thought that this ego psychological approach was not such a good fit for this particular patient. His view of the supervisor as "down-to-earth" made it easier for him to make use of her ideas without feeling that he was joining with the patient's "manicky ways" by "flying off" into speculation and theory.

The candidate liked the patient, but he felt less empathy with her problems than he had with his previous analytic patients; "her stuff" was very different from his. He felt a greater similarity between his own conflicts and those of his other patients; this had enabled him to apply his own analyst's view of himself to them. (He had terminated his own analysis during the early part of this patient's treatment.)

There was, however, some personal resonance with her; the patient saw herself as an outsider, and he could relate to that. In addition, like the patient, he had experimented with other psychological modalities before becoming interested in psychoanalysis. His experimentation had never gone as far as hers, however. Both he and the patient wanted to see themselves as "nice"; the patient thought of herself as "sweet." While he thought that he was "not as nice as I like to think of myself," his patient was really "out of touch with how she can be mean and angry." He was aware of his resistance to seeing this aspect of himself.

His supervisor was "not sweet." She was more comfortable with her aggression. Her tactful presentation of her personal comfort with aggression enabled the candidate to be more accepting of his own and of the patient's aggression. He became increasingly tolerant of being "put down" by the patient without feeling defensive and without turning back on himself a form of counteraggression. He recognized that the patient made him feel he "had to compete with all her other helpers; she made people feel dismissed." Over time, he was able to help her see her competitiveness and aggression, and he felt it less personally.

The supervisor's perspective on the candidate was similar to his own, but she viewed herself as more like him than he realized. She saw herself as "not a star," but rather, like the candidate, as someone who made slow, steady progress. They shared "a diligent, hard-working devotion to the task." She liked these qualities in herself and in the candidate. She thought he took criticism really well, learned from it, and changed. She saw him as "resilient, likable, teachable." The patient was "vivid, hysterical"; she showed off. The candidate and she were quieter and less vivid in personal style, more "slowed down and muted" in affect display. She might be "a little more affectful" than the candidate, but they were much more like each other than they were like the patient. The use of a particular theory seemed less important to her with this patient than the awareness of countertransference feelings and the empathic bond in the supervision.

In this example, there is a smoothly working treatment. The candidate and supervisor are pleased with their collaboration, and their differences are primarily about how the supervision was facilitating. The patient induced the candidate to react with feelings of inadequacy. He believed that the supervisor's "quickness" and confrontative style supported him and opposed the patient's power. The candidate viewed the supervisor's "quickness" and theory as more important than the supervisor did. The supervisor did not see herself as her supervisee did, as exceptionally comfortable with aggression. Thus, the candidate saw new aspects of himself and learned new ways of working with patients. In his view, his supervisor's confidence and comfort with assertion helped him to be more confident and more comfortably assertive.

Discussion

Each of these examples was related primarily through the eyes of the candidate. Self-reports are always open to criticism on the grounds of personal bias, the wish to present oneself in a favorable light, the need to believe that the activities in which one has invested a great deal have been fruitful, and similar problems of subjectivity. Nonetheless, in a field like psychoanalysis where we can never be free of subjectivity and where candidates now do give voice to dissatisfaction in ways they often did not in the past, it is necessary to take candidates' perceptions seriously. These candidates volunteered to discuss these particular triadic matches because they believed they illustrated a particular effect on them of a particular quality of a supervisor in relation to a particular case.

The selection of supervisors: comfort versus challenge

Supervisors, like analysts (Petsky, 2000), are perceived as offering varying degrees of "comfort" or "challenge," and are sought out for these qualities depending on the stage of analytic training and the particular needs of the candidate. Similarities, when they are found in characteristics that candidates like and value in themselves, bring comfort. An atmosphere of safety is created in which the candidate may be freer and better able to listen and "take in" the supervisor's ideas. On the other hand, to be confronted with new ideas and techniques can be stimulating. The capacity to tolerate the tension in the challenge of new ideas accelerates growth.

For many beginning candidates, the main question in supervision is their own capacity and competence. A supervisor may best facilitate the candidate's growth by appreciating that in order to learn, the candidate needs external affirmation to develop self-confidence. While intellectual recognition of the importance of different factors at particular stages of training may guide supervisors in their choice of stance and intervention, supervisory styles are not infinitely flexible. On the contrary, character and conflict define the range over which shifts can occur. Furthermore, supervisor and supervisee may elicit different aspects of each other; the characteristics of a particular supervisee influence those characteristics of the supervisor that become manifest in their interaction. As an example, both patient and candidate may need affirmation as a condition for confronting specific conflicts and characterological issues. A supervisor who is able to provide a sense of affirmation to the candidate may help the latter allow the patient to discover strengths in him- or herself, contributing thereby both to the candidate's education and to the treatment process. Both the specific kind of "affirmation" sought and its meaning may differ for each pair and for each triad.

When candidates feel more confident, they are less prone to fear criticism or experience shame, and are more receptive to learning something new. Being comfortable enough is a necessary, but not sufficient condition for learning. And what is "enough" comfort is a subjective, not an objective, state. Too great a convergence over time may fail to provide enough difference in perspective and may result in intellectual complacency. Blind spots may go unheeded. Potential growth in the candidate's thinking and potential depth in analytic work may be lost if comfort is sought at the expense of challenge. But if the candidate becomes too anxious or narcissistically vulnerable, all efforts are likely to be directed toward tension reduction and self-protection; little energy or attention will be left over for learning. An inevitable tension exists between these pulls.

The selection of supervisors: conscious and unconscious fantasies

When candidates select their supervisors, they may or may not have a conscious idea of the relative balance of comfort and challenge they seek. Choices may be determined unconsciously. Choices based upon fantasies that idealize the supervisor and his or her perceived characteristics, however, may lead to frustration and disappointment when the reality does not correspond to the idealized image. Candidates often speak informally of their selection of a supervisor to compensate for perceived deficiencies in their training analyst and their general analytic education. Candidates often select a favorite teacher or someone who is favored by other candidates. Sometimes the conscious attempt to balance perceived needs and to compensate for problems succeeds; at other times, it does not. A realistic wish to learn and identify with a supervisor may be successful, but it may also be superimposed upon the avoidance of a more personal struggle. Conscious selection of a supervisor for particular characteristics fails to take into account the dynamic interaction between the two participants and the unique nature of what may evolve between them. "Characteristics" are all imbedded in character, but which ones predominate in any given relationship is a function of the dyadic interplay.

Candidates may be unprepared for how their interaction with a supervisor may cause a particular experience to differ from their expectation. But they may also be unprepared for the effect that the patient's characteristics have on the supervisory dyad. For example, one candidate described the selection of a supervisor who had been both affirming and stimulating in supervision prior to her candidacy. The candidate had particularly appreciated the supervisor for teaching her new ways of hearing patient material, and illustrating techniques that deepened the level of the material. The analytic patient she brought for supervision, however, had much less tolerance for affect, was less well organized, and more narcissistically vulnerable than the previously supervised case. The supervisor's theory and suggestions for technique, when tried by the candidate in the context of this patient, seemed to disorganize the patient further. The candidate felt that the supervisor was disappointed in her as well as irritated with the patient, and she became anxious and less able to think flexibly in the supervision. The supervisory situation progressively deteriorated as patient, candidate, and supervisor each came to feel that they were not getting what they had hoped for from the experience.

The effects of the particular patient

Since in many instances supervisors are chosen before cases are selected, it may be difficult to anticipate such occurrences. While sometimes supervisors recognize that a particular case may not seem suited for analysis (at least for an analysis that they are supervising), often these interactive difficulties do not emerge until the work is under way. A "difficult case" may be more "difficult" for some candidate-supervisor pairs than others, depending on the nature of the match.

Patient selection is based primarily on patient suitability for analysis. Ideally, candidates will treat diverse patients and thus have a wide range of experience. But patient selection, like the selection of a supervisor, does not necessarily predict what actually happens. The dynamic interplay of patient and candidate may yield surprises. Patients may evoke conflicts in candidates that were insufficiently analyzed or that did not emerge in their analyses. The extent to which these conflicts either impair treatment or serve as an opportunity for growth (for patient and candidate alike) often depends on the supervisor's ability to help the candidate work with the conflicts that have been evoked, especially when the candidate is no longer in analysis.

The effect of the particular supervisor and the supervisory perspective

From the supervisor's perspective, matching candidates with particular patients is difficult, and so is any supervisor's task of assessing his or her match with a given candidate. This is because detailed understanding of the candidate, such as would be available about a patient in analysis, is lacking. When problems in learning occur, it may be hard to evaluate such factors as the candidate's resistance and anxiety. The supervisor may not have understood the candidate's abilities or psychological readiness to take in the supervisor's views, or the supervisor may not have conveyed these views with sufficient tact or sensitivity. The supervisor may also not want to cope with confronting a resistance or the anxiety that may be stirred thereby. Candidates' anxiety about being evaluated may also interfere with their ability to ask questions, integrate ideas, and openly express their concerns (Cabaniss, Glick, & Roose, 2001). A particular supervisor's capacity to recognize and then address effectively resistance or anxiety in a particular candidate with regard to a particular patient may be facilitated or impeded by the interplay of their characteristics and conflicts. A supervisor's capacity to help a candidate explore countertransference issues depends not only on supervisory talent, but also on the supervisor's being sufficiently free from the specific kinds of anxiety and conflicts that have been evoked to explore them with the supervisee. In addition, because the supervisor-supervisee relationship is different from the analyst-analysand relationship, the supervisor may not focus sufficiently on countertransference toward the supervisee and its influence upon him or her.

It is inevitable that some conflictual issues will affect the triadic interplay, though they may never become prominent enough to disrupt the process and therefore may never be directly addressed. But when they do, there is an opportunity to learn. Competition is likely to play some role for all patients, candidates, and supervisors. When it is a central feature for the patient, it may exacerbate the candidate's conflicts in this area. The supervisors' own competitive issues may influence the degree of tension surrounding this issue. Addressing this constellation in the context of the supervisor-supervisee relationship may enable the candidate to cope better with it in the analysis of the patient.

Awareness of interactional effects raises questions about supervisor selection. Some institutes assign supervisors. Increased appreciation of the effect of the supervisor-candidate match among institute education committees would seem likely to benefit assignments. However, it is not likely that the effect of a match can be assessed from the outside. The effect of the supervisor-candidate match may only become apparent during the process of the case. If a candidate seems to be seeking comfort at the expense of challenge, this perception could be raised at the time of progression to later cases. But ultimately the balance between comfort and challenge seems best decided by the candidate.

The effect of shared areas of difficulty between candidate and patient

One particular difficulty in supervised cases arises when the patient has problems similar to the candidate's. A candidate in early stages of training may do better to take on a patient whose conflicts and character are not too similar to his or her own, since the candidate's personal concerns are less likely to be activated through their work together. Almost inevitably, beginning analysts, still in analysis themselves, identify with their analysands; sufficient dissimilarity in their conflicts and defenses reduces the likelihood of an overidentification with the patient's struggles and a loss of the boundary between self and other. As a result, the candidate may have greater freedom to learn.

In a survey done by the candidates at the NYU institute, candidates reported that the most painful and stressful part of candidacy was work with patients who had difficulties with which the candidates identified, and which had not yet been sufficiently understood or resolved in their own analyses (Stuart & Haseley, 2000). Reports of parallel process in treatment and supervision have been understood to reflect the supervisee's enacting with the supervisor a process, not consciously comprehended, that is being enacted by the patient (Arlow, 1963; Doehrman, 1976; Ekstein & Wallerstein, 1958; Gediman & Wolkenfeld, 1980; Sachs & Shapiro, 1976; Searles, 1955). These authors view the enactments as a communication of what cannot yet be formulated in words.

When candidates are not conscious that their distress, conflicts, or defenses are similar to the patient's, these problems may be enacted in the treatment and the supervision. The supervisor's perspective, his or her attitude toward the particular struggle, his or her discussion of theory and technique, may in displacement be therapeutically beneficial or it may generate too much anxiety. Emphasis by the supervisor on analytic skills may lead the candidate to understand the importance of curiosity and understanding in balancing and replacing the tendency to emotional reaction and enactment. By maintaining his or her own individuality and not identifying with the candidate, a supervisor may demonstrate the advantages of avoiding overidentification, gaining a greater emotional distance, and offering a steady interest and perspective.

Practical implications for institute policies

Discussion of theory and technique may in displacement be therapeutically beneficial or it may generate too much anxiety. Emphasis by the supervisor on analytic skills may lead the candidate to understand the importance of curiosity and understanding in balancing and replacing the tendency to emotional reaction and enactment. By maintaining his or her own individuality and not identifying with the candidate, a supervisor may demonstrate the advantages of avoiding overidentification, gaining a greater emotional distance, and offering a steady interest and perspective.

Gediman and Wolkenfeld (1980) and Strean (1991) have focused on the negative aspects of these triadic interactions. The examples in this paper, in contrast, illustrate the beneficial aspects of the match. Three of the examples show how differences in character and style, sometimes recognized only retrospectively by the candidate—and in these instances not consciously perceived by the supervisors—may compensate for an area of need in the candidate that was stimulated by the particular patient. These differences occurred in the context of a supervision in which the candidate felt liked and respected. These compensations do not seem to have been specifically acknowledged or discussed by the candidate in the supervision itself even when they were recognized. Yet some aspect of the supervisor's behavior toward the candidate—some attitude, stance, or style—influenced the candidate, consciously or unconsciously, and its influence was reflected in the candidate's work with the patient.

Considerations about prediction

The data from this study and from other reports cited in this chapter suggest that candidates who perceive themselves as liked and respected by their supervisors will experience the supervisory situation as conducive to learning. Some degree of affirmation by the supervisor also seems beneficial to candidates' self-esteem; it too may aid in the acquisition of knowledge and skill, since anxiety is lessened. It seems to be more difficult for candidates to learn when their conflicts, defenses, or character are too similar to the patient's; interference is especially notable early in candidates' psychoanalytic education, when they have not yet had sufficient personal analysis to understand these issues in themselves. Once candidates are familiar enough with their own psychodynamics, they may conclude that certain supervisors have styles not compatible enough with their own for maximal learning to occur. Ideally, such conclusions will not be based on a defensive avoidance of intellectual challenge. Candidates may also know enough about supervisors (from having had them as teachers or from the reports of other candidates who have been supervised by them) to assume that some supervisors will be more helpful with certain kinds of patients than with others.

Having made these general observations, I want to reemphasize that the nature and helpfulness of the match cannot be predicted in advance for several reasons. One is that what is manifest in each of the participants does not reveal all that potentially may emerge; different people bring out different aspects of each other.

Another reason is that interactions among the three participants and their specific characteristics evolve and change over the course of the work. Supervisors who are helpful early in a case may be less so later on, and the reverse may also be true. Patients and supervisors who are difficult to work with may also turn out to be the ones from whom the most is learned.

The role of the candidate's analyst

The role of the supervisor in relation to the candidate's analyst also needs to be considered. Some candidates consciously select supervisors whose theory, technique, or style is similar to their analyst's, and some choose supervisors who are different in these respects. The nature of the candidate's feelings about the analyst cannot be assumed from the manifest choice. Choices of similarity may reflect positive feelings about what has been gained in analysis and a wish to learn more actively what the candidate assumes will be similar skills. Sometimes, however, these positive feelings reflect an idealized transference to the analyst, a wish to minimize different views, or the potential stirring of conflict or negative feelings in the analytic relationship. Choices of similarity may also be protective of the candidate's narcissistic vulnerabilities or the narcissistic vulnerabilities that the candidate attributes to the analyst.

The choice of a supervisor who is dissimilar in theory, technique, or style may reflect a wish for something different from the candidate's own analytic experience, even when this has been beneficial. A choice of difference may express the candidate's wish to increase his or her autonomy, expanding analytic skills different from the analyst's in order to facilitate a separation process. Sometimes, however, the choice of difference becomes a way to split the transference.

In these instances, either the analyst or the supervisor may be perceived as the "good" or "bad" one, depending on the transference at the time. A choice of difference may also reflect a temporary protest over some specific disagreement that the candidate is having with the analyst. Whether the manifest choice is for similarity or difference, if the motivating factor is rooted primarily in conscious or unconscious conflict, the supervisory process is burdened with tasks beyond the learning of analytic skills. When a clash between the analyst's and the supervisor's ways of analyzing is a central focus for the candidate, one arena or the other, or possibly both, may become hotly charged. If this happens, it may provide an opportunity for exploring and resolving conflict. Alternatively, it may lead to a supervisory or analytic impasse.

In the best scenario, candidates learn more about themselves and the analytic process through their work with their patients. What is stimulated in the treatment is brought to supervision. The supervisor offers a fresh perspective. The candidate understands something more deeply, or discovers something new about the patient and him- or herself. The personal aspect of discovery is brought to the candidate's own analysis. In analysis, the candidate expands this new self-understanding and develops a deeper appreciation of personal conflicts and defense as they are stirred by the analytic work and amplified by supervision. Less encumbered by the blind spots engendered by personal conflict, the candidate can be freer to hear and respond to the patient. The candidate returns to supervision able to refine or extend the supervisor's observations and ideas. It is a reverberating process. Every step augments the others. While in reality the process rarely proceeds this smoothly, it is a model to be aspired to.

When a candidate has terminated analysis, the supervisor's role may be broader; in fact, supervision may be the situation in which the candidate most actively continues personal analytic work. To the extent that the candidate feels safe and comfortable enough to discuss personal issues (while maintaining appropriate boundaries) and the supervisor can find a respectful way to address the candidate's struggles in the context of the analytic work with the patient, the candidate can use the supervisory experience to continue his or her personal analysis.

In summary, supervisory styles, like analytic styles, have considerable variation. Even when training and theory are similar, every individual contributes a unique aspect to analytic work. When two individuals work together, the interplay of their characteristics creates a process that will differ from the process that either of the two would develop working with another person. When the focus of their attention is on the interaction of one of this pair with another person, as the supervisory pair focuses on the candidate's interaction with the patient, the characteristics of the third individual will also influence the process. The particular gains candidates derive from working with particular supervisors is a function of the specific needs arising from their stage of training, their previous experience, their character and conflicts, and their interaction with the character and conflicts of their patients. The complex nature of these interactional effects makes it increasingly apparent that no one model of supervision is applicable to all situations.

* * *

Analysts continue to need a perspective that enables them to step outside of the dyadic relationship with their patients. After formal training ends, many analysts continue supervision, but over time they are more likely to find a peer with whom they undertake a mutual supervision. The degree of structure and regularity of these supervisions varies, but the person selected is almost invariably a trusted, respected colleague, often a very close friend. Since in-depth exploration of countertransference is part of the process, these mutual supervisions also provide the analyst with continuing personal self-discovery.

The mutuality of reciprocal presentation reduces the transference. Both participants understand that this relationship is as confidential as a treatment. I have found it beneficial to present all my analytic patients throughout their treatment—not just those with whom I note a difficulty—and to begin to do so as early in the work as possible. We must value our patients' privacy, but to keep our work totally private may seriously limit our ability to be helpful; sometimes it may do outright harm. Of course, no format is entirely free of side effects. While making peer supervisions mutual may help reduce transferences, mutual idealizing transferences can develop, increasing the likelihood of mutual blind spots.

Glen Gabbard (personal communication) advocates ongoing mutual presentation of analytic work as a safeguard against boundary violations. When the treating analyst begins to lose the role of guardian of the treatment, the analytic peer can sound the alarm before the process has gone too far. For some analysts, once they are caught up in an erotic countertransference, it is very difficult for them to halt the loss of an analytic stance. Perhaps if signs of slippage are recognized earlier, the outcome might be different. Perhaps not.

While I do not think we are all vulnerable to the specific pitfall of living out sexual boundary violations, I do believe that we are all prone to some form of loss of distance that can pull us from our professional roles. Alternatively, we may be in danger of being too distant from the patient and the process. In either instance, discussing our work with a trusted colleague is apt to reveal aspects of our patients and ourselves of which we are less aware and allows us greater freedom to speak of what we come to see—to our patients, when it is relevant to them, and in writing when insights may be a professional contribution. Continual recognition of our patients' effects on us and ours on them leads to a deepening and expansion of the analytic work, and reminds us of the importance of the analytic stance. While some analysts do really lose their sense of boundaries and of what is and is not acceptable to the extent that they are cannot retrieve a professional stance, most are likely to respond once they see how their personal vulnerabilities are conflated with the patient's.

An analyst I interviewed for "The Patient's Impact on the Analyst" (Kantrowitz, 1996) told of the pleasure he experienced, and his horror at himself for it, when a woman patient cried with frustration about love and erotic longing for him. Exploring his reaction with a colleague and friend with whom he had long been meeting weekly for mutual "confessing and confiding," he revived memories of himself as "an intensely wanting and frustrated child." He saw that his "satisfaction" in the patient's wanting something from him that he would not give was his way of not identifying with her—a defense against painful reawakened feelings of longing for something from someone that would never be forthcoming. "Better to have someone crying over... something I couldn't do [for her] than to face the experience of unmet need that was in me." Talking with his colleague left him better able to face and tolerate these feelings and to feel empathy for both his patient and himself, which facilitated analytic work.

Group peer supervision may be helpful, but we are less likely to reveal personal and conflictual aspects of ourselves in a group setting. Even though confidentiality is maintained, the conditions are more public. The presenter is less likely to feel confident that he or she can read how listeners are responding. Fears of being misunderstood, criticized, judged, or shamed may limit full exposure of reactions of fear, anxiety, shame, competition, envy, anger, hate, lust, wishes to rescue, longing, or love. When the presenting analyst has not already recognized a loss of perspective—if it is perceived first by others—he or she may feel caught in shameful surprise and then tend to hide and keep private what he or she has seen, lest still more be inadvertently revealed. If the analyst is aware of the intrusion of personal issues, the loss of distance needs to be understood as well as interrupted. It is often difficult, if not impossible, to achieve such a detailed examination in a group. Anxiety is likely to be stirred in the members that they too could be in the presenter's place.

Sometimes, such identificatory anxiety leads to compassion and empathy, resulting in help that enables the analyst to extricate him- or herself from the dilemma; however, often the reaction is to distance oneself and respond harshly, leaving the presenting analyst to feel shamed, alone, and less likely to reveal more of his or her struggle. Nonetheless, it may be that if the group is small enough and together over enough time, real trust, and therefore openness, may develop.

Still, one-to-one relationships are more conducive to the conditions of safety and trust that facilitate expression of what is personal and may be unrecognized or unspoken. These communications are more intimate and more private. They replicate some of the qualities of a treatment setting and allow the analyst to see him- or herself more fully and clearly through the eyes and thoughts of a respected colleague. If the symbolic realm of "as if" is forgotten, the trust placed in the colleague's view more often enables the analyst to regain perspective by seeing how he or she has been in danger of acting on, rather than owning, some form of countertransference experience. The analyst colleague is also likely to be freer in exploration and in response when listening one-on-one than when concerned about how much personal material the presenting analyst is revealing to a group, or how the group members will react to it. He or she can also suggest a return to treatment for the presenting analyst, if this seems desirable, without the recommendation becoming public to peers.

A patient, relatively new in treatment, though objectively accomplished and intimately engaged, experienced limiting inhibitions. She was very likable and interesting. So I was surprised when I found that my attention waned. I presented her twice to my analytic peer. Nothing changed. I suggested to him the next time we spoke on the phone that I talk only about my associations. Somewhere far into this hour with my colleague, I was thinking of my grandfather, whom I had never met. I was told of a certain impulsivity of his only in my adult years. My colleague spoke of intergenerational transmission. While neither he nor I could specify what exactly this meant for me, it riveted my attention. I found that I was not again inattentive with my patient, and she began to explore anxiety connected with her increasing awareness of her competitive feelings. The exchange with my colleague stimulated a process for me that worked consciously and preconsciously to further my availability to, and understanding of, my patient. My understanding of myself was affectively alive before it was explicit and conceptual. We now are aware that registration of affective understanding may lead to change prior to any insight. Eventually what I came to understand is that I had joined my patient in her state of affective inhibition, which led to my diminished attention. My patient's inhibition related to her fear of loss due to her competitive strivings, an impulse she defended against; the impulsivity I defensively inhibited also related to a fear of loss, but was less connected to competition and more to the consequences of indulging one's desires, as I had learned my grandfather had.

Training analyses pose special problems around confidentiality. Ideally, the training analyst has a colleague in another city whom he or she knows, trusts, and respects enough to discuss the work. I have been fortunate over the years to have several colleagues far from home with whom I have felt it safe to pursue peer supervision of my analyses of candidates. Not everyone has this good fortune. To avail oneself of the help of an out-of-town colleague means either being willing to travel to another city as frequently as needed, or being (or becoming) comfortable with working on the telephone. Either way works, but not for everyone. If the training analyst cannot avail him- or herself of this solution, the choice is to confide in a local colleague, with all the attendant anxiety, or to remain alone with the difficulty.

If one's analytic colleague is in the same city, as most often is the case, he or she may recognize the patient. Under these circumstances, the colleague would recuse himself from being this candidate's supervisor and from any evaluative role on progression in analytic training. Maintaining the privacy of the dyad, even, or perhaps especially, with candidates, is potentially hazardous to the participants. Both patient and analyst may be deprived at the least and endangered at the extreme, if the analyst believes he or she cannot, or must not, discuss the process that unfolds. If already caught deeply in countertransference enactments, the analyst may find it preferable to go to a trusted colleague, but someone who is not a personal friend and is paid for the help. Shame over the loss of one's professional self is likely to create a greater need for privacy (Kantrowitz, 2009).

Notes

1　This supervisor stated that it was a recommended procedure at his institute for supervisors to review their supervisory relationships with their candidates and recommend a change if there seemed to be impasses that did not resolve themselves after they had been addressed.

2　This candidate was "rather surprised" to read a rendition of events by her supervisor that she perceived as very different from her own experience of them, and very different from what she believed her supervisor "knew [her] experience of his actions and opinions had been." She thought he had told her that he thought the treatment was going well when he clearly did not think so. She did not believe that it was possible for her to have missed any major explicit or implicit messages in his communication to her. She believed that she had "utilized what seemed good about [his] approach, and rejected the rest out of clinical judgment rather than unconscious resistance."

Chapter 8

The external observer and the lens of the patient-analyst match

In the course of analyzing patients, certain phenomena catch analysts' attention and make them wonder what they are not seeing and why this is occurring. The most notable of these occasions are when analysts become aware of intense countertransference reactions, when they find themselves repeatedly caught in enactments and when analyses become stalemated. Sometimes analysts have not understood an aspect of the patient's difficulties, but for experienced, skilled analysts most often the problem resides in the transference-countertransference (Chused, 1991; Davies, 1994; Ehrenberg, 1992; Hoffman, 1983, 1994; Jacobs, 1991; Kantrowitz, 1992, 1993a, 1995, 1996; Mclaughlin, 1981, 1991a, b; Poland, 1988; Renik, 1993; Sandler, 1976; Schwaber, 1983, 1992; Spillius, 1994). At these times, analysts often, formally or informally, seek the view of a colleague to illuminate the situation.

Overlapping conflicts between patients and analysts that emerge in the transference-countertransference are interferences that analysts most often recognize. The effect of characterological overlaps are apt to be subtler and their disruption to the work less easily detectable. Therefore, they may stay unrecognized unless something external forces them into conscious attention. When analyses seemingly are going smoothly, analysts are not as likely to discuss them or seek the view of colleagues. After formal training ends, there is no built-in expectation that analyses will be discussed. Analyses then may remain totally private communications between patient and analyst, subject to the strengths and limitations of the particular pair. Unless analysts find a format to discuss their cases, such as a peer supervision group, a mutual supervision with a colleague on a regular basis, or an ongoing consultative relationship, there are likely to be areas of blind spots in some aspect of their analytic work. These blind spots may or may not impose a significant impediment to analytic progress, but in some more nuanced way they are likely to influence the process.

This chapter focuses on the important effect of reporting clinical experiences to a colleague or a group of colleagues. The reporting of this material, which in all other respects remains totally confidential, is undertaken to obtain an outsider's perspective. The outside view is sought so that the analyst can acquire awareness and insight into what otherwise would likely remain removed from consciousness. The concept of the match between patient and analyst may provide a particularly useful lens in this process. I will define my understanding of match as a perspective for insight about the effect of the patient-analyst dyad on the analytic process. I will offer three illustrations of its beneficial value in the context of a third party's perspective on the analytic pair.

Considering the effect of match between patient and analyst provides one way of conceptualizing the impact of their interaction on the analytic process. I am not trying to define a "good" or "bad" match, but rather to clarify how considerations of the nature of the match can illuminate aspects of analytic work. Focus on the match calls attention to specific aspects of character, defense, or conflict elaborated in the transference-countertransference interaction. Match highlights the similarities and differences between the participants. Similarities may lead to understanding, but also to blind spots and defensive collusion. Differences may lead to curiosity and exploration, but also failures in empathy and engagement; either may facilitate or impede the process. The effect of the match may change during the course of treatment. Factors that initially benefit engagement in analytic work may later impede it.

While my definition of match includes all the multifaceted ways that patient and analyst overlap in conflict, character, and experience, it is in the area broadly called character that the concept of match may prove most useful. Attitudes, values, beliefs, cognitive style, and strategies of adaptation and defense are components of character that are likely to influence the course and depth of the work. A focus on similarities and dissimilarities alerts the colleague, supervisor, or consultant to manifestly non-conflictual or at least non-anxiety charged areas of overlap or disjunction between patient and analyst that may affect analytic work.

When the countertransference reaction has its roots in the analyst's character and conflicts, then whether or not the match is impeding will depend on how much the analyst's character is modifiable. However, unless they are aware of an obstacle, analysts cannot begin to modify habitual characteristics or dynamic conflicts that interfere with analytic work. Sometimes patients point out these interfering factors to their analysts. And sometimes analysts listen, pay attention, and change (Hoffman, 1983). But analysts cannot rely on their patients providing this feedback. Even when invited, not all patients will do so. In addition, the areas I am considering are ones which analysts are less likely to enquire about since they remain outside of their view. Therefore, an invitation for feedback from a party external to the analytic dyad affords an opportunity for a fresh analytic perspective. Making analysts aware of "blind spots" can make them a focus of analytic scrutiny that may then decrease countertransference intensity or enactments and reopen the process if a treatment is stalemated. It may also lead the analyst to more extended self-scrutiny, greater self-awareness, and potentially to psychological growth.

Thinking about the patient-analyst transference-countertransference, and especially characterological issues, in terms of the match between analyst and patient provides the colleague, supervisor, or consultant with a particular lens for focus on the interactions. The external observer can view how their conflicts, their characteristics, their styles, and the meaning of them mesh or clash. Match offers an overarching perspective that can be used to evaluate the effect of the distance between patient and analyst in terms of their similarities and differences. Since, depending on the phase of the analysis, matches of similarity and dissimilarity are sometimes beneficial and at other times obstacles within the same dyad, considering the effect of the match permits an assessment of whether it is useful or detrimental for the analytic process at any given time. Awareness of the consequences of overlap or divergence affords the analyst the opportunity to make a correction in attitude or stance.

An analyst's awareness that a "blind spot" results from the effect of overlapping characteristics creates a Janus-faced problem. Too vigilant a focus on the uniqueness of the patient's experience may result in the analyst's distancing from an affective resonance. The same analyst might spontaneously provide such emotional attunement for a patient whose history was less similar. For example, an analyst whose parent was overstimulating may resist an empathic identification with a patient who experiences him as an overstimulating parent in the transference. Resistance, both to being identified as the hurtfully overstimulating parent and to re-experiencing the pain of being overstimulated in identification with the patient, create a countertransference reaction. The analyst may then affectively distance himself in a way that the patient experiences as a rejection. This pain goes beyond the inevitable pain of frustrated yearnings since it is based on a perception, albeit preconscious, of what Racker (1968) has called the analyst's countertransference predisposition. In other words, the analyst was predisposed to react in this manner to this situation with any patient.

The other danger is too great an immersion in an affective resonance; it may prevent an awareness, and then exploration, of important dissimilarities. Taking the same example, an analyst, rather than resisting identification with a patient who has been overstimulated as he was, may empathically join with this state. Then, for example, he may erroneously assume the intensity of experience was similar. This assumption may result in his failing to understand or explore a traumatic state. The patient's more blatant or subtler experience may be obscured. In these instances, the transference-countertransference blind spots that develop may limit or even prevent important areas of analytic work.

The effect of overlapping characterological factors can best be illustrated when an analyst's work with several patients is considered. For example, a now graduate analyst was described by three of her four supervisors as talented. They specifically emphasized her working like a more experienced analyst in her awareness and monitoring of her countertransference. The fourth supervisor, who had supervised the third case, also praised her work. However, this supervisor noted one area of countertransference interference that considerably impeded the analyst's work with this patient.

While overall the analyst had a well-conceptualized understanding of the patient's difficulties, and in many ways a tactful and sensitive approach in her interpretations, she tended to side with and reinforce the patient's self-critical approach, which was severe. The patient had been helped therapeutically in many areas and had grown in self-understanding. The analysis, however, seemed slower and more labored than with her other patients. The analyst was open and welcomed most supervisory observations and suggestions, which were usually smoothly incorporated and increased her analytic skill. However, this was not the case with regard to comments about her approach to her patient's self-criticism. The analyst did not become defensive; she listened; she seemed ready to "accept" criticism and become self-observing, but for a long time she also seemed unable to significantly modify her approach with this patient.

The supervisor and this analyst had an open, respectful relationship. They talked about the difficulty the analyst was encountering. The supervisee acknowledged that self-criticism had been an area of considerable work in her own analysis. While she was much less self-critical than previously, she could easily believe that she was joining her patient's self-critical stance; she knew she still tended to be this way in relation to herself. The analyst seemed always to be on the side of the critic whether against herself or the patient. She treated the patient as she treated herself because she identified with her. The problem was that it was so seamless that she usually didn't see that it was occurring until after the fact, when it was pointed out. The supervisee continued the supervision on this case after graduating. She was consciously aware she needed help in lessening her own harshness with herself as well as monitoring its impact on her work.

In the discussion of the committee prior to her graduation, the other supervisors were very surprised about the analyst having this difficulty. They each then reflected that the cases they supervised were patients who did not suffer from excessive self-criticism. Under these circumstances, the analyst's residual conflict and characterological defense were not stimulated in the analytic work. While it seems a significant area to remain so clearly activated in her work, all who knew and worked with her believed her to be a very competent analyst and capable of further growth in this area. However, the implications are that unless or until she works out this issue, there are certain patients with whom she will be mismatched.

The second example comes from a series of supervisory consultations, during which an analyst became aware of the different impact of her assertive style on two patients who had patently dissimilar characterological adaptations to their conflicts around aggression. In the course of this work, the analyst increased her understanding of her own characterological conflicts and modified her style in a manner that facilitated the work.

The first patient came from a relatively stable family where all the members were successful in their ambitions. She was alone and felt adrift. She sought treatment for her long-standing depression.

The analyst began this case with high hopes. Her patient was bright, in pain, and seemingly motivated to understand herself. A history of small but painful early disappointments emerged. For example, she had not been chosen for a part in a school play; a friend preferred another's company to hers. Later, boys who liked her were never the ones she liked. Her current life seemed similar. What she wanted she did not get. What she had seemed unsatisfactory. The analyst empathized with her disappointments and they gradually traced her hurts back to her sister's birth when she was four and how hard she had taken losing her role as the youngest and only girl. They found and elaborated their understanding of slights the patient felt from the analyst. But nothing seemed to move or change in the patient's life or her mood.

The second patient came from a family where there had been little emotional support. The father drank heavily, was erratic in his employment, and was occasionally abusive to the patient's siblings. The mother was seen as depressed and ineffectual. Having worked from an early age to contribute to the family income, the patient had dropped out of college several times due to financial pressures. She had boyfriends, but did not speak of any special relationship. She too sought treatment for her long-standing depression.

The analyst began this second case with great trepidation because of the patient's chronic deprivation and unstable family history. This patient also recounted many stories of hurt and disappointment, but her focus quickly shifted to her attempts at mastering situations. The analyst interpreted her move away from dysphoric affects. The patient could acknowledge moving away from painful feelings. The work continued with deepening exploration of her feelings of anger, hurt, fear, and longings to be taken care of. Her backing away from these painful feelings by throwing herself into outside activity was continually addressed. The underlying conflict was explored. Her dysphoric experiences became more fully and intensely expressed in the analysis. Over time, the patient began to describe more enjoyment in her life. She got a better job, thought about returning to school, and began seeing a man who interested her.

It seemed to me from her presentations that this was a competent, well-trained analyst. She was attuned to her patients. What she said conveyed a clear understanding of her patients' states, affects and defenses. She understood the first patient's retreat from narcissistic vulnerabilities and the second patient's retreat from painful affect. With each patient, she was also able to shift and focus on issues as they surfaced. The first patient did seem more difficult to treat. But was it only the patient's entrenched stance that created the problem?

As I listened to the analyst describe her patients, I was struck by her style. She was forthright, direct, pulled no punches in how she conveyed her thoughts, but was still tactful. She could be described as feisty. Clearly, she enjoyed being assertive and feeling the power of mastering with her mind. Her style had a similarity to her second patient's who also met troubles head on. If her problem was that she hadn't been staying with her painful feelings, this patient was now going to try to do this. In contrast, her first patient tended to retreat from assertion. Her aggression was turned on herself; she maintained a muted kind of victim stance. With this kind of patient the challenge was to analyze rather than accept the invitation for sadomasochistic interactions. The analyst did not seem to get caught in enactments, but the work did not deepen as it had in the second case. She did not seem as fully affectively engaged in the process with the first patient. In a subtle way, she maintained a greater distance. Her work lacked the zest she conveyed with the second patient.

The assertive style of the analyst seemed to fit too well the first patient's underlying fantasies that she was someone who could and would be pushed around, which she unconsciously extrapolated to not being treated well or respectfully. The analyst's manner allowed her to be seen as one more person who would bruise the patient. Perhaps the patient identified the analyst with her competent and disappointing mother whom she, in turn, wanted to disappoint. By failing to use the interpretations actively, she could disappoint her analyst. The fact that they analyzed these occurrences meant less to the patient than the "feeling" that they were continually happening in tone. Once I shared this observation with the analyst, she became aware of it herself.

After several consultations focusing on this aspect of her style of intervention and its impact on the patient, she felt something ease between them. When she returned for a consultation several months later, she described an hour in which the patient saw herself as less helpless. The analyst then began more actively to question her contribution to incidents in which the patient felt injured. She began to see more clearly the countertransference that she enacted.

The analyst stated that work with this patient made her aware of how little tolerance she would have for being in a passive, victimized position that her patient described and put the analyst into. It had led her to wonder whether unconsciously she been impatient with her analysand for being willing to remain in this role and thus frustrating the analyst. She wondered if she had become even a little more assertive than usual, as if to say, "Don't ever think I will join you in that passive position." Now, more conscious of her style through the consultations, she thought her approach may have softened somewhat.

The analyst's comfort and even pleasure in her assertive style may be in part a defensive use of her aggression, a possible reaction formation to her own masochistic tendencies. If this speculation is correct, there still was no evidence that this difficulty interfered with her effective professional work or enjoyment of life. The conflictual aspect of her aggression seemed bound in her character in a way that became manifest in my contact with her only when stimulated by this particular kind of interaction. Once the analyst recognized the presence of her countertransference, she was able to shift her tone. Her self-reflection enabled her to respond to the patient in a manner that was sufficiently different that the patient also was able to make some shift in her stance. The patient-analyst match with the first case illustrates an initially problematic overlap that was eased by the analyst's becoming aware of the difficulty and being able to alter her stance somewhat.

The analyst's comfortable assertive style seemed to facilitate the second patient's work. She used her technical skill to direct the focus of the treatment, but her particular manner also resonated with and supported the patient's own assertive push for mastery. Listening to her report the hours, I could hear them enjoy the "toughness" in getting to work. Yet this was not a toughness that took them away from facing dysphoric affects; rather, it was employed to help confront and withstand it. Perhaps at a later point in the treatment, the patient's and analyst's similarity in style will prove an impediment to reaching softer affects, but at this stage of the treatment it seemed an aid in deepening the treatment and freeing the patient in her life.

An example of a match that was beneficial for the major part of an analysis but became problematic in the latter phase of treatment was brought for consultation to a group of which I was a member. This was a small conference in a city distant from the place where this analysis was occurring.

The patient was herself a gifted clinician. She was sensitive and articulate. Both her personal and professional life seemed rich and engaged. She never had any treatment until well into her thirties. When she sought analysis it was manifestly to enhance her skill as a therapist. However, the patient was aware that she did not feel the confidence in herself that her functioning would seem to deserve. Shortly after beginning analysis, she recovered a memory of a traumatic occurrence. The trauma was not of the magnitude of a sexual abuse, but it involved feeling unprotected and betrayed in a way too painful to allow into her consciousness until the analysis. Both her fear and her fury had been repressed and she had developed a reasonableness in her approach to life.

In analysis, she freely moved among the past, her present life, and the transference. She experienced and expressed affection, and desire, and annoyance, and anger both toward people in her life and toward her analyst. She made good use of dreams and actively explored the real world. She loved her husband, enjoyed and struggled with her children, had good friends, and seemed gifted in her work. She seemed not only an ideal analytic patient, but remarkably adapted in her life.

However, like Stein's (1981) patients who hide the fullness of their passions behind an unobjectionable positive transference, this patient was "too reasonable." The analyst addressed this issue steadily after the early years of analysis. From this focus emerged a realization of how thoroughly the patient's precocity hid her anxieties. She had described panic reactions as an adolescent, but there had been no hint of this in her adult years. While she could be angry with her analyst, this did not precipitate great anxiety. The only hint of real distress was shown in how quickly her competitive, rivalrous feelings that stimulated aggressive impulses toward the analyst were dispelled as they were balanced by homosexual desires and attendant anxieties. It was hard to know which conflict was central as each was employed as a defense against the other. The alternating focus kept her from going too deeply into either conflict. The analyst interpreted all these shifts and explored and helped her to expand her affective experiences.

After the analyst presented this material, one of the conference members believed that the patient was suffering from "annihilation anxiety." He thought the patient was very fortunate to have an analyst who had stayed so closely attuned to her state. While he agreed the patient was psychologically well organized, he perceived there was an underlying terror.

Two years later, the analyst again presented this case to this conference group. In the year following the first presentation, the patient began to have terrifying dreams; memories of childhood nightmares were revived. Panics around separations were then remembered with the accompanying affect. However, separations from the analyst, while always some source of distress, actually seemed less, rather than more, troubling. Throughout this period, the analyst retained the same stance of reflecting, interpreting, and generally staying closely in resonance with the patient's state as the patient's conflicts became more fully apparent and affective experience intensified.

On this occasion, her colleagues were much less sanguine about the analyst's stance. While there was an understanding that the analyst was being sensitive to the patient's vulnerabilities, most of the group now believed that she was too closely joining the patient's state. There was not enough "asymmetry" in her stance. This position deprived the patient of the transference experience of aloneness that was essential to analyze her anxiety and panic in relation to separation.

The analyst's first reaction was to be surprised, having thought the work was slowly but progressively deepening. However, she quickly grasped the point her colleagues were making. She recognized her characterological tendency to assume a stance of "joining" rather than standing at a greater distance from the patient's state. While she had been aware that she was employing this stance with the patient, the fact that this joining might be preventing rather than facilitating analytic work had not occurred to her. She saw this as a striking "blind spot" on her part.

Later, the analyst reported what had then occurred. On returning from the conference, she was able to subtly shift her stance. Rather than beginning her interpretations of the transference with statements such as "It sounds as if you feel" or "think that I feel," she stated, "You imagine that I feel that..." The analyst described the patient immediately registering the difference and experiencing a painful and frightening sense of aloneness. With the analyst present but less emotionally holding her hand, the patient relived her sense of having been abandoned to overwhelming intense anxiety; she recovered memories and feelings of childhood terror. In her fury with the analyst for affectively leaving her alone to face this state, she revived her childhood fury as well as fear.

Fantasies that she would be the only person left on earth as well as panic that she would disappear were then linked with her fury and destructive impulses. Her fury then was understood to be at the heart of her terror. Her destructive fantasies became the basis for her unconscious construction of why she had been abandoned. As she worked her way through these painful and frightening feelings and fantasies, she also understood that "joining" and being in resonance with others, something that made her very good at her work with patients, had served a protective, defensive function. It had kept her from the experience of being alone and facing the anxiety embedded in this lifelong conflict. Her joining had been a way to reassure herself that she was a person others would want to be with, a caring, empathic person, not a competitive, destructive one. Following this analytic work, her freedom of feeling was greatly increased and the analytic work moved into the termination phase.

From the description, it is apparent that the analyst and patient had similar therapeutic and personal styles. They both tended to join the affective experiences of others, especially their patients. One could speculate that the analyst identified with the patient. Their similarity in style as well as their choice of profession may have increased this affinity. For the patient, a central conflict lay hidden behind this characterological adaptation. The deeper layers of meaning of this style for the analyst were not presented. However, in reporting back the changes that occurred in the work following the shift in her stance, she indicated that her increased awareness of their similarity led to insights that had personal reverberations.

In this example, a similarity of style and its defensive function facilitated the analytic process during the earlier part of the treatment by creating a feeling of affective resonance and an atmosphere of safety; later, this similarity impeded analytic work. Recognition of the blind spot enabled the analyst to see the masking effect their overlap created and to shift her stance. The analyst's conscious focus on understanding this area of similarity expanded not only the patient's analytic work, but also the analyst's self-understanding and experience of conflict and affect. Attention to the blind spot then resulted in the psychological change for both participants.

Taking an aerial view, as if in a consultation, analysts may use the lens of the match with their patient to explore how similarities and differences between them may be affectively charged in ways that the analyst was not aware of. Analysts may use the idea of patient-analyst match as a device for furthering their self-analytic work. But there are limits in this focused pursuit, as there are in all self-analytic enquiries. The analyst's view of their dyad with the patient will necessarily be restricted by the analyst's own blind spots and other countertransference phenomena.

As analysts, we no longer believe in the perfectly analyzed analyst (Abend, 1986). No analysis is ever complete, though some are more far-reaching than others. There is always more to learn about both personal strengths and limitations. Patients help analysts expand their self-knowledge (Kantrowitz, 1996, 1999, 2009). But patients are part of the dyad and subject to the same potential blind spots in interactions. The introduction of an outside point of view can more reliably broaden understanding and bring insight. If it becomes a focus of attention, a match between patient and analyst that an analyst has been unaware of as an impediment to the work may thus become an opportunity for growth in both participants.

In the past, experienced and skilled analysts were thought to seek consultations only when they believed there was an interference in their analytic work. Contrary to this public perception, many analysts have always maintained some form of ongoing dialogues with other analysts (Kantrowitz, 1998). These discussions take place in many different formats. Some analysts have peer groups that have met for many years. Other analysts engage in a mutual supervision, which over time may have many similarities to mutual analysis, in that they focus on each other's blind spots. Many other analysts prefer to maintain a more formal consultation relationship; this may be a planned, ongoing arrangement or a more infrequently initiated contact.

The introduction of an external observer provides a lens of objectivity not possible from within the dyad. For this feedback to be meaningful, it must, like an effective interpretation in analysis, resonate affectively as well as cognitively with the analyst. No matter how many colleagues concur on a view, unless the analyst is receptive to the perspective offered, it will not be assimilated. Ideally, the analyst will not be too defended to take in this information. Under these conditions, the new view will serve to increase the analyst's self-awareness, which in turn will lead to deeper analytic work.

The views of external observers, of course, are also influenced by their own subjectivities. Their characteristics and conflicts will interface with the analyst's, just as the analyst's does with the patient's. Therefore, the mesh or clash of character and conflict for the analyst-consultant dyad is potentially liable to the same conditions of blind spots as the patient-analyst pair. In addition, who the analyst selects as a peer supervisor, peer group, or consultant will be influenced by the analyst's own proclivity for comfort or challenge in relation to her way of working (Kantrowitz, 1999). Experienced analysts know the views and approaches of their colleagues. To a large extent, they are choosing how much similarity and difference in theory, technique, and personal style they wish to encounter when they make their selection. In other words, even with a conscious motivation to be vigilant about self-deception, the possibilities for its continued occurrence remain great.

It is easy to be lulled into thinking that continued discussion of analytic cases with one person or group will protect against blind spots. While reporting one's work in this manner certainly increases the likelihood of expanded self-awareness, it is not a guarantee. Analysts who present in such forums need to feel both safe enough and motivated enough to expose their work, their countertransference feelings, thoughts, and fantasies. They also need to stay alert to the effect of the feedback, both on the analytic pair and on themselves personally. Too little or too strong a reaction that does not lead to self-reflection, insight, and some shift in ideas, attitude, or stance might suggest the need for a different external observer. New eyes and ears may discover something still hidden.

Neither patients' nor analysts' comfort nor discomfort with their engagement is a reliable indicator of analytic benefit. A longitudinal study of analytic outcome showed the match of patient and analyst to be the single factor that illuminated the areas of analytic impasse (Kantrowitz et al., 1989; Kantrowitz, Katz, & Paolitto, 1990c). Sometimes neither party was aware of the blind spot. Both believed the analyses to be very successful, but comparison of pre- and post-psychological tests showed a major area to be unchanged. For example, their mutual valuation of creativity led to an analyst's interpreting a patient's fantasy of "pouring molten lead" on people as "free expression of fantasy"—and failing to recognize or analyze the aggression.

The efficacy of the match can change during the course of analysis. Therefore, feedback offered at one point of analysis may be very different from that offered at another phase. The same study illustrated how an analyst's calm, accepting attitude helped a very anxious, skittish patient gradually to feel safe enough to begin to explore her feelings and fantasies, but later permitted her to avoid actively grappling with her sexual conflicts. These findings make clear that analysts need to keep discussing their cases with others over time in order to remain aware of the effect of the dyad.

In addition to helping the practicing analyst become aware of blind spots, a focus on the patient-analyst match is a useful tool in teaching. Listening to candidates present their cases, it is often possible to discern how similarities or differences in the dyad may be enhancing or limiting of the analytic process. Currently, young analysts are open to recognizing the inevitability of their personal influence on analytic work. They do not seem so burdened by ideas of personal perfection nor do they seem to expect that their own analyses will remove all traces of personal conflict. As a result, they appear to be less narcissistically vulnerable in discussing their countertransference reactions and are more comfortable with observing newly seen aspects of themselves than candidates have been in earlier eras (Kantrowitz, 1999). These newly discovered aspects are usually manifested in their attitude, style, or stance toward the patient, as it is reflected in their presentations in seminars and supervision.

Often candidates' professional and personal curiosity about the dyad and themselves increases as the overlap in the analytic pair becomes clear. Once an awareness of an underlying conflict emerges, the transference-countertransference is revealed and can be understood by them. This perspective aids them in their appreciation of the effect of unconscious factors and of how conflict can be embedded and hidden in character. For example, one candidate was aware he was uncharacteristically reluctant to change the time of a patient's hour and took a seemingly "tough" stance in relation to all issues of the analytic frame. In contrast, during the actual analytic hours, he often seemed to work with an affective resonance in relation to the patient that bordered on a merger. In the course of presenting this material, he came to recognize that while his conflicts and their intensity were far less than his patient's, he and the patient shared a yearning for intense closeness that they both defended against with a "tough guy" stance. This awareness seemed to allow him to be both less "tough" in relation to the frame and to maintain more distance during the actual analytic hours.

Still another use of the perspective of the match is in the evaluation of candidates' learning needs. As the first example in the paper illustrates, reviewing a candidate's work with more than one patient may make it apparent that a personal difficulty interferes with some cases but not others. This discovery can be brought to the candidate's attention by supervisors. Then, together, candidate and supervisors can be alert for the manifestation of this problem in clinical work. With greater awareness, the candidate may then be able to integrate this insight in a manner that allows some shift in the analytic process.

In summary, different people bring out different aspects in each other in life, in analysis, in consultation/supervision, and in teaching. Analysts need to keep in mind that ego-syntonic ways of organizing experience may conceal aspects of their interactions with their patients that impede analytic progress. Some peers and consultants may provide a new perspective, while others whose outlooks are too similar may not. The same is true of supervisors and teachers. On the other hand, third-party views that are too different may not be able to be integrated and therefore are not of use. Too little or too much similarity or difference affect both the course of analysis and of learning. However, when an external observer can use the lens of the match to stimulate an analyst's curiosity about overlapping areas between patient and analyst that have led to enmeshment or clashes, then previously overlooked aspects of the analyst may become available for self-analytic scrutiny. The concept of match points out meaningful overlaps and disjunctions that can be used to increase awareness of similarities and differences and how they may affect analytic work in different ways at different phases of treatment. This awareness can help us better assist ourselves, our patients, our students, and our colleagues when we serve as their consultants in relation to analytic work.

Chapter 9

A different perspective on the therapeutic process

The impact of the patient on the analyst

Over the last decade and a half, a shift has occurred in the way analysts view the analytic process. While many analysts have always seen analytic work as interactional, for many years there was a school of thought in the United States that considered psychoanalysis an enterprise in which analysts functioned as "blank screens" on whom patients could project their conflicts. Analysts were thought to be relatively interchangeable, their principal contribution the offering of interpretations. In this context, countertransference reactions were seen as intrusions, something to be analyzed by the analyst and controlled, or a reason to go back into analysis. Countertransference was not regarded as providing data for exploration, an opportunity for greater understanding of the patient through greater understanding of what has been evoked in the analyst in the interaction. Increasingly, analysts have recognized that they are active participants in the process, influencing and being influenced by what occurs with their patients (Gill, 1982; Hoffman, 1983). In studying the impact of the patient-analyst match on the outcome of psychoanalysis (Kantrowitz et al., 1989; Kantrowitz, Katz, & Paolitto, 1990c), it became apparent that analysts frequently believe that they, as well as their patients, change during the process of an analysis. This belief seems consistent with the current way of thinking, with its greater attention to the impact of the patient on the analyst's functioning as a way of providing more information about the patient (Dorpat, 1974; Dorpat & Miller, 1992; Gedo, 1979; Gill, 1982; Goldberg, 1979; Goldberg, 1993; Greenberg, 1986; Greenson, 1967; Hoffman, 1992; Kohut, 1984; McLaughlin, 1993; Mitchell, 1993; Modell, 1986;

Natterson & Friedman, 1995, Skolnikoff, 1993; Stolorow & Atwood, 1992; Stolorow, Atwood, & Lachman, 1988; Stolorow, Brandchaft, & Atwood, 1987). Once analysis is viewed as a process influenced by and impacting on both participants, it would seem expectable that the analyst, as well as the patient, would be affected by participating in it. Yet analysts often resist openly discussing and describing such changes in themselves and how they come about. There are, of course, notable exceptions in which analysts openly describe their counter-transferences and elaborate their self-analytic process (Calder, 1980; Eifermann, 1987, 1993; Gardner, 1983; Jacobs, 1991; Kramer, 1959; Margulies, 1993; McLaughlin, 1981, 1988; Natterson & Friedman, 1995; Poland, 1984; Silber, 1996; Sonnenberg, 1991). Nonetheless, when analysts discuss the phenomenon of their continuing personal change among themselves, there seems to be an uncertainty about how representative or unique their own experiences are.

While only in the last decade has the view of analysis as an inter-actional enterprise become a mainstream belief in the United States, the idea that the practice of analysis has a therapeutic effect on the analyst is not new. In response to Glover's survey (1937), which in-vestigated analysts' views on psychoanalytic practice, a majority of analysts considered the dominant effect of analysis on the analyst to be therapeutic. It was recognized that the analytic situation was one in which there was continuous stimulation of conflict for the analyst; therefore, most analysts assumed that there would be temporary ex-acerbations of conflict that would require self-analytic work. Glover termed this effect "countertransference therapy," which occurred for different reasons for different individuals (p. 79).

In recent years, the analyst and his or her role in the analytic work has become a focus of study (Baudry, 1991; Kantrowitz, 1986, 1992, 1993b, c; Kantrowitz et al., 1989; Kantrowitz, Katz, & Paolitto, 1990c). Countertransference (Agger, 1993; Jacobs, 1991; McLaughlin, 1981, 1988, 1991a, b; Schwaber, 1992; Spruiell, 1984; Weinshel, 1993) and enactments (Boesky, 1982; Chused, 1991; Renik, 1993) increasingly engage analysts' attention and interest. Hoffman's social construc-tivist model (1991, 1992, 1994) tilts the balance of relative contribu-tion and participation still further with his emphasis on analysts as knowing no more than patients and their co-creation of meaning and understanding.

I am going to discuss the effect of the analytic experience on the analyst in the context of thinking about one's role as the analyst and its maintenance. To preserve this role, the analyst must apply a consistent self-scrutiny. Affects, thoughts, or behavior provoked by patients require that analysts continue to find an effective means to rework their own history of conflict. A concern heard from some analysts is that with this new emphasis, patients lose their place as the proper focus of analytic attention. Despite this increased interest in the analytic process as an interactional engagement, however, most analysts retain their primary focus on the patient's inner world and use their countertransference awareness to monitor themselves in their work. The shift in emphasis, however, has meant an increased attention to exploration of the analyst's process. Particular life events, such as illness (Abend, 1982, 1986; Dewald, 1982; Engle, 1975; van Dam, 1987) or pregnancy (Beiser, 1984; Friedman, 1993), inevitably stir transference-countertransference reactions in treatment. These, in addition to illuminating aspects of the patient's conflicts, stimulate analysts to greater self-scrutiny and thereby, an awareness of previously unrecognized aspects of themselves. Nonetheless, relatively few North American mainstream analysts have described the reverberating effects their work has had on them. A notable exception is McLaughlin (1981, 1988, 1991a, b, 1993), who documents how his belief system has been changed as a consequence of self-discoveries emerging in clinical work.

Many analysts express a recognition of increased self-awareness growing from their analytic work (Gardner, 1983; Poland, 1984; Spruiell, 1984). Smith (1993) believes that the analyst is shaped by the nature of the engagement with patients. Whether or not this shaping is consciously recognized, "the analytic work itself is for the analyst a source of personal growth and development" (p. 427). Similarly, Goldberg (1994) states, "We do not leave an analysis the same person as we were when we entered" (p. 28). These statements, however, remain abstract and undocumented.

While it is unlikely that an analyst could undertake an analysis without gaining new intellectual information and personal insight, it is not inevitable that these new understandings result in psychological shifts. Analysts, like patients, can idealize their own changes. Nonetheless, if an analyst permits himself to become fully engaged in the analytic interchange with all its intensity, the probability that some personal shift will occur is great. The nature and extent of such changes, however, depend on the interdigitation of the characteristics and conflicts of the particular patient-analyst pair.

Studying how analysts perceive changes in themselves over time allows for a longitudinal view of the impact of the analytic process on a group of people who have devoted themselves to this process as their lifework. For most analysts, this means that the psychological issues explored in their personal treatment are not re-repressed, as they might be following termination, but rather are kept actively alive in their work with patients. As a result, the analyst has the continuing opportunity to rework these issues on a potentially deeper level. Every analysis an analyst undertakes is in this respect potentially a reanalysis for him- or herself.

A brief report of a survey

In order to obtain data more extensive than personal anecdotal information, a national survey was undertaken. Eleven hundred questionnaires were sent to psychoanalysts who were members of the American Psychoanalytic Association. All 550 training and supervising analysts and 550 graduate analysts from each institute were selected as the sample. The training and supervising analyst group was selected because they were presumed to be the most experienced of the analysts.[1]

The purpose of the survey was to explore (1) whether and to what extent analysts believe that their analytic work with patients has led to personal change for themselves; and (2) when analysts do believe that such change has occurred, (a) what in the patient-analyst interaction triggered it, (b) what method, if any, the analyst employed to continue his or her personal work, and (c) what kind of change they believe has occurred.

The survey provides three kinds of data: (1) a series of items that have been checked and therefore allow comparisons among analysts in relation to gender, age, and institute position; (2) brief written examples that supplement the more general answers and provide data that allow comparisons about the kinds of triggers for self-inquiry, the nature of the process, and the definitions of psychological change among analysts; and (3) telephone interviews with a smaller number of analysts, selected on the basis of the varying degrees of depth and complexity in these illustrations, which allowed a more intensive examination of the analysts' process in all the areas described. Three hundred and ninety-nine analysts responded to the questionnaire; 206 provided written examples, and 26 from the latter group were interviewed. (Complete results of this study are presented in Kantrowitz, 1996.)

The current chapter uses one analyst's interview to illustrate the impact of the patient on the analyst. I will demonstrate the parallels between the effect of the therapeutic process on the patient and on the analyst. I will investigate the nature and extent of the influence of the analytic process on the analyst to illuminate the contribution of various factors as agents of change. I hope to show how we can extend our understanding of how psychological development builds on analytic work and continues after formal analysis ends.

Studying the effect of patient-analyst match provides a means to consider the factors that impede or facilitate psychological growth (Kantrowitz, 1986; Kantrowitz et al., 1989; Kantrowitz, Katz, & Paolitto, 1990c). Overlapping characteristics or conflicts, a similarity of values, attitudes, or beliefs in patent and analyst, often result in "blind spots" that prevent certain areas from receiving analytic inquiry. Differences along these same dimensions may pose another kind of interference. Too little resonance can result in an experience of affective distance and a failure of understanding and communication. Fortunately, when these similarities and differences become the center of analytic attention, both participants may learn a great deal. For the analyst, the recognition of areas of overlap or tension offers the opportunity to reconsider and potentially rework previously neglected or partially resolved aspects of the self (Kantrowitz, 1992, 1993a, b, c, 1995).

What evolves in any analysis, although this is to some extent shaped by the character and conflicts of the two participants, is not predetermined but context dependent. The interaction of the specific character and conflicts of the two participants will bring out different aspects in each. Since the patient provides the material that is to be the focus of the work, it is likely that an analysis conducted by a skilled analyst with no blind spot in the patient's central area of conflict will address the most troublesome areas. The depth and range of exploration and development in other arenas, however, will vary depending on the particular patient-analyst pair. For the analyst, however, the areas of personal conflict or distress that are revived and explored are dependent more on the overlap with the particular patient; therefore, some analyses more than others contribute to the development of further self-understanding and growth.

It is in the context of countertransference reactions that the analyst's participation in the analytic process most parallels the patient's. Examples of transference-countertransference engagements therefore provide the best illustrations of the therapeutic impact of analysis on the analyst.

In the example that follows, an analyst recounts his experience of self-discovery, the impact his patient has had on him, the reverberations of his insights, and his perceptions of the psychological changes in himself, both professional and personal, that have emerged as a result of his work with this patient. The analyst describes how primitive rage and terror in his patient led to similar experiences in himself. These powerful feelings when unearthed in the analyst helped him toward a new understanding of his past and a new sense of security and confidence in himself.

One analyst's account

The patient was an "intimidating," "explosive" man of powerful intellect and temper. The analyst described him as being much smarter than himself. He treated the analyst with "a narcissistic indifference" to his state and expressed an explosive rage toward him. The analyst, after a long period of distancing himself from the patient's anger by an "icy" withdrawal, because initially he felt unable to withstand its intensity, found himself able to allow the patient's fury to build without "interrupting or defusing it." The analyst knew he had a tendency to "become cold inside" and not let himself feel in response to fear, and he worked consciously to not deaden his own response to the patient. When he would start to feel this "coldness," he would ask himself why he was needing to do this. The questioning helped him not to withdraw.

Once able to overcome his icy response, he came to feel a rage and terror in response to his patient's behavior that he had "never knowingly experienced anywhere else." He found himself going to the mirror after sessions with this patient and realized later that he was "struggling to feel if [he] existed in the face of the [patient's] total refusal to see and accept [him] in any way as a separate person." The analyst was literally checking to see if he was still whole and still existed; he was experiencing the power of the patient's rage as shattering and fragmenting.

The analyst had not had this kind of patient while he was himself in analysis; the level of intensity was greater than anything he had previously known. "Most of the initial working through was done running [jogging] and obsessing and thinking" about why he was "wasting [his] time with this patient. And working it out over and over again until it became more powerful and less fragmenting personally."

As he became better able to tolerate this experience, he could begin to think more about what went on in the patient. He came to understand that this "terror" was what the patient had experienced growing up. The patient had long used his explosive rage to keep others away. Now, as he became aware that his analyst was less "blown away by the rage," the patient too became less afraid of destroying everyone and everything else and became better able to stay with his feelings.

The analyst realized that it was only by facing his urge to disconnect that he could stop himself from "going cold" with the patient. When he did go cold, he had no idea what was going on for his patient. Once able to let himself feel the terror, he gradually found himself able to bring in pieces of his own history. "Whatever... the experience would be filled in with, either a memory, more genetic material, a kind of fuller understanding of something [he'd] done all his life, it got filled in mosaic-wise over time." He came to the realization that "disconnecting and becoming cold" were "habitual ways" in which he had dealt with conflicts similar to those he experienced with this patient. Having reached these understandings about himself, the work with the patient proceeded without these intense reactions on the analyst's part. Toward the end of this patient's analysis, the analyst's father died.

During the first phase of the patient's termination process, the work had seemed unremarkable to the analyst, and he was feeling complacent. Then the patient "began to talk about being very angry with [him] in a way he hadn't been." He talked about the analyst "not being with him." At first, the analyst listened "relatively complacently." He thought he knew that what was going on was a repetition of an aspect of the patient's early experience with his mother; it was an expected part of the mourning process. But as the patient "continued to complain rather stridently" and "was filled with rage," saying the analyst "just wasn't with him," something about the nature of his complaint suddenly took on a different quality. "It wasn't just a repetition; there was something happening between [them] that made [the analyst] more curious about what was going on." He became aware that his complacency was "kind of peculiar"—he wasn't feeling empathic at all; it was "no big deal." That was not how he usually felt when someone was terminating. This recognition resulted in his feeling "something literally lift" inside of him, and he became "overwhelmed with sadness." Until that moment, he hadn't recognized the degree to which he had been fending off a lot of his own grief about his father's death and his own "sadness about this guy's terminating." They had been through an enormous amount together, and he had learned an enormous amount from him, "so there was this kind of dual hit." It struck him that in many ways he had a countertransference to the patient because the patient's way of relating was not all that different from that of the analyst's father—"so who had the transference and who had the countertransference at times was a good question."

Once the analyst had this realization, without his saying a word, the patient relaxed and said, "You're with me now." There followed from that a whole series of sessions about a person, very important to the patient, who emotionally withdrew whenever he disapproved of the patient.

In the course of describing his reactions and discoveries about himself through work with this patient, the analyst came to a new realization. He saw that he had had a father transference to this patient:

> I'm wondering if I have to retract my statement about never having had this kind of rage before consciously, because what I was just thinking is that maybe this was some of the rage I had with my dad, who in my eyes was very powerful and was built like this guy. He also carried a monumental intellect and there was no way I could hold a candle to him.

These factors made the analyst feel like a little boy in the patient's presence. The analyst had not consciously been aware of this aspect of his experience before recounting it in the interview. The link to the experience with his father when he was a child emerged as a new discovery: "This is something that has just come to me now. What I've become aware of is just how much of a transference I had to this person."

The analyst knew that something very important had shifted for him; after his work with this patient, "a kind of primal terror of the other is no longer so easily evoked" in him. He feels his sense of his "own separateness is much firmer now." He can now "sit with patients who want to obliterate [him] and not feel obliterated." He no longer needs to "disconnect" from this kind of patient in order to feel intact. He also has "a keener sense" of when feelings of discomfort are coming from himself, and so is less likely to incorrectly view these feelings as projected from patients.

Changes also occurred in his intimate relationships. He finds he has "much more tolerance" for his own affects and "more ability to reflect on them." When he was growing up, his "family had been unexpressive of affect," except for his explosive father, and "strong affective displays had been disquieting" to him. He now is "much less reactive to the emotionality" of members of his adult family. Subjectively, he feels he can be "more intimate." His wife notes the difference and appreciates that he is "less reactive."

The analyst was aware that analyzing this patient had made a very strong impact on him; this awareness of changes in himself was what had led him to volunteer to be interviewed. However, it was only in the process of reporting on these changes that he connected the experience with this patient to his childhood feelings in relation to his father.

Although this analyst made the particular discovery about himself in the context of talking to me for the purpose of my research, this kind of self-discovery is what analysts frequently find when they engage in mutual supervision or more informally discuss their clinical work with a trusted colleague-friend (Kantrowitz, 1996, 1999, 2009).

Discussion

In this transference-countertransference interaction, the analyst experienced his patient's impact on him. Several parts of a therapeutic process occurred for the analyst as well as the patient. I shall now trace the process of therapeutic action for this analyst.

Awareness of the analyst's personal engagement is most often ushered in by a recognition that a personal conflict has been stirred. Once the analyst becomes aware of an internal struggle or an area that requires deeper exploration, the analyst engages in a process that parallels the patient's—in both, a disquieting inner experience needs to be understood. For many analysts, familiar defensive operations are what first alert them to a need for self-scrutiny. This analyst first perceives his disequilibrium by the appearance of a familiar feeling of withdrawnness and becoming "cold"; it warns him that some old issue is diverting him from his work. This recognition is sufficient to decrease his defensive response of withdrawal.

The process of analyzing defenses is usually the first step undertaken in analytic work with patients once an atmosphere of relative safety is established. Sometimes, however, an intense affective reaction to the analyst comes to the fore more powerfully than does a recognition of defense. Under these circumstances, instead of a gradual unfolding, patient and analyst are plunged into an affective engagement that catches both by surprise. The transference rather than the resistance to the transference claims center stage. The patient has experienced or enacted the very thing in early development that was most frightening, but has done so before patient or analyst has enough information to understand what is occurring. Analysis of defensive retreats must take place at a later point. Although rarely is the analyst in a position that is exactly parallel to that of the patient, for this analyst the comparability is greater than usual. He recognizes that his frozen state is a defense against a potentially overwhelming affective reaction. Aware of his defensive retreat, he allows himself to be open to his affective response and finds himself flooded by almost overwhelming affects he at first does not understand.

Personal analysis should have informed analysts about their own conflicts and defenses. The reality is that some analyses have informed analysts more than others. Work with patients when they stir these conflicts may lead analysts back for further treatment, though many analysts find that "confessing and confiding" to a trusted colleague can be of sufficient aide to quiet the intensity of such reactions.

When intense reactions occur in relation to a patient, analysts most often have a familiarity with the personal historical sources that are being reevoked. Relatively quickly, memories of related past events or interactions can be brought to the analyst's mind. These reflections, along with insight previously achieved, provide a perspective that prevents the analyst from being as flooded or confused as the patient is when caught unawares by a transference reaction. Recognition of the activation of familiar defensive reactions also stimulates self-exploration. In this instance, the analyst recognizes as familiar the pattern of his responses to fear, but not until much later does he discover the early experience that shaped his fear. Caught in a countertransference reaction, analysts experience responses to their patients that are totally discrepant with their expectable analytic selves. They lose temporarily their position of empathy with the patient's struggle and respond instead as if the patient were a threat. This analyst, once he has relinquished his initial defensive stance, then faces such a situation, experiencing his countertransference rage and terror in relation to his patient.

In countertransference reactions or enactments, the analyst's cognitive control is diminished. The analyst must then affectively step back and reflect on what in the interaction has stirred this response. Stepping back and reflecting are skills the analyst employs to help the patient gain perspective on what transpires between them. Here the analyst needs to activate these skills on his own behalf. To deepen his insight, the analyst uses what he sees and what he knows about both his patient and himself. In exploring his countertransference, the analyst progressively gathers data: first from his response to the patient, next from the exploration of memories from the past, and then from the placement of what is learned against what he knows about himself and his mode of relating and working in the present. While the experience is affectively intense, the process usually remains cognitively controlled.

The recognition of defenses and conflicts (or other states of distress) is a cognitive aspect of analytic work. Insight into the motives and manifestations of their reactions enables patients and analysts alike to attain some perspective on themselves. Insights can both stimulate and consolidate psychic shifts. Perspective serves to decrease affective flooding and self-criticism. These factors are likely to modify systems of belief, but they are unlikely do so in any profound way unless other object-related affective conditions prevail. The containing and consolidating function provided by communication to an emotionally important person is a crucial dimension contributing to the power of analytic work.

New integrations can occur in the context of a relationship in which a person feels safe and understood. Our concept of therapeutic alliance is based on this assumption (Greenson, 1967). In their personal analysis, analysts have not only learned about themselves; they have also developed the skills to do analytic work, the most notable being the ability to associate freely. It is therefore not so surprising that they would be able to continue their emotional growth and deepen their understanding of themselves as new and different situations arise, such as the affect-laden issues with which their patients confront them.

Analysts are aware of the necessity to establish conditions of safety for their patients. If their patients are to be free to hate, love, and fear them, they must be able to trust them enough to do so. The situation for the analyst again is different. Analysts may well come to trust their patients, but they expect and, in the context of wishing an increased freedom of expression for them, welcome the openness and intensity of the affects, both negative and positive, that are directed toward them. The analyst expects the patient to contain actions, but not the expression of feelings. In contrast, the analyst expects to be able to contain both actions and the shape and intensity with which his or her own feelings are expressed to the patient. Once less defended, this analyst was initially "blown away" by his reaction to his patient and believed that his patient was preconsciously attuned to this fact; however, he did not enact this response to his patient in any blatant way. Nonetheless, the analyst's "coldness," the suddenness of his "feeling overwhelmed," and his unawareness of the connection of his experience of his patient to childhood events with his father all indicate a relative loss of control on the analyst's part. At moments of the analyst's countertransference enactments in this case or others, the analyst's loss of control may not initially be beneficial to the patient. Under these circumstances, patients may not feel safe enough to proceed with their work. Only if the analyst can use the enactment to inform himself about himself, his patient, and their interaction is the enactment of therapeutic benefit. Ultimately, this analyst was able to keep the treatment "safe enough" for his patient, though it took considerable time and self-reflective work before the analyst felt safe.

Caught by intense affective reactions, patients often talk with others about what they are experiencing in analysis. Often they do so to dilute the intensity of the analytic work. For the patient, this may be a resistance to something developing in the transference; looked at from an adaptive perspective, it may be a way to enable the patient to remain in analysis without becoming overwhelmed by its intensity. The relative weighting of defensive and adaptive aspects undoubtedly varies both for each patient and for each situation.

It is not surprising that analysts have similar experiences. For the analyst, too, talking with others may be a way to dilute the intensity of transference-countertransference interactions and to gain some perspective on them; at times, however, this may detract from what might be experienced and learned in the analytic involvement with the patient. When countertransference reactions are very intense, confiding in a trusted person may be an ongoing accompaniment to the analytic work. All the analysts interviewed who offered examples of countertransference as the source of personal recognitions describe discussing their self-exploration and discoveries with at least one other person. Most communications of personal struggle stimulated by analytic work (or by self- discoveries attained from it) are initiated to help the analyst contain the affective reaction, gain perspective on the experience, or provide a reality check on self-perception.

This analyst reports the containing and sustaining function of describing his frightening experiences to the two people he believed knew and understood him best. Finding a means of diluting his response of feeling "blown away" was essential, if he was to manage his affect. He actively reflected on what was occurring within him; in addition, he talked with his wife and a close friend. His patient was not the topic; his reaction and state were what he described and tried to understand in their presence. They knew him intimately, and their listening presence meant he was not alone with his intense affect. Sharing his experience enabled him to contain it, to reflect more deeply, and to be able, now somewhat less flooded by what was stirred in him, to refocus his understanding of his patient. Later these same confidants provided confirmation of his own sense of personal change.

Working through issues involves a process of making unconscious experiences conscious, lessening affective charge, and gradually reintegrating previously unacceptable or disavowed aspects of the self.

This process occurs in different ways and with different degrees of intensity and depth for different analysts. The two steps described so far are (1) the analyst's private self-reflections and (2) the sharing of conflict, affect distress, insight, and work in progress with a colleague or psychologically informed friend. Some analysts engage only in the first step, and some are more systematic in these explorations than are others. Some, but not all, analysts find that the shared exploration of their self-scrutiny promotes and consolidates their understanding. A third step occurs in the actual work with the patient. It is likely to occur simultaneously with one or both of the other methods for attaining understanding and affect management.

Many of the analysts interviewed describe a process that involves a reverberation between the patient's and the analyst's issues that occurs during the actual analytic work. Since each analyst has his own specific constellation of characterological and conflictual issues, of which only a particular array will be stimulated, depending on the nature of the "match" with the patient, the content that is reworked will vary for each analyst. The safety of the analytic setting permits a regressive process enabling usually suppressed or repressed affects and fantasies to become available for both patient and analyst. The "play" that becomes possible in the context of such safety creates an opportunity to rediscover identifications and to become more conscious of their formation. Then, in relation to a new and different object, shifts in self- and object representations become possible. Concomitantly, shifts occur also in defense, in availability or tolerance of affect, and (more consciously) in attitudes, values, or beliefs.

For this analyst, affect availability/tolerance is worked through directly in the analysis with his patient. Once the analyst interrupts his defensive reaction, he experiences powerful and frightening affects parallel to those the patient is struggling to understand and master. The analyst not only allows himself to experience intensely frightening affects but also learns to tolerate and not be "blown away" by them. This change in the analyst's capacity is then paralleled by the patient's increased capacity to stay with his affects as his own rage and terror abate. Both patient and analyst learn more about each affective state (and what triggers it) in the course of this exploration of self and other in which they are powerfully engaged. As the process evolves, rage and terror are experienced alternately by each participant in relation to the other. Although the analyst does not detail the process between them, what occurs seems to be a mutual exploration of what each could tolerate from the other. This exploration was affectively enacted, not just put into words. The analyst's experience in the treatment, if not as powerful as the patient's, was close to it. While the patient's reactions are re-embedded in their historical context, the analyst's at this point are not. For the analyst, it is a "here and now" reworking that takes place.

The psychological changes that attend successful analysis occur in areas that are embedded in the process. Broadly defined, these areas are intrapsychic, interpersonal, and work-related. In each of these areas, shifts in defenses, availability, and tolerance of affects, and self- or object representations, as well as more conscious shifts in attitudes, values, or beliefs, play a role.

To understand the curative aspect of psychoanalysis, it seems necessary to tease apart two foci of this work. One involves affect availability and tolerance, the other object relations. The non-interpretive aspects of the analytic work that revolve around these two variables are experiences of the patient that have many direct parallels for the analyst.

The analysts in this survey all describe slightly different content or foci when considering the question of therapeutic action; nonetheless, there is a commonalty in their approaches. Most analysts agree that it is necessary to reengage repeatedly with painful or disappointing experiences or states from the past and to reexperience over and over the consequences of unconscious conflicts, fantasies, defenses, and affects in the context of the present relationship with the analyst. Most, but not all, analysts place a value on insight; they believe that cognitive clarity, an intellectual appreciation of unconscious determinants, provides increased freedom. Most, but not all, believe it is important that the patient be able to articulate these insights. All analysts believe that for analysis to have an impact, what is learned must be emotionally alive. Most analysts believe also that reopening painful past experiences requires a regression.

Learning to self-regulate, to tolerate frustration and modulate affect, is a developmental task most often mastered during the latency years. It is not infrequent that intellectual precocity interferes with a fuller development of this capacity. The precocious child, for whom many intellectual tasks are easily and quickly grasped, is spared the frustrations usually encountered in mastering them. As a result of this decreased exposure to enduring frustration, the skills involved in mastering and containing tension and intense affects are less developed in such individuals. Analysis offers these analysands the opportunity to attain these skills (Gedo, 1979; Kohut, 1984). This is accomplished by what Kris (1990b) has called an alliance of self-control and what Modell (1986, 1993) has referred to as affect retraining. We think of this as the analyst helping to provide containment for intolerable affect as the patient comes gradually to tolerate increasingly stronger affects without fleeing or becoming flooded.

Analysts generally can be assumed to be considerably ahead of their patients in the acquisition of the capacity for affect availability and modulation. They have had their own analysis, in which, even if self-regulation has not been a direct focus of the work, the experience of frustrated wishes must have been endured. So even if, in the most idyllic (and unlikely) scenario, life circumstances or choices have limited the amount of frustration the analyst has had to withstand, practice with tolerating disappointment and frustrated wishes is not entirely lacking. In addition, in the current analytic situation, the degree of frustration and disappointment experienced will likely be much greater for the patient than for the analyst. Although the analyst, like the patient, may experience disappointment and frustration during the course of their work, these occurrences are not part of the treatment design; the material to be the focus of attention is properly the patient's. All of these factors contribute to making the analyst's tolerance of frustration and affect modulation much less an issue in the analytic setting than they are for the patient.

In the analysis being discussed, the analyst more deeply experiences the intensity of affective distress than is commonly the case. The analyst permits himself to regress in this manner in order to help his patient. He knows that if he maintains his defensive distancing, he will not become flooded—but he will also not be able to understand or help his patient. He therefore faces and overcomes his affect inhibition and gives himself over to the process. He trusts himself enough to take this risk. The patient began analysis with a transference in which he perceived his analyst as an enemy to be destroyed. He was the kind of patient Winnicott (1965) described as ruthlessly aiming to annihilate the analyst and Bird (1972) described as having wishes to actually, not symbolically, inflict harm on the analyst. At first, it seemed that the patient might be able to destroy the treatment, if not the analyst himself, because his analyst backed out. The analyst's ability to acknowledge his defenses and face himself reversed this outcome.

The analyst believes that the patient had been able to perceive that his analyst had backed away from him in response to his powerful rage. The analyst believes also that the patient preconsciously registered both the analyst's terror and his ability to withstand it. Once the analyst no longer retreated, the patient was no longer "blown away" either, since he could then be less afraid of the effect his rage might have on the analyst. The patient found, it seems, that the analyst was neither destroyed nor about to destroy him. The patient was then able to experience and express feelings other than rage and to explore and come to understand these affect states.

The analyst, for his part, powerfully revived, though he did not cognitively register, early childhood experiences of terror and rage. He reacted and recognized his reactions, but did not know the origin of his terror. Now a grown man with the physical, intellectual, and emotional strength he lacked as a child, he was determined to face and not flee his terror. Why was he willing to do this? Both professional and personal factors contribute to the answer and in this instance may not be totally separable.

He is committed to helping his patient, a commitment based on professional ideals. These ideals, of course, are shaped by the personal values that led to his choice of profession. This analyst has an ideal of personal honesty and courage that is reflected in his determination not to withdraw in the face of his experienced terror. Undoubtedly, based on his later understanding that this experience was a repetition of early terror and retreat, his determination also reflects his unconscious need to master this childhood trauma. The wish to master is a powerful motive in shaping behavior.

In their transference-countertransference engagements, this patient-analyst pair struggled with their mutual terror and rage. The analyst, to be sure, was much more in control of its expression. Patient and analyst emerged changed from a combination of insight into their defensive maneuvers and a sense of safety and trust achieved through having survived their intense emotional entanglement. The power of the treatment was in their interaction. In their work, the analyst was overcome by an intense affective reaction that paralleled the patient's, and both participants learned to withstand and ultimately regulate their affective experiences. The analyst "feels" the familiarity of his affective distress and reactive pattern of coping, but does not recover its historical context until the interview. He withstands the affective intensity by focusing on his understanding of personality organization, by recognizing his defenses and their repetitive nature, and by a determination to master his fear and help his patient master his. Most important, his sense of increased strength and ability to cope come from seeing that he is doing so. His patient perceives his increased strength and is calmed by it. This gradual calming of the patient further increases the analyst's sense of strength, effectiveness, and mastery. He illustrates the idea that changed behavior precedes insight.

Increased tolerance of painful affect is not something that occurs outside the context of a relationship. Shifts in affect availability and tolerance may precede or follow shifts in self- and object representations. A change in the analyst's capacity to tolerate and modulate intense affect and a change in self-representation are related. A greater sense of one's ability to be self-regulating increases a sense of competence and self-esteem. A new integration, which includes changes in self- and object representations, occurs after the analyst confronts and struggles with the modulation of his aggression.

Change in the analyst's affect availability and tolerance facilitated a change in his self- and object representations. Not only was there a mastery of early terror, there was also an unconscious reintegration of his sense of himself in relation to his identification with his father. The analyst, in choosing to become an analyst, has selected a field of work in which he actively seeks to help others ease their pain and fear—again suggesting he has selected a career that supports a mastery of early pain. Unconsciously, this choice may have also been based on a negative identification with his representation of his father: he, the analyst, would ease fears by analyzing and mastering them, rather than creating them, as he believed (unconsciously) his father had created them in him. As the patient explored the feelings that lay behind his rage, the analyst was able not only to feel less afraid but also to consciously empathize more with his patient and, unconsciously, with his father. Once the analyst perceived his patient differently—no longer as just a terrifying bully—he must also, unconsciously, perceive his father differently. An interpersonal terror then became understood as an intrapsychic terror, and paralyzing fear was replaced by anxiety that could be grappled with and understood.

The transference-countertransference is viewed as the dynamic pivot facilitating psychological change. Psychoanalysts have a theory of why the affective reliving of dangerous or disappointing relationships in the context of a new relationship with the analyst creates the opportunity for psychological change in the patient. We have theorized that the understanding of past fears and disappointments, through both their reexperience and their interpretation in relation to the analyst, permits an internal reshaping to occur. All this is contingent on the analyst's becoming an emotionally important figure in the patient's life.

While analysts are usually deeply involved with their patients, we do not assume that a patient is likely to have the centrality in an analyst's life that the analyst has in the patient's. Indeed, if this should occur in any sustained way, there are likely to be untoward consequences for the treatment. However, the degree of personal involvement an analyst feels with a patient varies with each analytic pair. The more areas of personal overlap, perhaps especially when these overlaps are in areas of shared difficulties, the more intense the analyst's personal involvement is likely to become.

Under the conditions of this increased emotional engagement, transference-countertransference interactions are likely to be more heated and to have a more powerful impact on the two participants. While it is the patient whose difficulties are the focus, the analyst becomes a participant in the struggle as the patient's transference intensifies. The analyst increasingly feels, not only understands, what the patient has been describing. Sometimes this affective understanding is in empathic resonance, but sometimes it is not. Both the position of being "inside" the patient's experience and the position of being "outside" in the role of "the other" provide data about the patient and oneself. Allowing oneself to actively participate in the affective life of a patient means being open to one's own affects, fantasies, hopes, and fears.

Although the asymmetry of the relationship means that the analyst is by definition in a "safer" position than the patient, the former, once this emotional openness is permitted, engages in an emotional risk.

Without this emotional risk, no psychological change can take place. To be truly engaged is to allow oneself to be vulnerable to another. The relationship benefits the analyst beyond the cognitive recognition and clarification of personal issues. Once engaged, the interaction that occurs between patient and analyst provides the analyst an opportunity to change.

Such engagement is not lightly undertaken. It requires trust in one's capacity to withstand the intensity of the patient's affects and the intensity of what these fantasies, wishes, and fears evoke in oneself. The degree of freedom the analyst can permit is dependent on the extent of this trust and also on the extent to which the analyst believes the patient can be trusted. The analyst's spontaneity and emotional openness are likely to increase the more the analyst believes in the patient's capacity to express freely the thoughts, feelings, and fantasies stimulated by the analyst, the analyst's interventions, and the analytic situation. And while it is not the patient's obligation to maintain confidentiality in relation to anything learned directly or indirectly about the analyst or in relation to what transpires between them, the manner in which the patient deals with such material undoubtedly affects the analyst's sense of safety and freedom in the analytic setting.

If the patient's psychological change comes about, at least in part, because what goes on between analyst and patient is different from what the patient has previously experienced—that is, frightening or disappointing expectations about the other and/or oneself are not repeated, or if repeated are reworked, re-understood and then relived with a different outcome—then something parallel is likely to occur for the analyst. The patient may become an old/new object for the analyst in parallel with the analyst's being an old/new object for the patient.

If the analyst is really emotionally engaged, and if this engagement is around an area of mutual difficulty, the interaction between patient and analyst entails a mutual reworking of past expectations. The analyst not only sees and experiences his patient's reliving of these expectations in relation to him, but has the opportunity to be in both roles and to appreciate affectively, therefore, the complexity and ambiguity of these experiences. At one moment the analyst is identified with the patient, as in this instance the analyst's countertransference terror and rage become understood as his patient's earlier states, at another moment he is experiencing himself as the perpetrator of this pain. When he experiences himself as on the "outside," he sees himself being represented as causing all this distress. The analytic situation allows him to see, and experience, both points of view—the patient's perspective and the perspective ascribed by the patient to "the other." This analyst's fluctuation between the experience of rage and terror ultimately facilitates his developing empathy for his patient and perhaps for himself as a child, which deepened as he was more fully able to move back and forth between these states.

The analyst's trial identification with the patient, which enables the analyst to explore empathically the patient's difficulties, also provides a vicarious experience of these issues for the analyst. When an analyst enters a patient's world in this way and tries to understand and grapple with the patient's experience, if the issues the patient is struggling with parallel issues for the analyst, the process that results offers the analyst a chance to work on these difficulties in a once-removed fashion.

The analyst holds the patient's construction of self, of the analyst, and of the analytic relationship and juxtaposes this against his or her own perspective on self, the patient, and the relationship. The analyst does this not to determine which is "true" but rather to understand further each of these different views. The discrepancies are likely to be the areas where important work occurs for both participants.

What is being played out interpersonally is also intrapsychically represented; these two perspectives—of patient and of analyst—are externalizations of intrapsychic representations. What we see as an interpersonal struggle is also an intrapsychic conflict. Therefore, as patient and analyst become more empathic, understanding, and open to these multiple and at times conflicting points of view, complexity and ambiguity increase and the sense of conflict diminishes. Disowned aspects of the self are able to be reintegrated because they are no longer experienced as so frightening; they are experienced as less dangerous because they are no longer seen as so black and white. The reintegration creates a new synthesis, with slightly expanded capacities for self-acceptance and the acceptance of others and their differences.

Self- and object representations shift and consolidate during the course of working with patients. For this analyst, only in the termination, which coincided with his father's death, did he affectively experience how deeply attached and sad he felt at the prospect of his patient's leaving. In parallel, he experienced how attached he felt to his father and how sad he was at his loss.

This analyst is one for whom sharing his thoughts and feelings, being open with his intimate experiences, is not a rare occurrence. He talks freely with his wife and with a close friend. The insight he attained in the course of the interview may have emerged because he discussed the patient in greater analytic detail than he might have with his wife and friend, who were not analysts.

While the analyst does not know me well, we have discussed some mutual interests previously, and he views me as someone who would understand, respect, and respond positively to the ideas and experiences he conveyed. Before the interview he had the powerful experience of shifts within himself, but during our talk they became newly understood in an historical context. It was in the context of feeling trust and safety in relation to recounting the example that he made the cognitive link between his experience with his patient and with his father, and recovered the memory of early terror. While it is reasonable to conceptualize his response to me as "transferential," I am not sure that such a conceptualization enhances or is necessary for an appreciation of his discovery.

In the context of sharing his strong affective experience, the relational aspect came more into focus for him. What occurred for this analyst in the interview is not a psychological change—based on his description, the shift in him had already occurred. What he achieved in the interview was a deepened understanding of what had taken place for him and why it had been so emotionally gripping. This insight will further consolidate the changes that have occurred, helping the analyst to more fully reintegrate past experiences with present ones.

The analyst reports that his experience of working with this patient changed his tolerance for affect, in both his professional and his personal life. In relation to his work, he no longer finds himself becoming cold inside, disconnecting, or experiencing primal terror in response to patients' rage. He is better able to recognize and own his discomfort and less likely to assume it is a projective identification. In his personal life, he is no longer so disquieted by intense affect and volatility. He finds himself much more comfortable with the emotional expressiveness of his family, much more tolerant of his own affects, and much more able to experience a sense of intimacy. His wife has spontaneously corroborated his observations about his decreased re-activity to the expression of intense affect.

Although it is not possible to know how deep or far-reaching the transformations are when analysts report shifts in their attitudes, values, or beliefs, these phenomena have a conscious representation; at that level, we can accept that in this instance the analyst has changed. But whether earlier attitudes, values, or beliefs continue to persist un-consciously and influence his reactions and behaviors in ways he is unaware of cannot be assessed from this material.

I am not suggesting that when patient and analyst share an area of difficulty the analytic work will result in identical psychological changes in each or even changes in the same general areas. For all the similarities and overlaps, the differences between the two mean that each will make use of the work in his or her own way. What a particular interaction means for the patient and what he or she learns from it may be very different from what the analyst learns from it, even if there was some similarity in their initial construction of its meaning. In this instance, both patient and analyst experienced terror and rage. We know that the analyst came to both master and understand his response in the context of his personal history. The patient likely has learned something similar, but he may also have learned something very different, something more relevant to his particular history and dynamic organization.

In every analytic situation that succeeds, some form of intense emotional engagement occurs at some time in the analysis. When the affective intensity is high, as occurs in analytic dyads in whom mutual erotic transference-countertransference is deeply experienced, or, as in this instance, where the terror and rage of primary aggression are shared, the mutual change and growth may be very striking. How much of this the analyst allows to occur in him- or herself would seem to depend not only on similarity of conflict areas but on similarity of values. This does not mean that the patient must actually resemble the analyst but only that the analyst is able to find a place of respect and regard for the patient. Most analysts report that the longer they work with patients, the more these feelings of regard increase as they come to better understand what their patients have struggled with and why they have come to the solutions they have chosen. The more the analyst comes to know and respect the patient, the more the analyst trusts the patient and is able unconsciously to move closer and to be more open and vulnerable. I am not suggesting that this is expressed in the content of what the analyst says, though at times it may; rather, I am alluding to something nonverbal that is communicated in subtle ways. This is an area of our work that deserves further consideration.

In our attempts to elucidate the nature of therapeutic action, it becomes clear that many factors play a role, though their relative importance remains to be determined. The recent emphasis on the experience of analysts during analysis has allowed us to begin documenting how the analytic process affects both participants, to the extent they open themselves to it.

Note

1 Many experienced analysts have not chosen to become training and supervising analysts.

Chapter 10

The role of the preconscious in psychoanalysis

Currently there is theoretical debate over whether psychoanalysis is a one- or two-person psychology and whether interpersonal or intrapsychic factors are central to psychic change. Here I will propose, as have a few other analysts already (Ghent, 1989; Hoffman, 1983, 1994), that these are false dichotomies. Both the individual intrapsychic dynamics of the patient and the interplay of the intrapsychic organizations of both patient and analyst, as given expression in affective, behavioral interchanges, influence the shape and nature of change. I will discuss the relationship between intrapsychic and interpersonal factors and demonstrate their linkage in the preconscious attunement between patient and analyst. This preconscious connection provides a segue whereby the intrapsychic experience of both participants becomes manifest and conscious in their interaction. I will illustrate the inevitability of countertransference and subjectivity that become conscious for the analyst once he or she is open to preconscious experience. I will argue that the creative use of this mode of working requires a self-discipline and continuing consciousness of maintaining one's role as analyst in order to keep the treatment safe and facilitate the process of change.

Analysts have increasingly come to view the therapeutic action of psychoanalysis as occurring in transference-countertransference interactions. The recent focus on these engagements has heightened our awareness of the impact of interpersonal factors. As has occurred often in the history of psychoanalysis, however, a tendency toward polarization has developed, giving rise to groups of opposing theories. Some analysts (Dorpat & Miller, 1992; Greenberg, 1986;

Mitchell, 1993) view the relational aspect as central, while others (Natterson & Friedman, 1995; Stolorow & Atwood, 1992) concentrate on the intersubjective aspects of the work. Still other analysts (Gill, 1982; Schwaber, 1990, 1992) stay more rooted in intrapsychic phenomena, emphasizing the internal shifts in patients that result from their responses to the analyst's communications.

While Freud's focus was on intrapsychic conflict, he did not ignore the influence of external factors in the development of character. Freud (1912a) proposed that characterological adaptations, the methods one employs to obtain what is wished, and the particular nature of what is desired are all shaped by a combination of constitutional and environmental factors.[1] Today many, if not most, analysts (Colarusso & Nemiroff, 1981) would add that external factors occurring later in development have an ongoing influence on both the mode and method of conduct and the goals and desires of any person. What I wish to emphasize is that a person's character and conflicts are the consolidation of a history of relationships and experiences as they were amalgamated on the basis of the individual's innate disposition. Environmental factors and goals that initially were external become internalized; in the process of internalization they are transformed, based on the innate characteristics of the individual, into the particular character and conflicts of the person. This individual's character and conflicts are then expressed in way of experiencing, processing, reacting, and responding in relation to later events and engagements.

Although Freud emphasized the constant repetition of the template established in early years, he too allowed for the impact of later experience. The transferences that develop to an analyst are capable of being modified, because patients create them based both on their own character and conflicts and on the real characteristics of the analyst. In the transference, patients play out their intrapsychic conflicts and/ or express their resistance to involvement with the analyst through their characterological patterns. They are transferring an intrapsychic representation into an interpersonal arena. The patient first treats the current situation intrapsychically as if it were from the past, and then experiences this construction as related to the analyst. In the replay, the analyst most often assumes the role of some aspect of important childhood figures. But such aspects are the representation not of actual figures from the past but of those people as internally represented by the patient based both on experience with them and on a particular innate disposition. While this aspect of the representation (say of the mother or father) might bear many characteristics that could be verified by others in the patient's world, there is also always the unique and specific way they are made part of each child. Transferences express and reveal the way in which affectively powerful interactions have been internalized. They convey a representation of a past way of relating, not the actual or whole figure from the past.

Identifications are formed through the child's taking in experiences of the self via interactions with caretakers, in which a sense of self is modified by how others see the child and reflect that view back. When these identifications are positive, the internalized characteristics are most often expressed in the individual's attitudes, values, and behaviors. But the situation is in fact much more complex, since a child might consciously admire some aspect of a parent but, because of some characteristic of their interaction (say a competitive aspect), be unable to take it in as part of the self. When the identifications are negative and conscious, they become models toward which the individual exerts active opposition; these negative models have qualities that the person consciously rejects as part of any self-representation.

Sometimes people are unaware that some of their attitudes, values, or behaviors are repellent to others. They blindly recreate previously distressing interactions or experiences of others, now with no conscious sense of distress or pain; they do not know or assume that things could be different, and the painful affect associated with these situations in the past is repressed or isolated. When these identifications are negative and unconscious, disavowal of unwanted, negative parts of the self may also occur. Then the individual may be critical or disdainful of these characteristics as observed in others, but may remain unaware of fighting any awareness of these aspects in oneself. Here I emphasize the projective aspect of transference.

In the treatment situation, the analyst is unconsciously scanned for whatever characteristics might be gleaned that support a view of him or her as similar to some internally pressing representation, owned or disowned by the patient. Thus the patient transfers intrapsychic aspects of the self to the interpersonal field. Part of what unfolds is conscious. The patient is aware of certain kinds of distress and frustration that are mobilized and given expression in relation to the analyst. Most often the patient is conscious, too, of some important sources of satisfaction previously known or sought that occur also in the analytic relationship. But alongside these consciously recognized patterns of pain and pleasure are the buried unconsciously representations of past, multifaceted interactions that are contained in what is transferred onto the analyst. In the course of analysis, if it is successful, these unconscious representations—the fantasies, affects, and ideas buried in repression—can resurface and eventually be understood through the associations stimulated by the present-day interchange with the analyst. The possibility that past experience in its conscious and unconscious aspects can be reevoked, reunderstood, and reworked toward a different psychological outcome pivots on the extent to which the analyst can be experienced as both an old and a new object for the patient (Loewald, 1960).

Patients bring with them a specific life history that through conscious and unconscious means they will try to relive and rework in the analysis. This replay is the invariant aspect of the transference, the characteristic that applies to all analyses, which would occur with any analyst. The variable aspect of the analysis is shaped by the character and conflicts of the particular analyst with whom the patient has chosen to work. Just as the genetic disposition of the child processes and reacts to the environmental influences in unique and specific ways, so the impact of the particular approach and style of the analyst, shaped by his or her own character and conflicts, influences the course of treatment. With the analytic pair, though not to the same extent as with parent and child, we see a constantly evolving, two-way system of interaction.

The analyst has a double role. There is a procedure to carry out, but the analyst too has an inner life. Though focused on patients' affects, ideas, fantasies, and interactions, and trained to keep one's own concerns off center stage, the analyst nonetheless, as someone with a unique set of personal characteristics and conflicts, will experience, process, and react to patients in a particular way. It could not be otherwise. Analysts' own training analyses have made them aware of their struggles and their typical means of defense and adaptation; their analyses have helped them rework and ameliorate the most troublesome aspects. Their analyses have also taught them a method by which to monitor and learn about themselves. Their formal training, especially supervision of analytic patients, has provided instruction and practice in the use of theory and technique to facilitate an analytic process.

With this experience comes an awareness of when their own issues intrude and interfere. These elements together place a constraint on the expression, in the treatment situation, of the analyst's inner life. But no training, however rigorous, eliminates the real characteristics of an analyst. Subjectivity is inevitable, as are residual conflicts. These factors affect perceptions, choice of focus, scrutiny of one area and avoidance of another, and tolerance of intensity around specific affects or affects in general. Responding to a patient on the basis of one's personal characteristics occurs in varying degrees with different analysts and, for each analyst, with different patients.

Development and repeated life experiences reinforce characterological strategies, defenses, methods of adaptation, and unconscious beliefs that may become adhesive. Nonetheless, our belief in analysis is based on the conviction that the psychic system is malleable if we can create certain conditions—for example, forces favoring the lifting of repression. When patient and analyst are affectively engaged, when the patient has come to trust in the analyst's basic benevolence, and when in this context the patient feels safe enough to lessen defenses, the modification of intrapsychic organization becomes possible. Resistance to engagement may at the outset be due to a socially expectable caution requiring that trust be earned, to a characterological wariness, or to unconscious fantasies that express an initial transference to the analyst.

If patient and analyst are able to overcome resistance to engagement and enter the exploration of the patient's central organizing difficulties, an intense affective engagement takes place. When analysis is successful, patient and analyst are able to see and understand previously unrecognized aspects of the patient. They see this change played out in their interactions; this is the interpersonal, relational aspect of analysis. Powerful emotional discoveries occur most often in the context of the analytic relationship. The patient does not just remember and reinterpret; the patient relives. But what is relived interpersonally is an expression of what has been consolidated intrapsychically, now modified by the impact of the analyst's real characteristics and skill in helping patients to understand their compromise formations and to tolerate previously unacceptable and unrecognized aspects of themselves. Thus, the current experience is different from that of the past. Because the analyst has come to be so affectively important, the patient must find a way to integrate these new characteristics within the self. In the interpersonal experience, the analyst has been given the role of an aspect of the self, an intrapsychic self- or object representation that may be positive or negative, avowed or disavowed. The role, played out with similarities and differences vis-à-vis the earlier representation, requires the patient to confront that representation and reconcile the cognitive and affective discrepancies. Because what is revealed and understood in the interpersonal context may be viewed as an externalization of intrapsychic conflict, it needs to be reintegrated intrapsychically.

It is not that the relationship is only an externalized repetition of the patient's internal conflicts. Were this so, the real characteristics of the analyst would have no bearing on the work. And were we to believe that, we would have less reason to be hopeful that change can occur. But neither is the analyst only a new object, different from the patient's frustrating and disappointing objects in the past. Frustration and disappointment, though most often represented as contained in the objects, are also invariably representations of aspects of the self. An image of oneself as disappointing contains within it an experience of one's having felt to have been a disappointment to another, even if that feeling was based primarily on fantasy. The analyst has been called on to give form to these representations so that the patient may better see and come to tolerate these aspects within the self. In light of all this, what occurs in an analysis must be discussed in terms of both interpersonal and intrapsychic representation; it is meaningless to consider one to the exclusion of the other. Both are ever present and intermingled. What is intrapsychic began as an interaction and then is replayed interactionally. This is what we mean by reliving in the transference.

Patients deeply engaged in analytic work have allowed themselves to be less defended, which means that in relation to the analyst they have modified their usual ways of hiding their vulnerability. Defenses less strongly maintained facilitate the emergence of associations that lead to unconscious material. Freud (1912b) stated that the analyst uses "the derivatives of the unconscious which are communicated to him to reconstruct that unconscious, which has determined the patient's free associations" (p. 116). To the extent to which analysts allow themselves to become emotional participants in this process, they also allow an increase in their own vulnerability in relation to the patient, at least during the analytic hour. Then analysts, like their patients, relinquish the usual defenses and resistances to facing and experiencing aspects of the other or of the self that are frightening or disappointing. This fuller acceptance of the analyst's self allows for a fuller view and acceptance of the patient (Kantrowitz, 1996).

Once it is granted that there are two characters and two sets of conflicts engaged in the analytic work, and that there is both intrapsychic and interpersonal impingement, we need to consider further the question of how change occurs. If it is inevitable that analysts are, like their patients, affectively stirred by the work and may develop countertransferences to them (Hoffman, 1992, 1994; Jacobs, 1991; Kantrowitz, 1996; McLaughlin, 1981), how does this affect our theory of therapeutic action? Attunement and Resonance?

Considerable attention has been given to the role of insight, of making the unconscious conscious (Arlow & Brenner, 1964; Blum, 1979;Eissler, 1953; Gray, 1990), and to affective cognitive discoveries (Blatt & Behrends, 1987; Chused, 1991; Loewald, 1979) that come about through transference-countertransference engagements and enactments. I wish to focus my attention on the preconscious aspect of this process, which, probably because it is difficult to describe, is seldom addressed. It is in the realm of preconscious communication that the interwovenness of intrapsychic and interpersonal phenomena becomes most apparent. Here the intrapsychic experience of the patient registers and is responded to by a correspondence or resonance in the intrapsychic experience of the analyst.

In designating this form of communication preconscious, I am referring to an area of experience in which phenomena, though not yet organized or consciously observed, are no longer repressed. I do not mean phenomena that are just temporarily out of awareness, such as a phone number. Rather, I am describing experiences that are registered without awareness but that can be brought into consciousness once attention is directed to them. Preconscious intrapsychic attunements provide segues between conscious awareness of affective, behavioral, and interpersonal engagements and unconscious affects, fantasies, and reactions intrapsychically represented in both patient and analyst. While these preconscious phenomena are not yet consciously shaped, their occurrence is based on some interpersonal engagement, which, should it become the center of analytic scrutiny, can usually be given conscious form.

Thus, preconscious experience forms the bridge both between conscious and unconscious phenomena[2] and between intrapsychic and interpersonal phenomena. The impact of the personal characteristics and conflicts of the analyst on the patient is often registered by the latter only preconsciously. Such recognitions, which are inevitably constructed preconsciously, or interpreted through the filter of the patient's intrapsychic representations, may have profound reverberations on the course and outcome of the treatment.

The mutual lessening of defenses by patient and analyst allows them to dip into preconscious aspects of themselves not usually accessible. When the work is going well, there is a resonance and flow to the process. Analysts such as Hoffman (1992), Gill (1982), McLaughlin (1981), and Schwaber (1981, 1987) have identified factors interfering with the development of this state and have suggested analytic stances likely to facilitate its occurrence. Some analysts have always been more open than others to the intrusion of their more undefended, primitive responses and work more readily with their preconscious. Preconscious attunement undoubtedly occurs more often with some patient-analyst pairs than with others, and occurs more often during some periods of the analytic work than in others. I have suggested that factors of patient-analyst match—temperament, character, conflict—may also facilitate or impede this work (Kantrowitz et al., 1989).

As the analytic process deepens, preconscious fantasies emerge. These are fantasies that are not directly in the individual's awareness, or that occur within it fleetingly, only to be suppressed. In contrast to unconscious fantasies, however, which remain outside of awareness even when attention is turned to them, preconscious fantasies become, when focused on, consciously available. The telling of a preconscious fantasy, which embodies derivatives from unconscious fantasies (Kris, 1950), makes it possible for the latter to be exposed.

How do we understand what happens in unconscious attunement? Freud (1912b) described the phenomenon as involving a transmission from one unconscious to another. However, I think this transmission of unconscious content is mediated through behavior that is pre-consciously registered. I am assuming here a developing attunement between patient and analyst in treatment that makes this kind of understanding possible. Even in our outside lives, when we feel safe and intimate, as in love relationships and some close friendships, this phenomenon can also occur. Under conditions of safety, emotional risks are taken which otherwise would not be. Each time the patient experiences greater freedom and closeness without an attendant experience (consciously or unconsciously anticipated) of danger or disappointment, the courage to risk again is increased and the willingness to expose and explore is strengthened.

But how can we illustrate what is not consciously represented? In a discussion of intuition, Kohut (1959) maintained that in situations in which analysts believed they had intuitively grasped some aspect that had not been made explicit, careful review revealed the presence of actual data on which they had built their understanding. These data, however, were not consciously registered. Since patients are always presenting more of themselves than we or they can recognize and understand at the time, this construction seems well-founded. Illustrating the unconscious reception of what is transmitted, however, poses a task which, though daunting, is essential that we attempt.

It is possible to offer examples of attunement and resonance that facilitate the patient's sense of being understood and the flow of associative material, but out of context it is unlikely to convey why this synchrony has developed. A patient mildly complains that her husband is urging her to dress in a more sexy manner. He wants her to wear lace underwear and sheer nightgowns. She rather likes the idea, doesn't really mind his slight pressure, but... Here the analyst, sensing the patient's state and the quality and extent of her discomfort, spontaneously speaks the line of the sentence left unspoken: "Where will it end?" The patient sighs, "Exactly," and then elaborates, with greater nuance and detail, the worries that are stirred, the memories revived.

Responses of this sort have referents that are recognizable. What had been registered that led me to complete my patient's thought in this manner? I had a context much greater than the words recorded here, from which my response immediately emerged. My detailed knowledge of my patient meant not only that I had much more information than was provided at the moment, information enabling me to contextualize her material, but that I also was familiar with the forms and nuances of her expression of affect. I had been attuned to a certain tone and timbre in her voice suggestive of tension, anxiety, possibly excitement. But none of these thoughts were consciously present when I spoke. Only in retrospect, on reflection, could I account for what seemed at that moment to be my spontaneous completion of her thought. At the time, my comment might have been described simply as empathic.

Could the patient have reached all that material without the analyst's comment? Possibly. The intervention was not formally analytic and might be viewed as primarily supportive. Not all analysts view such "spontaneous" occurrences as desirable, but they do occur in almost all analyses, though the analyst may not think about them in this way.

In retrospect, as I have suggested, what seems simple becomes more complex. The patient has left a sentence incomplete, and I have finished it. The incompleteness may represent a subtle pressure on me to respond. By taking over the part the patient has not finished, am I giving voice to the part the patient doesn't wish to express? What exactly am I empathizing with? I am highlighting a particular sense of fear. By offering an affective, but global, expression of what I sense as her state and concern, have I, at least at this moment, allowed her to evade more specific fantasies and fears about where her husband's sexual interests might lead? Perhaps to some loss of boundaries or control, or to unbridled, unforeseen sexuality? Or to some version of fantasized, exciting, submission that she might not want to acknowledge? Perhaps my patient preferred that such masochistic thoughts not be admitted to consciousness. If so, was the sentence left incomplete so that I might bring up the thought rather than she? Did my patient know more specific details of her fantasies or discomfort? Was she caught up in the shame of it, unable to say it, before another woman gave voice to it? Had she previously known and then forgotten these details, or were the fantasies still inchoate? From my perspective, was my response an attunement, or was I preferring to be the mother with whom she was in alliance, rather than the one with whom she was competitive?

As it happened at the time, these questions were not consciously articulated for me. My "Where will it end?" was a global resonance with her affective state and seemed to make less shameful, and therefore to facilitate, her exploration of more detailed fantasies and fears she had not allowed to become fully conscious. The rapidity with which she was able to bring them to consciousness suggests that they were already preconscious. My preconsciously generated response was to her affect and to the general tenor of her discomfort, rather than to the specific content of her fantasies.

Less clearly identifiable resonances also occur. A patient enters the office and lies down on the couch, but does not speak. In the silence, I recall for the first time my own dream from the previous night. When the patient speaks, he begins talking about a topic directly connected to my dream. It is so close; it feels uncanny. I become focused on my patient's material and return to this striking occurrence only later, at the end of the day. At first I feel mystified, but further reflection makes my experience more comprehensible. I assume that in the previous day's hour my patient must have been talking about this material or something related to it. This likely stirred in me some similar issues, not so conscious, that then surfaced in my dream. When I saw my patient the next day, the memory of the dream was evoked because of its link to his material from the day before. The dream had not been actively available to my memory earlier, undoubtedly because of my own resistance. My patient's presence, then, was the stimulus for the recovery of my dream and for bringing this material into consciousness. His similar thoughts were not really connected to mine, but rather were a continuation of ideas and affects from his last analytic hour. A review of some notes confirmed the presence of issues of my patient that had been expressed in the previous day's session that had a preconscious resonance for me, but there was nothing mystical about what had transpired.

In this example, a train of thought is started in my mind that seems to tap unconscious material. The patient's material the previous day had stirred an unconscious conflict for me that surfaced in my dream, was re-repressed, and was recovered only by the stimulus of my patient's presence. What was missing at its recovery was my awareness of the preconscious segue, the fact that the patient was the stimulus for this material to emerge. I had had a preconscious recognition that, in some as yet unspecified way, I was in a place similar to where he was. This feeling of similarity might have arisen, but need not have, from a shared conflict. It might have been stimulated instead by a transference to the patient's transference to me, or by some similarity in our defensive and adaptive strategies. The point is that the unconscious nature of my intrapsychic process may be connected to, but is also distinguishable from, the preconscious element. Something that was stirred in me was from my unconscious, but the link to my patient was preconscious. I had not been aware that some aspect of my patient had stimulated my dream, which was neither manifestly nor latently about my patient. Once I reflected on why my dream was recovered in the presence of my patient, I was able to bring back into my consciousness the reason why he was the stimulus for this material. However, it took considerably more self-reflection before I uncovered the affective link between his material and my own.

While in this instance it was possible to trace the data that explained the phenomenon, often such experiences of preconscious attunement are more difficult to link to describable events. The analyst remains less able to define what is stimulus and what is response. A fluidity of related associations between patient and analyst occurs that deepens the material without any conscious reflection about the source of resonance. Later, the analyst may pursue further the personal affects or ideas evoked in the interchange with the patient and become more conscious of the overlapping aspects between patient and analyst.

In the actual work with the patient, this process usually remains more seamless. The analyst dips empathically into the patient's experience and then puts words to what is found. When these words give shape to something the patient is on the verge of seeing, the patient may respond with still more intense or more fully elaborated associations. The analyst is likely to listen while the patient spins out memories, fantasies, dreams, affects, and ideas and if still finely attuned, intersperses an observation, echoes an affect or idea, possibly offers a synthesizing comment, all of which serve to further the patient's associations. There is a back-and-forth, a dance, which while not undisciplined is nonetheless more spontaneous than carefully thought out. A working through of previous frustration and disappointment is occurring as new understandings are arrived at in the context of safety in connection. This is the experience of the analyst as new object. It is where hope grows for something different from the past.

Enactments

Enactments are another source of analytic data that reveal how we participate in behaviors with our patients that are not always so fully under our conscious control. In enactments, analysts unconsciously bring in an aspect of their real selves that has a confluence with the transference. This multi-determined behavior Sandler (1976) has referred to as role-responsiveness. The analyst's participation is a compromise formation shaped by both the internal push of personal issues and the external pull of the patient's transference. The ratio of these forces varies from one patient-analyst pair to another and with the nature of the particular situation. Enactments give form to preconscious phenomena. Experience not yet within the conscious awareness of patient or analyst, and therefore not yet verbalizable, is revealed through the actions of the participants. Once these inchoate phenomena are given shape in actions, patient and analyst have something to examine together in which they can discover previously hidden aspects of themselves and their impact on each other.

In the analysis, the focus is on the patient, but it is unlikely that the analyst will be unmoved. Enactments most often represent moments when the analyst's preconscious attunement is disrupted. Consciously, the analyst does not intend to act out the role of frustrating or disappointing other, of seducer or seduced. While rejecting the idea of role-playing where positions are consciously taken to counter the patient's fears and expectations that the analyst will be manipulative and ultimately unhelpful (Alexander & French, 1946), the analyst does make a point of not intentionally repeating behaviors that have pained the patient in the past. Yet when analyst and patient give themselves over to engaging in a preconscious process, what is not yet consciously understood may first be given form in enactment. Then, within the preconscious representations, the unconscious sources may begin to emerge.

Often when the analyst plays a part that in some way fulfills the patient's fearful expectation, the role represents an aspect disavowed by the patient. In these instances the analyst is putting into action something the patient cannot yet consciously own. While the analyst must have some personal issue that hooks into the patient's issues if it is to be given form, how the preconscious transmission takes place most often remains unspecified.

Let me offer an example. My patient was complaining how rest-less, bored, and frustrated she became when she spent extended time in her retirement home. It was beautiful and she had everything she could wish, but she felt totally stultified. Her grandchildren were adorable, and at moments she could really take delight in their pres-ence, but all too soon she would feel herself imprisoned by their need for engagement. She described sitting with a grandchild at mealtime, listening to him chat, and finding her mind drift away. Forcing her-self to attend to the child's patter, she responded in pro forma ways. Her heart and head were not present. She longed to be able to go off by herself, to be able to read without interruption. She ached to be able to get back to her work. It was all painfully reminiscent of when she had small children of her own and felt trapped by them and by having to accommodate herself to suburban life as she thought she should as a "good mother.".She had thought her analysis had freed her from being bound by these "shoulds." Having raised her children, she thought she would no longer feel such a need to accommodate to what she experienced as the tyranny of their needs, but here she was again in this soup. Yet there were moments when she did not feel like this, when she could really enjoy her surroundings and her grandchil-dren, without this sense of stultification.

As I listened to her, I felt I could grasp the sense of claustrophobia she was feeling. I felt for her in her discomfort, which she had pro-vided for me to sample, but in which I did not feel myself immersed. Though caught by her affect, I did not yet understand the conditions that triggered it as fully as seemed necessary. There were moments, she had said, that she experienced differently. What made them dif-ferent? So I asked her about the times she could enjoy. She spoke of carrying a grandchild who didn't want to step on the prickly grass. The child was really too old to be carried, and the weight made her tired. Still, the child continued to beg to be held, and my patient had complied. As they returned to the house, her granddaughter stroked my patient's hair, tenderly running her fingers through it, and snug-gled her head in the crook of her grandmother's neck. The feeling of intimacy and connection was delicious, and the sense of burden dissolved. I felt affectively carried by her account, at first burdened and then suffused with the pleasure of another's offer of intimate ap-preciation. I remembered how it felt to hold a child that way and feel her melt into you. It enabled you to tolerate a lot that was not so pleasurable. Later, on reflection, I saw that there were two different ways I was attuned to her. I felt carried by her, as if I were her grandchild, but also identified with her as a grandmother or mother.

My patient continued. Another thing was the garden. While most often she felt it a burdensome chore to keep it up, weeded and newly planted, she could at times really get into it and enjoy the process. She had designed the garden herself and bought a variety of flowers. She began to recount the digging and the placement of plants. Then, abruptly and rather urgently, she was asking me if I was going to answer her. I was thrown and startled. I was quite certain I had not fallen asleep, but I also knew I had no idea that she had asked me if I was familiar with balloon flowers. Had I heard the question? Had she lost my attention? I acknowledged she had.

Understandably distressed, she wondered what had happened. I answered that I was not sure and would certainly try to figure out my part, but that together we could try to explore the part between us. I repeated the last thing I had registered and asked her if she could reconstruct what she had next said. It was about arranging delphiniums. She was sure I knew about them. She had seen them in my garden. Then she had begun to describe buying balloon flowers and wondered if I knew what they were. But I hadn't answered. She couldn't imagine why not. I almost always responded to direct questions, and when I didn't she could usually see the reason. This had made no sense. She realized she had lost my attention. But why? She was talking about something that she was sure would interest me. I always had flowers in the office, and she had watched my garden grow over the years. Was she being boring? Going into needless detail?

Only once before in the analysis had I left her like that. On that occasion, we had eventually understood that her part had involved being so affectively detached from what she was saying that I had ceased to be engaged. That was boring. But gardening! How could I have left her? That was something for me. I asked what she meant that her talking about gardening was for me. She said gardening was my interest, not hers. So she was telling me about something I would enjoy. I said I thought she had begun to tell me about moments that had not felt like obligations, ones where she had not felt trapped by expectations, but ones that felt pleasurable and were for her. She was puzzled; indeed, that had been her intention. She had conveyed just that in her story about carrying her granddaughter. But she didn't think I had grandchildren and so hadn't been at all sure that the story was something I could relate to. So she had told me about the gardening, an area she thought I would respond to, but instead I left her. She was angry and hurt. I said I could understand that.

As she continued to reflect on what had happened, she began to realize that perhaps she had not really enjoyed the gardening as much as she had thought. I wondered, I said, if in the process of her describing it, it had come to seem as if she had undertaken something burdensome. In recounting the details of her gardening, had she been carrying me, as she had her grandchild, with some at least dim expectation that she might be rewarded with a show of appreciation and intimacy? I said I wondered if she had been trying to please me but had instead lost my involvement. She pondered this a bit, now seemingly more curious than angry about what had occurred. She could see now that what she had been involved with was more the idea of pleasing me than of having actually enjoyed the gardening. I said, "So it was more like sitting with your grandchild while he was eating and talking about what he was interested in when you were not really engaged, with it." She agreed. As much as part of her wanted to be engaged, I said, we both knew how deeply resentful and angry she became when she felt compelled to attend. Again she agreed, but said she had not been aware of her anger or resentment as she had said all that. I wondered aloud if she had turned the tables and unconsciously created a situation in which while consciously trying to please, unconsciously she had trapped me in something she experienced as tedious, enabling me to feel, as she had, the sense of being caught and trapped by detail that was not engaging. I suggested that unconsciously she might be trying to get me to feel what she had been describing. But again she expressed wonder at how this could be, since even if she could be bored with gardening and its detail, I would not be. I said, "But my interest was in your interest here, not in the gardening, and it was your own interest that you abandoned and then I abandoned you."

My patient then returned to thoughts of her growing up, of her recently deceased mother, who had been so trapped by how she thought she had to be. Her devoted mother had been so giving, but in so many ways not really affectively present. My patient's identification with her mother's self-sacrificing ways had been greatly modified during analysis but had re-intensified since her mother's death. She saw how she was trying to hold on to her mother and how she had been doing to me something that had been done to her. There was something mean in that kind of loving attention that cost the giver so much. Still later, as she went over what had occurred between us, she saw that she had the fantasy that she could control my attention. If she did the "right thing," she could hold my gaze. But it meant she constantly had to be performing, and that was exhausting. She began to see how large she made herself in the picture and how great she must have assumed her powers are in believing she could control the responses of others. This was the other side of how helpless she had felt as a child. She began to understand that the consequence of believing herself so powerful was that she felt so responsible all the time. Then, paradoxically, she felt so helpless and inadequate because she could never make things come out as she wished or make people respond and behave as she wanted. She sobbed as she thought about my not answering her, echoing the repeated abandonments she had felt growing up.

While I did not convey my further thoughts about this incident to my patient, I realized that I had not only withdrawn my attention from her, but also abandoned my conscious intention to try to stay with, to identify with, her experience. My unconscious resistance to allowing myself to be trapped in her experience of being captured had led me to withdraw my attention from her words. Despite my conscious wish to know her experience so I could help her understand, in the countertransference I had come to a place where I unconsciously rebelled. I had lost my connection and resonance with one aspect of her conscious and preconscious experience, but had tuned in to another, disavowed part of her. I had unconsciously refused to join her in her identification with her self-sacrificing mother, but in doing that I had enacted another part, that of her abandoning mother. I regretted causing my patient more pain, but over time I have come to understand that the depth of participation makes me vulnerable to such enactments. If the alliance with my patient is strong enough, I have always found it possible to learn from these occurrences.

But let us reconsider this example, now trying to tease out what is preconscious and what is unconscious in both my patient and myself. When I missed what my patient had said, something unconscious was transpiring for me. But why was my patient so upset? She had learned to expect that I would respond to a direct question, but if at this moment I hadn't, why did she so urgently need me to do so? She must already have been upset with me to be so concerned that I didn't respond at once, for she did not yet know she had lost my attention. And there is data to confirm this. She had previously offered a subtle reproach: she thought her analysis had freed her of being bound by "shoulds," only to find now that "shoulds" still constrained her.

Here is an earlier indication that she wanted me to have done something for her that I hadn't. She had expected something from me in both instances that had not been forthcoming. So in the transference I seem to be her weak, incapable mother. Yet I am also the mother who longs to return to her "work," her reading, her own self-absorbed world, and she has the painful sense, which comes from earlier experience, of not being enough to hold my interest. I have a double identification to her; she has a double tie to me. I am both her ineffectual mother and the powerful mother who, if pleased, will both give to her and make her feel powerful in turn. I am also my patient herself, as both inadequate and powerfully withholding.

She had reacted as if I had asked her to talk about what interested me, as if she expected me to be grateful that she had. She believed I would like her if she did this. If she met what she assumed were my unspoken wishes, she hoped I would reciprocate by meeting hers. She did not directly own or ask for what she wanted, but wanted me to know and give it to her. This was a preconscious structuring of our relationship. If I were to present this construction of what she had done to my patient, she would recognize and acknowledge it. She also is aware that she has a need to please me as she needed to please her mother. But she couldn't get her mother to be really interested in her. She counts on my being attentive. Because she lacked attention from her mother, she even feels entitled to it—though she is ashamed of feeling such entitlement.

She is also identified with her mother as someone who deprives a child of attention. Her mother, she assumes, felt burdened by trying to please her. She knows she has felt burdened by trying to please her own children and her grandchildren. What is preconscious is that she had previously felt burdened by trying to please her mother and currently felt burdened by trying to please me.

There is a boundary problem for her. Who is pleased and who is doing the pleasing? When I don't respond, I have broken an unconscious bargain she has unconsciously constructed about what we will do for each other. We are also in a preconscious competition about being good, as well as about pleasing and not being manipulated. Unconsciously, this is about which of us will hold the aggression. Unconsciously, by not responding, I have felt like I am a bad child. While I am able to recognize this aspect in myself sooner and more readily than does my patient in herself, I designate it as unconscious rather than preconscious—I would likely have explored her urgent need for a response more directly had I not unconsciously felt guilty about not responding.

Most often, enactments that are this clear occur at pivotal points in a treatment, points at which the patient is ready to face and begin to reintegrate a part of the self that has been disavowed. The unconscious and disavowed aspects, as well as the preconsciously conveyed representations of each of our intrapsychically contained histories, are given interpersonal expression in this enactment.

This patient and I have already done a lot of work together. The process between us can usually be teased apart, as it was here. The disavowed part exerts a pressure that taps into and creates a synergy with an independent but related aspect in me that is also pushing for expression. But how that pressure is transmitted is less clear. In this example, I think, I tuned out because I was suddenly swamped with guilt about aggressive wishes and tried to ward them off by becoming unconscious of them, a disconnection from my conscious experience and usual cognitive controls. Pressure such as I experienced in this example bypasses the analyst's usual cognitive controls, tips the participant-observer balance to the far side of participation, and overrides the analyst's trained intention to maintain an analytic stance.

Concluding remarks

Taylor (1996) has pointed out that if analysts indeed develop transferences to patients, we must rethink our theoretical commitment to analytic neutrality and anonymity as facilitating the development and interpretation of the transference. Certainly the patient is neither anonymous nor neutral in relation to the analyst, and yet the analyst may develop a transference to the patient. On reflection, of course, it is clear that we form transferences not only to people about whom we have limited data, but also to people in our real lives about whom we have abundant information. Clinicians who treat couples in therapy are acutely aware of the role transference plays in difficulties partners have with each other. Analysts recognize the way their patients play out past conflicts in their current relationships. Indeed, analysts work in displacements as well as directly in the transference. Some (Ehrenberg, 1992; Hoffman, 1994; Renik, 1993) would even argue that neutrality and anonymity are never really possible and are not necessary for the analysis.

Granting that they are, of course, never fully achievable, I would argue nonetheless that analysts should try to preserve them, not to facilitate the transference but to maintain the analytic stance, which is always at risk. Maintenance of the analytic stance facilitates a safe setting and may open these very enactments to further analysis. Chused (1992) has cogently pointed out that a patient's accurate perception of an aspect of the analyst does not preclude that aspect's having a transference meaning. When a patient observes such an aspect, and the analyst recognizes the perception as accurate, the analyst may find this dimension difficult to discuss.

In psychoanalytic treatment, the analyst is placed in a position of authority that is an inescapable aspect of the analytic situation and that inevitably engenders certain kinds of transferences. By virtue of the structure of the analytic relationship, including the fact that the patient seeks help and pays for it, it is inevitable that the analyst will be experienced as an authority. Hoffman's (1994) description of the psychoanalytic dialectic between the analyst's discipline and spontaneity speaks to a central tension in the work. If, as most analysts now seem to believe, the power in analysis emanates from what is affectively learned in the interaction, then the extent to which the analyst can allow affective engagement sets a limit on what can be achieved. However, if the analyst permits this tilt to become too pronounced, the role of analyst will be lost. When an analyst becomes self-revealing, it is not the patient's knowledge of facts about the analyst that endangers the process. The patient may learn any number of things about the analyst outside the office and may infer all kinds of personal information from what the analyst says and does. All of this material, in terms of its meaning to the patient, becomes part of the analytic investigation.

The danger in self-revelation lies not in the patient's having information about the analyst, but in the analyst's own deepening involvement with the patient. Self-revelation tends to intensify the analyst's personal engagement. When the patient has become not only an affectively meaningful person in the analyst's psychic life, but a person the analyst, however unconsciously, uses to meet personal needs, the danger is in the extent to which this is enacted with the patient. Once this shift in the relationship occurs, the analyst's ability to step outside the process and observe is diminished. The relationship at best becomes more like a friendship, but one that is unequal because the previous transference of authority is likely to remain; at worst, it may occasion a violation of boundaries and abuse of the patient. The analyst's conscious attempt to maintain anonymity and neutrality in the work with the patient helps to maintain abstinence.

Trying to adhere to anonymity and neutrality, as inevitably compromised as they may be, helps the analyst to maintain an equilibrium between being an observer giving oneself over to preconscious processes and what spontaneously may occur. The safer the analyst feels, the more freely can the analyst participate in the regressive aspects of the analytic process, thereby creating a greater openness to the preconscious material within both members of the analytic pair. Like many analysts, I believe there is great potential benefit in analysts opening themselves to the spontaneous use of preconscious responses to patients. But along with the benefit comes the danger that in this spontaneity the analyst may cease being an analyst. The consequences of this loss of analytic role are not always harmful, but they may be. At times they are disastrous for both participants. We need to find ways to be both creative and safe in our analytic engagements.

Keeping the patient as the focus of the work, while simultaneously making use of personal transference-countertransference reactions for the benefit of the patient, is more reliably achieved when analysts maintain self-discipline. Self-discipline involves trying to keep personal attitudes, values, beliefs, conflicts, and characterological tendencies from intruding on the work. I do not think it a contradiction to believe, on the one hand, that it is impossible to eliminate the effects of the analyst's character and conflict on the patient and, on the other, that it is incumbent on the analyst to keep the analytic work as centered on the patient as possible. The fact that it is impossible to eliminate the effects of subjectivity does not mean that the attempt to be objective should be abandoned. Any personal benefit the analyst may derive, however considerable, is a private matter, though the fact that there is such a gain may well be acknowledged.

In conclusion, I am suggesting that the analytic process inevitably involves the interdigitation of the intrapsychic structures of both patient and analyst. This interplay is expressed in transference-countertransference interactions. The safer both patient and analyst feel in relation to each other, the more freely will they relax their customary cognitive controls and permit the emergence of preconscious responses. Preconscious resonance between patient and analyst is likely to facilitate the lifting of repressive barriers and the emergence of unconscious material for both participants. The integration and reworking of old conflicts then becomes possible. In the context of such an affectively intense and meaningful connection, the analyst needs to find ways to balance this profound involvement in order to maintain an analytic stance in relation to the patient and to keep the patient's concerns as the central focus. Although objectivity, anonymity, and neutrality are all impossible to achieve, the analyst may use these concepts to maintain an emotional equilibrium. To try to adhere too strictly to objectivity, anonymity, and neutrality may lead to a sterile environment, in which neither patient nor analyst can freely explore affects, ideas, fantasies, or engagement. To pay too little attention to these concepts in favor of spontaneity, however, may imperil the analyst's role as analyst through the loss of an analytic stance and the sacrifice of the ambiguity possible in analytic space.

Enactments may provide the basis for understanding the past and how it lives on in the present, or may be the first steps in an ever-increasing violation of boundaries. Patient and analyst have a "real" relationship with each other, but it must be used as a vehicle for understanding, not for direct gratification in interaction. Analysts must remain keenly aware of how what patients experience in relation to them is both about and not about the analyst. Maintaining a focus on the reality and unreality of the patient's affective attachment to the analyst helps us to maintain our analytic role and to allow the spontaneous emergence and subsequent use of preconscious responses to the benefit of the patient's treatment.

Notes

1 Although his attention was directed specifically on erotic life, the same elements of constitution and early external influences combine to shape methods that are less directly instinctual, though Freud considered them to be aim-inhibited expressions of erotic life.
2 The bifurcation between unconscious and preconscious is not usually as stark as this statement may suggest, since it is from the patient-analyst relationship-transference-countertransference as well as other manifestations, which are the topic of this book, that most insight is derived, rather than the emergence of a preformed unconscious fantasy.

Chapter 11

The patient-analyst match in a second analysis when a patient returns

When we have engaged with our patients in the intense exploration that analysis affords, we, as well as our patients, experience feelings of loss when the treatment ends. In addition to whatever particular meaning the specific patient holds for the specific analyst, there is always the loss of knowing what the future will hold for our patients and what part our analytic work will play in life after we no longer meet. We are curious. That's part of being analysts. We do not initiate later contact. That's also part of being analysts. We try to monitor our personal needs. Some patients would welcome our contacting them, but others would not. My follow-up studies tell me that we are not always so accurate in predicting whether this later contact will be welcome. Patients themselves may think one thing at termination and another later on. It is up to our former patients whether we learn about their lives. So I have pursued my curiosity about what happens later by conducting follow-up studies (Kantrowitz, 1993c; Kantrowitz et al., 1986, 1987a, 1987b, 1989; Kantrowitz, Katz, & Paolitto, 1990a, 1990b, 1990c), in an attempt to understand what works well, what doesn't, and how it plays out in the specifics of the particular patient and particular analyst. Most recently, I have been exploring how former patients think about the termination phase of their treatment and what happened afterward. We know a lot about what analysts think, but we don't so often have the voices of former patients.

What I would wish is to have the voices of both patient and analyst on their experience together, but the intrusion on the analysis, including the possibility of the analyst's saying something that was not said at all to the patient, or saying something in a way different from how it had been understood during the analysis, could be disruptive. So probably the closest we can come to knowing both parts of an analytic experience is when our patients return, tell us about what has happened since we've last seen them, how they have thought about us and our work together, and what has led them to return. We can see how they have changed, but we also learn how we have changed. Some patients we never hear from again. We don't know whether this is from satisfaction or disappointment. Others keep in touch with a holiday card, sometimes with a brief recounting of where they are in life. Others return briefly around a specific issue. But those who return for another intense period of work enable us to reflect most deeply about our understanding of them, ourselves, and the nature of our analytic work. They are our best teachers about development, both emotional and intellectual, theirs and our own.

The patient I am going to describe, I will discuss again in the next two chapters. She has given me permission to write about our work without needing to read the material. She is not in the mental health field, but appreciates the importance of illustrating our work. In these three chapters, I will be illustrating elements of the patient-analyst match with a particular patient, showing its day-to-day relevance to our work as it unfolds.

When she first came to see me, she was a graduate student in her late twenties. She sought analysis to calm her anxiety on the eve of her marriage. She was a star student; her husband-to-be she described as average. These relative positions were to continue throughout their professional lives. She was a competent, attractive woman who took pleasure in mastery and prided herself on her self- sufficiency. She viewed herself as the special, favored child among her three siblings, toward whom she expressed positive feelings. She thought her mother was her best friend. A history emerged of idealization, admiration, and unconscious envy toward her glamorous mother, and a relative lack of feeling toward her father, whom she saw as a bland, improbable mate for her mother. During her childhood, her parents would frequently travel abroad, sending postcards that detailed delicious meals they were eating. The children were left with a housekeeper whom she spoke of with great warmth. As an adolescent, my patient pursued boys, was viewed as "fast," was shunned by girls, and seemed indifferent to this reputation. Drugs and alcohol accompanied social and sexual behavior. She had one long-term boyfriend, but she ended the relationship, frightened by sexual games they had begun to play, where food treats were rewarded by sexual acts. Her future husband was different. He didn't want to have a sexual relationship with her until they were more personally intimate. She regarded him as her best friend but, nonetheless, feared dependency on him.

She was one of my first analytic patients. In analysis, she seemed able to speak freely of thoughts, feelings, and fantasies. Only later did I learn that she forced herself to do this, primarily as a kind of mastery. It was not until late in a six-year analysis that the picture of a neglected and overstimulated child emerged. Her mother would take her on shopping expeditions to buy herself clothes and get nothing for my patient. She described her parents as totally absorbed in each other. Her sister had a closeness with her father, and her mother was most attentive to her brother, she decided. She then remembered her mother flying into rages and her disdain for her mother's lack of control. She came to realize it had been her sustaining myth that she was the special child.

While her outer life had appeared relatively smooth, her inner world was often in a turmoil that she tried to control with her mind. For example, on the way to her hour, her dog had gotten out and wouldn't return when she called. Ultimately she left him, rather than be late, but felt guilty. She was being selfish. Her feelings of guilt mounted as she drove to her hour. She began fantasizing that he would be hit by a car and die. She was a murderer. No wonder she didn't want to have children. Then, recognizing her escalation, she reversed course, saying to herself she was being ridiculous and had done nothing at all. We could see how she rebelled against her harsh self-criticism with a denial of any responsibility. She absented herself from feelings that distressed her. This was also true in relation to her feelings about me. She wanted my help to ease her self-criticism, but she denied she needed or wanted more from me than insight.

Several years into analysis, in the last hour before a planned week-long interruption initiated by me, she asked, as she was walking out the door, where I was going. This was unusual. Previously she had expressed almost no curiosity about me or my life. Wanting neither to leave her feeling injured for an entire week before we could explore this new turn, nor to shut off her curiosity, I chose to simply state the name of the city I was visiting.

In her first hour back, I returned to this incident and wondered about the question and its timing. After much exploration, it became clear that my patient had been less interested in information about me than in keeping me present longer. She came to recognize that she had thought that I would remain "strictly" analytic and not answer her question. An unconscious fantasy emerged that I would tell her to return to the couch and continue her session. Her question, then, would have controlled my presence and prevented me from leaving her. My answering her question had warded off her feeling injured, as she had felt with her mother, but she had been unable to control me and keep me present as she wished and, unconsciously, had believed she could. At the time she asked the question, I was unaware of the aggression in it that had put me on the spot.

While this incident opened up some awareness of her need for me, she resisted experiencing dependency and exploring her need for control. I, in parallel, was not in touch with her aggression. Over time, she began to allow samplings of pain and sadness in her need for me, but her fear of her feelings kept them minimal.

During the sixth year of analysis, she introduced the idea of terminating, ostensibly because of time constraints, simultaneously acknowledging that much had changed. By then she had several children and was established in her profession. She was working full-time, fearing she would mother as she had been mothered and providing a devoted nanny like the one she had had. Only when she faced termination could she explore her intolerance for her affect and her clinging to a belief in her own omnipotence and omniscience. She understood more deeply that her defensive isolation of affect also maintained a belief that if she experienced sadness it would be endless. In the last phase, she found herself able to risk a new intensity of anger, yearning, disappointment, and engagement with me and to tolerate feelings of grief.

The termination phase facilitated work on her defensive use of her self-sufficiency, implicitly challenging her continued belief that she did not "need" others. At the time, I think, she felt satisfied with the work we had done. We had unraveled a defensive view of herself as special to her mother and others, her need for self-sufficiency and control. Yet in my view, we had only begun to touch on the anger and intolerance of affect that I suspected made her need to keep a distance in life and with me. Given the extent to which she had felt neglected, I worried how she would manage her feelings as a mother as her children got older. Yet in reality, she had accomplished a lot. I felt it best to accept her wish to stop.

In retrospect, I believe we had colluded in avoiding sufficient notice and exploration of her feelings toward me, both of us unconsciously fearing the intensity of her dependent longings. I may also have unconsciously feared that her disappointment in me, and the rage that might have come in its wake, would be retraumatizing rather than healing. Although I had terminated my own analysis years before, where modulation of my own affect intensity had been central—though in the direction of too much rather than too little—I think the depth and impact of affect in myself and others remained more of an issue than I was aware of then. For both of us, fear of her aggression had remained unconscious. At the time, I don't think I knew how to recognize, work with, or tolerate the extent of her underlying rage. I also was less familiar with concepts of dissociation, though we spoke of her isolated affects and states as her living in separate, disconnected stripes.

After she terminated, I saw my patient twice over the years for brief periods, once in relation to a health scare, the second time when her mother was dying. She told me she thought of me and our work together, would recall things I said, and remained aware that she kept herself and her feelings at a distance. But basically, she felt her life was going well. Each time, she quickly settled down after a month or so and left. Then, over 20 years after ending her analysis, she returned to engage in another intense period of work.

My patient had developed the reputation of being a maternal and supportive teacher, yet suddenly she found herself blurting out hostile responses to a student. She felt alienated from herself and out of control. She recognized that the rage she had protected her children from was occurring in her work. She was shaken and frightened. She knew she needed help. Her dreams were violent in ways she had never known. People hurtled objects at others, who were terrified. There were images of people being hollowed out inside, reminiscent of a frightening image of being in a white room, never sufficiently understood in her analysis. These images were disconnected from anything in her awareness. She was unable to trace what preceded these experiences.

Her parents had died. While men had always been significant in her life, she now had a close female friend. She also felt very warmly toward her sister. Neither of these women had professional lives; both were motherly toward her. Her children were grown and lived in different cities. She spoke with her son daily; her relationships with her daughters were cordial but more remote. She felt very close to her husband, except that she no longer experienced any pleasure in their sexual relationship. She was unclear when this had changed. She had pleasure in masturbating, with masochistic fantasies that she related, and about which she felt a great deal of shame. She began a twice-a-week treatment, the two of us sitting face to face.

In our renewed work, my patient's associations centered on feelings of being unseen by her mother. When she, her husband, and children would visit her parents, she realized she had been in a fog; she could not allow herself to know herself as, or act, as a mother in her mother's presence. She started to realize that as long as she and her mother were merged in her mind, as long as she didn't have any known needs of her own, they were in harmony. Her mother took the limelight. My patient became furious as memories reemerged of the shopping trips on which her mother, but not she, got clothes. Then, she had a recollection of taking a walk with her toddler daughter, who kept crying until my patient discovered she had placed the wrong shoe on each foot. She was aghast and felt guilty about repeating such neglect. Over time, she began to put some pieces together. She had experienced the woman student toward whom she had expressed uncontrolled hostility as showing off.

One day, she was sick and asked if we could do the hour on the phone. During the session she described a sudden impulse to put her hand on a hot plate. It frightened and humiliated her that she would want to hurt herself. She recognized that this was a reaction to not seeing me and feeling unconnected. The next hour she wanted to use the couch to face what she feared. The images she evoked were horrific—walking on hot coals, being trapped and feeling claustrophobic, people holding out morsels of food she desired and not letting her eat, cannibalistic fantasies of chunks of a person's body being fed to someone, her mother being forced to have sex with her.

I listened, trying to contain and not feel engulfed by her self-inflicted torture and the fury it represented. I said that she was letting me see and begin to appreciate the extent to which feeling disconnected was torturous for her. Disconnection was a defense against fury and the grief underlying it. She took control of her pain, bypassed her rage, and inflicted her fury on herself. She thought my interpretation was right. If she did this to herself, no one could do it to her. But it frightened her that she felt compelled to seek pain. She knew she had chosen to go to the couch, but she felt I was her enemy forcing her to do this.

The hour was up. She sat up and said she would see me in two weeks. I was totally shocked. I knew she had told me she would be away, but I had remembered it as a week later. I acknowledged my error and said that had I remembered, I would have suggested she postpone using the couch until her return. I told her I regretted her leaving with a last hour that was so painful, a kind of apology after the enactment. In retrospect, I saw we had colluded. My not remembering and her going to the couch put me in the role of sadist, while she was free to express her unmitigated fury in the role of victim.

When she returned, she told me she had been very angry, hurt, and disappointed with me. It wasn't that I hadn't remembered that she was going away then. It was much bigger. She realized that she had imagined that I knew everything that went through her mind without her telling me. She hadn't known she had this fantasy until it had been shattered. She saw she had repeated with me the fusion she had had with her mother. While this realization was very important, I said I thought she was doing with me what she sometimes did with herself— by focusing on an expectation of me that she knew was unreasonable, she was not letting herself acknowledge that I actually had abandoned her after she gave vent to her fury. I thought that rather than being critical of herself for wanting so much, she was afraid of being really angry and disappointed with me, frightened of my being her enemy, if she did not idealize me.

In the following weeks, she noticed that she became sexually aroused when she wanted a response from me—something previously out of her awareness. This was in the context of talking about lack of feeling in sex with her husband, rage at what she saw as his generic desire, not focused on her. Still later, she realized she felt desire also when she felt close to me and wished to be closer. At these moments she thought of shopping. She recognized this was a way of reassuring herself that she could now satisfy her own desires. One day, she began a session terrified of how hostile she had been to me. I was totally puzzled, not having experienced her hostility. She repeated that she had said her daughter's therapist was the best thing in her life. It took most of the session to get clear that she was furious about the pain she was experiencing in treatment because I had become so important to her, the best thing in her life. She was blaming me for her suffering, but she had expressed this in a way that displaced and undid her aggression about her unrequited desire for me. What she said to me had not conveyed her longing for me, nor how she felt furious that it was not reciprocal. Her fury terrified her. She imagined she had harmed me, but then saw how she had kept me from knowing or feeling her fury and turned it on herself. Although excruciating, it felt better to her to be a victim than release what felt like murderous rage at me. Following this, in her outside life, she began to have more feeling.

The depth of the work in this second period reflects developmental growth in both my patient and me. She had become more confident, more able to tolerate feelings that she feared could have disrupted and directly harmed her children or her mother in fantasy. That her mother was now dead made it easier for my patient to explore her fear of her own omnipotence, a fear that she could and did harm others. Just as she believed she had devastated me, she believed she had demolished her student. Affect, expression, and idea were all separated. I had not appreciated the depth of her masochism or fears of her sadism in the earlier treatment. The content was familiar but the intensity, the traumatic nature of her experience of frustration, of unmet desire and the vicious attacks against herself, against feeling itself— to prevent expression of her sadistic wishes—were beyond anything I could then imagine, and I think beyond what I could have tolerated at the time of her first treatment.

Between my patient's first and second treatments, I had many more years of clinical experience, as well as years of working with colleagues in peer supervision, exploring my own issues as they were stimulated in me by my patients. Now with my patient, I did not worry that she couldn't tolerate intensity, and when I was aware of her rage, though at times it stirred my own uncomfortably, I also felt a conscious pleasure in being able to find ways to make it alive between us. In the first treatment, I missed the depth of terror and horror because I didn't yet know enough about these feelings in myself. My patient and I had had a similarity in our ability to recognize and acknowledge a wide range of feelings and fears, but neither of us wished to dwell in them too long. This time I stayed with affects longer. Also, instead of interpreting her generic intolerance of feeling, I was more specific and drew it to what went on between us. I focused less on the past. My tolerance for both sides of a sadomasochistic polarity had stretched. I could experience myself as someone I would hate and fear, and so could tolerate being hated and abused in transference-countertranference engagements. While not yet active in our interactions, I am also more aware of the presence, as yet unexpressed, of homosexual desire. Now I can both better recognize and tolerate all these feelings, as well as feeling helpless, and contain more affect without withdrawing. My forgetting that my patient would be away seems like an unconscious sadistic abandonment of her and an unconscious wish to distance myself from fear and desire in myself—regrettable but tolerable by both of us and very informative to our work. It was a turning point, following which she could recognize and stay with her frustrated desire for me, and I could tolerate being a frustrator, believing we would both survive. Our work is ongoing.

Theory is personal. It supports our conscious beliefs or provides useful correctives. My personal proclivities are/were relational—in a personal sense—and a focus on adaptation. My training in the late 1960s and early 1970s provided me a useful self-discipline, an attention to what was not seen, what was darker, but there was a great deal that I was taught that did not make sense to me. In the last two decades and a half, psychoanalytic theory has changed. Gone is the idea that analysts could be blank screens or interchangeable—ideas I could never accept. Analysts now believe that two people are always involved in the process and that the character and conflicts of the analyst inevitably influence the process.

There is an increased understanding of narcissistic vulnerability, an awareness that a focus on defenses without an appreciation of the adaptive function they serve can be humiliating and increase resistance to self-exploration. These changes in theory gave support to my personal proclivities. I believe the increased external, intellectual support for emotional convictions of my own actually helped me look more deeply and incisively at the darker aspects of my patients and myself.

I think something similar may account for patients' returning. They have some memory of us, their therapists, holding a confidence in positive aspects of them that at times they could not hold for themselves; it enabled them to find and face more negative aspects of themselves. When their self-esteem becomes destabilized, they come back, hoping they can again find a view of themselves as people they can like and value through us, and our work together.

I think my patient returned to see me because her sense of herself as someone she liked and valued was destabilized, perhaps even lost, when she perceived herself as aggressively out of control with her student. I suspect she retained an inchoate memory of my liking and valuing her, even when she relinquished the myth of herself as being special that had previously sustained her self-esteem. I, or our analytic relationship, held a positive view of her in her memory of our previous work that she had lost and now hoped to rediscover in our working together. Being in my presence again, with my holding a view of her as a complex person, likable and valuable even when there were aspects of her that could stir my fear and aggression, could offer her a hope of once again finding value and goodness in her view of herself. Our later work enabled her to refind this more positive place, while simultaneously becoming more accepting and less afraid of her own competitive feelings, anger, and aggression.

Chapter 12

Reflections on mortality

A patient faces death; an analyst grieves

> Go out of this world as you entered it. The same passage that you
> made from death to life, without feeling or fright, make it again
> from life to death. Your death is part of the order of the universe;
> it is part of the life of the world.
> Greenblatt (2011, p. 248)—Lucretius—"That to philosophize"

Stephen Greenblatt finds these words of Lucretius a therapeutic me-
diation on the fear of death. To spend one's life anxious about death
is to deprive oneself of the fullness of life and its enjoyment. But if
one is afraid of dying, as was my patient, newly confronted with a
life-threatening illness, how do you overcome such fear?

My patient had been diagnosed with a cancer, a prognosis that statistically limited her lifespan to two more years at best. "It's just a
statistic," she would say in her characteristic manner, trying to counter her depressive proclivities with an artificial brightness. Then she
would weep. "I don't want to die. I'm too young. It's not fair." She was
60 years old—a very youthful, energetic, productive 60-year old. At
the height of her profession, she had just embarked on another creative endeavor.

I had known my patient for more than 30 years. She had sought
analysis in her 20s while a graduate student, unsure about her future
vocational direction. Her six-year analysis revealed a woman who had
had to rely on herself to make her own way in the world both emotionally and professionally. While financially well provided for, her
mother's self-preoccupation and need for admiration left my patient
feeling primarily unseen. She organized her self-esteem around her

own achievement and ability for mastery. Her analysis enabled her to face and grieve some of what she missed growing up, but she and I didn't dwell in that place too long. She felt optimistic about the future and ready to just live in it. It was early in my career as an analyst. I chose, wisely or not, to assume her insight would spread (Poland, 2013a) and would lead her to greater growth over the years. To some extent it was true. Overtime, she was increasingly successful in her career. She married a man she loved, had children she also loved, though these were not feelings she could consistently inhabit.

However, there were limitations in our work that revealed themselves over time. She returned when her mother was dying to talk about her unfulfilled need to find a place of centrality in her mother's heart and mind. She remained for only a brief time. As we later understand more fully, she needed to assuage her unconscious guilt about the rage and disappointment she felt in relation to her mother. Years later, she returned to do an extended and intensive piece of analytic work, when her rage became manifest. We then explored and experienced her frightening aggression in our transference/countertransference interactions. Anger, minimal in her analysis, took center stage in relation to her parents, husband, children, and me. Her longing for her father and disappointment in his not rescuing her from an engulfing closeness with her mother was new to her. The work freed her to experience her loving feelings with new depth and to pursue her creative work with expansion of her ideas. So at the time of her diagnosis, she felt more fully alive and engaged than ever before. The irony and unfairness pained us both. But it also confronted us with an unresolved psychological issue:

> I can't free myself from thinking that I have caused this to happen to myself. I know it can't be true, but I can't shake the idea that it is. Help me to understand this. I don't want to die so why should I do this to myself? It seems an extension of all we have understood about how I turn on myself to protect others from my anger. But this seems … I don't know. I don't understand, but I hate and am ashamed of myself for being so self-destructive.

What emerged as we explored her conviction that she had done this to herself was her belief in her omnipotence. Her need for self-sufficiency, to believe in her own powers to control what occurred was familiar territory, was one that we had addressed over the years. But now it took on a new meaning. If she was in control of her destiny, what would it mean that she had done this to herself. Could she be that self-hating and that self-destructive? She thought she had changed, softened in her feelings. I hadn't helped as she thought. She was angry and disappointed in me—and to feel that at this time when she needed me so much was frightening. Why hadn't I protected her? Or was I to blame? She oscillated between hating me and hating herself.

I said it seemed she was caught in a terrible dilemma. She needed to continue to believe she and I were able to control what happened to her, even an illness that she knew was beyond her control or mine, or she had to believe that she wanted to harm herself and I was refusing to protect and help her. Maybe I was even responsible for her being ill? She was silent for a long time. Then she began sobbing. It continued until the end of the hour. In the hours that followed, she was filled with grief and began to mourn her belief in her powers and mine. This mourning segued into the grief that she felt in relation to her illness.

Suddenly, her horizon was shortened in her mind. Thinking about the future introduced feelings of panic. What future did she have? She had to find a different way of thinking, a different way to create a sense of self-worth. It required a different kind of mastery. She now needed to live with uncertainty and still not become flooded by anxiety.

Time with her family became newly precious. Her husband would drive her to her treatments. They would talk about how this was time they might never have taken to be together and appreciate each other were it not for her illness. She didn't want to think about this as a compensation for her illness—a way she knew she tended to counter bad thoughts with good ones—but she wanted to be sure she was really allowing herself to appreciate that she had something of great value in their mutual love and her being able to depend on him. Similarly, her children were present and loving, taking time from their busy lives to be with her, express their love, something sensed but in their family not often put into words.

Her radiation and chemotherapy exhausted her. She did not have the energy to come to my office. Frequently we needed to rearrange our time to accommodate her medical treatment. We continued our sessions on the phone. I lost the opportunity to see what was happening with her body, to see how sick she was. She was familiar with SKYPE from her work, but never indicated a wish to use it. I believed I should follow her lead. I thought about going to see her at home, but she never suggested this. If she were dying now, I know I would have raised it. I think it would have scared her if I had suggested it at this time, interpreting my suggestion to mean her death was imminent. She worried that our sessions focused too much on her telling me how hard this all was for her and getting me to let her know I understood and was there for her. Could she permit herself to not be trying to learn something new about herself? Learning was her life-long way of being in control, defending against dependency, passivity.

This was not the first time I had worked with a patient who was dying. About a decade before, a former patient, who had by coincidence also been in analysis with me in her late 20s and whose mother had also been self-absorbed and inattentive to her daughter, had returned to talk with me when she learned she had a cancer that was likely incurable. This patient then lived far away and I spoke with her on the phone once a week until she died some eight months later. Although many of their conflicts were similar, their adaptations to life were quite different. My former patient overtly struggled in her intimate relationships. She had ambitions she was never able to actualize. But in this last year of her life, she became able to appreciate her love for and from her family and close friends. Her envy and anger with others diminished and then seemed to disappear as she let herself enjoy being cared for. In this period, she got the attention she had longed for throughout her life and stopped fighting her dependent wishes. What she didn't want to burden her family and friends with, she could tell me. It made her feel less frightened and less alone. I admired her ability to face her illness, let go of grievances, to let herself be loved. I've missed her and think of her often, even more so now with my other patient facing a life threatening illness. I ask myself whether I am muting the intensity of my pain and grief as this past threatens to become more alive. Probably so.

When a patient of ours faces death, we, their analysts, if we are to be of help, need to face and tolerate helplessness, fear, rage, and grief along with whatever other emotions our particular histories stir in us (Norton, 1963). The impending loss of someone with whom we have had such depth of experience evokes a special kind of grief in which we are alone, unable to share it with other loved ones in our patients' lives and only sparingly and confidentially with trusted colleagues in our own. As in all psychological treatments of depth, in the course of our work, we will learn much about our patients, but also about ourselves (Gardner, 1983). What we learn, need to face in ourselves, may be frightening and painful. Our devotion to our patients and commitment to, and belief in, analysis itself as a process that strengthens enables us to remain present. And when the patient who has a terminal illness is someone we have previously analyzed (Margulies, Orgel, & Poland, 2014), analysts are confronted with an impending loss of someone whom they have known intimately over time. When we have analyzed a patient at an earlier time in their life and our own and they return (Almond, 2013; Kantrowitz, 2013; Orgel, 2013), we have an opportunity to appreciate what we have and haven't recognized, understood, or analyzed previously. At a different, later stage of life, we each know more about ourselves and are better able to face our vulnerabilities. We are now older too and thoughts of other lost loved ones and our own mortality inevitably arise (Norton, 1963; Orgel, 2014; Poland, 2014, 2016). Their return provides us a chance to go further. But when their return is precipitated by the onset of a life threatening illness or this illness occurs in the course of this later work, as was true for my patient, we know there is likely to be a very limited future. What then is our task?

Freud (1926) proposed psychoanalysis as a method to help one better face and participate in the vicissitudes of life. But what if it is death and not life that we anticipate awaits our patient. Poland (2014, 2016) movingly writes:

> News of a patient's impending death awakens awareness of the end awaiting the analyst's own life. The analyst's belief in being an exception to the rule that all flesh is mortal is challenged. In a patient's dying, the analyst's own death is foretold.
>
> (2014, p. 902)

I am pulled to personal reflections:

> Dylan Thomas wrote that once we experience a death, that experience determines how we think of all other deaths. Looking up this poem, I see there are many different interpretations of

what he meant by this line. I have never before explored how others understood this statement. Many people think he intended to convey that the first death one experiences means taking in the reality of death itself, the shattering of a belief in immortality that changes one forever. I cannot remember ever having that belief, though surely I must have had it once. My mother told me that at four I had cried begging her to think of, and tell me about, someone who had not died. The power of my fantasies shaped by own wishes and fears must have had a strong impact on me as a child.

I don't want to die, but it is being alone without those I love—the loss of loved ones, not death—that I consciously fear. Of course, I do not know what I will actually feel when facing death. I had interpreted Dylan Thomas' lines to mean that the first time someone we love dies, we experience a grief that is deep and powerful and that is revived with every other death of a loved one that follows, shaping and containing all subsequent experiences of loss and grief. I don't know if that is what he meant, and I continue to think about whether I believe it is true. I do think each death leaves one with an experience of sadness that revives the emotion attending earlier losses, though ones not of death. These losses Shelley Orgel (2000) describes as "a revived necessity to face again the wounds inflicted by the developmental calamities of his or her own childhood—those we abbreviate as the loss of the primary object, loss of its love, oedipal defeat, castration, superego criticism, or awareness of death" (Orgel, 2000).

Orgel was writing about the analyst's experience that accompanies ending analyses with patients, which foreshadow death of loved ones and ourselves. The first death of a loved one concretizes these earlier wounds as one loses the part of oneself that has been invested in the other and ones relationship to them. There is an irrational, emotional expectation that when one loves deeply, those we love will always be with us. The loss of this conviction leaves something more than just sadness. It leaves an anxiety about allowing closeness, intimacy, dependence that can be evoked by separations, illnesses—an awareness of our existential aloneness.

With patients, one knows better, at least intellectually. Termination is expected with the possibility that there may never be a future contact. A necessary loss. With people in our lives who we love, who are not our patients, we don't imagine such endings—unless like our parents, they are much older than ourselves. And even then with people in our lives, there is a way when we love, we don't really anticipate loss until we need to face it. Though some people, depending on their early life experiences, lack this shield against traumatic loss. The death of older loved ones undermines a fantasy of protection—in terms of how they may have nourished us, cared for us in illness, mentored us in crisis, served as a model, and helped us grow. It also forces us to be aware that we too will die, of death approaching ourselves. As we age, more and more people around us who we love become ill and many of them die. We lose an intimate and comforting surround. When a beloved young person dies, we also lose our investment in the future that we anticipated they would carry forward even when we are no longer alive. Each emotionally felt death piles upon the deaths before, reverberates and echoes previous grief. This is what I took Dylan Thomas to mean. And while I think it is true, I also think something else seems lost in this construction.

For each loss is also unique and specific in terms of the meaning of the relationship we have to the loved one. We love in a particular way in each relationship, and so we lose and grieve for the particulars of that person and what it means for us to go on in life without them. What we lose, what we grieve and need to mourn, is highly specific even while the experience of grief is already familiar. Sometimes, particularly as we age, losses accumulate too rapidly to assimilate, and we need to find time and space and ways to facilitate our mourning. We need to cherish our memories of who each loved one was and what our relationship was, to impress this in our memories honoring them and their meaning to us, acknowledging the loss of a future while marking what it is in us that we retain—how the relationship changed us in ways we do not lose with their death. Such is the case for me when thinking of our deeply loved young adult son who died at the age of 31 of a brain tumor. Memories of him make me laugh and then make me cry. I return to them frequently, but I do not want to dwell there too long.

So all this, and of course much more, was stirred in me when my patient told me her diagnosis. She needed my help, my accompanying her through this physically and emotionally terrifying, painful time. My patient knew of my son's death and feared what her illness revived for me. Could I tolerate hearing about her pain and fears? Would I leave her as thoughts and feelings in me evoked a need to return to my own loss and grief? Can she tell me that she envies and resents me for being well while she is ill? Can she talk about the unfairness of her situation? Does she dare to do so while feeling so dependent on me to stay with her and provide a place where she can say to me what she worries will drive others away? I tried to help my now deceased patient do these things. I am trying to make it possible for my current patient to do so as well. We have a history from which she knows I can withstand her hate and aggression. She also knows I hold positive, warm feelings for her. But in her panic about her own mortality, I worry that all she "knows" could evaporate.

Her treatments make her weaker and more tired. It creates a crisis of her identity (Rando, 1993). She is someone who has been tireless. Even in the early stage of illness, she continued to be able to work creatively. Now she is forced to adjust to the reality of her situation, to confront that she cannot continue to be progressive in orientation (Rando, 1993). All our sessions are now on the phone. Not seeing me is a mixed experience. She cannot feel reassured by looking at me, but she also does not have to fear what she will see or what I will see. She tells me she has lost 20 pounds. She loves sweets but will not eat any having been cautioned they may cause her harm. I wonder with her about the severity of her regimen.

We have rearranged the time of our present session. I have momentarily forgotten and not hurried as quickly as I usually do to be available for her call. The phone is ringing and stops as I enter the room. (I do not keep a phone in my office. I do my phone work from a different room within my home). A moment later it rings again and I answer. I apologize, tell her I just missed the earlier call, that I had momentarily forgotten that we had moved the time earlier. Is my forgetting also trying to forget that the time of her death has been moved earlier? Immediately I worry that my countertransference wish to not cause her more pain will have shut off the opportunity for her to be angry with me.

She begins: "The last 24 hours have been hard. The hospital has been having trouble with their equipment. All treatments were delayed. It's hard enough to go through this, but to have to wait. And it is in my interest for them to like me. I don't want to seem like a difficult patient. I will be doing this with them for months. I told them that they were having a very difficult morning. As I was leaving I heard one nurse say to another, 'Aren't we lucky to have such lovely people as our patients'."

Her anger with me expressed in displacement is so blatant. I wonder if it is conscious for her. I let a few moments pass. Just before I am about to say that it would be understandable if she were to feel the same anger and fear of expressing it with me, she begins to speak.

"I have to admit, I felt angry with you when you didn't answer the first time I called."

I wondered with her what she thought and felt when I didn't answer.

"I thought you were angry with me. Maybe you didn't want to talk to me. It can't be easy listening to me going on and on about my treatments and my fears. You like to help people get better, to understand things. I think sometimes it must seem like all I do is say how hard it is and you let me know you understand. That can't be very interesting or satisfying for you. Why wouldn't you want to forget our time? But then you explained and I stopped feeling angry because I knew from what you said that you weren't angry with me, that you felt badly you had kept me waiting."

Me: "But you had imagined I didn't want to talk with you, that I was impatient or dissatisfied with what we are talking about together. You reassure me you were reassured, but maybe as with the nurses you feel a need to reassure me that you are understanding about my feelings, about what I am doing with you, so I won't be angry with you, so I will want to continue to work with you. So I will think you are lovely, caring person."

My patient cries. "I'm afraid I'm frightening you. My illness may make you feel frightened you can become ill. I make you think about your death. Why would you want to think about death? It will make you think of your son's death. It will make you think of your own. So why would you want to talk to me? You've lost a child and you're a lot older than I am—closer to death."

There is a long pause. After a while, I note that she stopped and wonder what she was thinking and why she had become silent.

"You're a lot older. You may be thinking about your own death. Maybe you are thinking you are glad it is me and not you who is ill. That would be natural."

Me: "And it would be natural for you to think because I am much older that it should be me and not you who has a life threatening illness. You've had those thoughts about older people before. And you worry I will turn away from you because your illness revives memories of my son's illness and his death. That I cannot bear a revival of this grief or fear about my future."

She sobs, "You must hate me for making you think about your son's death and for wishing it were you and not me. How can you stand being with me."

Me: "I think you hate yourself, and you said before, feel ashamed, when you wish it were someone older, now me, rather than you. And when you fear your illness revives memories for me of my son and his death, you are frightened I will leave you in anger about what you stir for me. Then as you said, you imagine I will hate you and not want to be with you. You are afraid that your thoughts can harm me and drive me away, so when I was a few minutes late today you imagined that was what had occurred. That frightened you and made you angry that not only were you the one who was ill but then you imagined I couldn't tolerate the fear you imagine your illness stimulates in me, that I would abandon you. Then you can be your own advocate, feeling the unfairness of being younger, having this awful illness, and be angry with me, but then it frightens you that I would leave you and you have to be empathic with me to keep me on your side." And I thought: Having said all this—and there are so many words—am I also trying to hide the truth from both of us? That I also do want to turn away, and that my forgetting is likely not only based on a reality, but that part of me doesn't want to be there with her, identified with her, unable to ward off the return of my own past grief.

She cries and says all I've said is accurate. But how could she bear to go on when she had reason to fear that all she had would be gone, that she would be gone. She could not bear it and did not see how I could. What had the purpose of all she tried to do been worth? I wondered what she had imagined. After a long silence, she said, "I guess I imagined it would go on forever just getting better and better if I tried hard enough." The vestiges of her omnipotent belief were clear to both of us.

The reality for me is sessions like the one I have just described are easier than others. I feel I am doing our work, and that it is useful to her. She is right that I find it harder to sit with her sense of help-lessness and pain, feeling all I can do is be with her and bear the grief and fear together. I admire her. She is brave. She has grown so much over the years. I have watched her growth, been part of some of it. She is one of my analytic children. Almost like my own child, I ask with disbelief how can she die before me? She is right; it's not fair. I am left by others as they die; the frequency of this increases as time goes on. It is painful. Sometimes the grief does feel unbearable.

In a later hour, she says, "I do not want to call myself ill. I am afraid if I say that other people hear it as I am about to be dead."

I say: "You are afraid that they will jump ahead in their minds as you do in yours."

I need to be with her. But what does this mean? To be attentive to her state—not too far ahead or behind? To monitor my own state so it does not obscure hers. I talk to myself, to a few trusted others, in order to keep my own feelings as clear as I can. I try to hear where she is. I know I need to be honest with her, not unrealistically reassuring, but also not depriving her of the hope for whatever pleasure she can have in the time she has.

It makes me treasure the time we have. We cannot know how long it is, but it is possible now. There will be a time when it won't be. My task, I think, is to try to help her feel this way about time—to cherish what we have, face that it's finite, and invest in the present while we have it and to let go when there is more suffering in holding on (Adams-Silvan, 1994).

Later: My patient is in the last months of her chemotherapy treatments. She is thinking about what comes next. Should she return to teaching, which she loves. She misses contact with her students. Perhaps she could do it less than full-time. But she worries about money. She also wants time to be with her children. Time? She still doesn't know what time she has left. Her husband has always wanted to live abroad. Perhaps this is what they should do. Take six months in Rome. Yes, this seems like a good plan. She seems settled into this idea.

I asked her how she imagines it. She begins to describe the meals they would eat, the things she would buy. She stops. Then she begins to sob. She can no longer eat what she wants because she is told her diet likely affects her health. Food and buying thing have been such a huge pleasure in her life. Clothes and jewelry always are connected with the delight of imagining wearing them in the future. But will there be a future? She is so grateful to her husband for all his care and attention. She wants to do what he would want, but... We have been here before. This is about her willingness to sacrifice all her own wants and wishes to someone on whom she has been dependent. She reminds us that she knows this and thanks me for helping her remember this and what it costs her. Actually I have done no more than ask her what she imagines it would be like. The rest is her evoking what she already knows about herself.

After the session, I am thinking about my patient and her willingness to be self-sacrificing out of gratitude. We know she hates being dependent. And with this thought I realize that I have not been thinking of something in my own history, something I know very clearly and have known as long as I can remember, but which amazingly has not come to mind in the context of my patient's illness. When I was five, I had typhoid. It was before antibiotics. I was home in bed for three months. My mother took care of me, reading me the whole series of the Wizard of Oz. I was critically ill. My memories of this time are only pleasurable—a sunlit room, the endless engrossing stories. My mother's attentiveness. Clearly that cannot be all, but memory is merciful. Perhaps it links my lifelong love of reading novels. But, of course, what I wrote earlier needs to be modified. I had been faced with the potential of dying and perhaps my question to my mother. "Think of someone who didn't die" occurred during or after my Typhoid. I am an only child; there is no one left to ask. I was very close to my mother as a latency child, pulling away as an adolescent with much guilt about the pain it caused her, not understanding until my analysis in my early 20s what I felt I had to sacrifice to her in my gratitude. But gratitude is from the word "gratis." It is meant to be something freely given, without sacrifice. My anger about what I relinquished was covered over.

My patient's thoughts of gratitude had triggered my preconscious link to these memories. I was so glad to now be the one who was depended on rather than the one depending. But with this thought comes the recognition that my Typhoid was 70 years earlier. If I do not die quickly, as I would wish, then I will inevitably become dependent again as age or illness is my fate like everyone's. No wonder I dread being alone, left by those who I love and love me. I know my dependence but I also fear it—what if I am alone? The dread that arises has parallels to my patient's dread of dying. I return to my earlier thoughts with greater poignancy and understanding. We cannot know the future. All we know and have is the present.

I was in my early 40s when my father died. He was in his 70s. He too had a painful course of cancer. Given a history of early deaths in his family, he had never expected to live that long. He felt he had had a good and full life. A year after he died I dreamed that I was walking with him. In the dream I knew he was dead, that I was dreaming, and that when I awoke, he would be gone. We continued walking and talking. I awoke in tears with a renewed and condensed appreciation that he was not mine to keep.

I have always loved Freud's paper "On Transience." I now think I better understand why.

Freud begins: "Not long ago I went on a summer walk through a smiling countryside in the company of a taciturn friend and a young but already famous poet. The poet admired the beauty of the scene but took no joy in it. He was disturbed by the thought that all this beauty was fated to extinction, that it would vanish when winter came, like human beauty and all beauty and splendor that men have created or may create. All that he would otherwise have loved and admired seemed to him to be shorn of its worth by the transience which was its doom" (p. 305). "I could not see my way to dispute the transience of all things, … But I did dispute the pessimistic poet's view that transience of what is beautiful involves any loss in it worth" (p. 305). "… the value of all beauty and perfection is determined only by its significance for our own emotional lives, it has no need to survive us and therefore is independent of absolute duration" (p. 306). Freud concludes: "What spoiled their enjoyment of beauty must have been a revolt in their minds against mourning. The idea that this beauty was transient was… a foretaste of mourning over its decease" (p. 306).

Mourning is easier to experience when one can imagine a future—other springs that will come, new loves or friends or lives to invest in. But when someone is dying, they have to let go of that imagined future time. Our own age also affects us, as does our responses to a patient facing death (Houlding, 2013). As we age, it is hard to accept that there may not be future loves, friends, no future analytic children, or new lives to replace those we have lost—though it is very hard to relinquish such a hope. But it makes us aware of what Freud is suggesting. That is, what we have is now. We need to appreciate it, not to deny that it or that we or those we love are only transiently present. We need to try to live in that space. And all I can do for my patient is stay with her to help her with the unfinished business (Nuland, 1993) represented by her omnipotent belief that she could control her destiny with her thoughts, to help her mourn her loss of omnipotence, to tolerate her helplessness, to grieve what is likely to be her premature death, and to live as fully as she can, while she can. I hope our work together will make it possible for her to enjoy and savor what she has now, to access reality, to appreciate the present. I try to convince her she can count on my presence for as long as she wishes it and for as long as I am able. We both need to know, but not be paralyzed by an awareness of the painful reality that our current life, all we have, can end at any moment.

Over the following months, my patient and I continue to talk about her fears of death, of her grief over anticipating never being with her loved ones again. Simultaneously, with increasing frequency, she talks of current pleasures. When her chemotherapy is completed, she selects a necklace to celebrate the event. Then she buys new clothes for her slimmer figure. She spends a weekend visiting one of her children. They laugh a lot and don't talk much about her illness. Another weekend, they visit old friends. The friends want to talk about her illness, to know what she was going through, but one of them had been ill too. Talking about her illness with them isn't so painful. She feels close to them, not so alone. It is harder when she is home; everything reminds her of her illness. Even so, as she begins to regain her strength, she feels better more of the time. She is no longer collapsing time as much. Her future, of whatever duration, is a time she can find some pleasure in for as long as she can. It is all we can hope for. And while today I am healthy, I know that most of my life is behind me. Together we face the heartbreaking reality that all we have is now and it is that what we must cherish and enjoy.

Chapter 13

The analyst

Disabled and enabled
by what's personal

How do we become analysts? In this final chapter, I will present the trajectory of my use of my self and my understanding of the mutual influences my patients and I have had on each other over my professional life. The use of myself and the mutual influences my patients and I have on each other, of course, are about the patient-analyst match. I believe our engagement reflects a process of working through for me as well as each of my patients. Events in our lives also affect who we become as people—sometimes only in subtle ways and sometimes more significantly. Changes in our selves have reverberations in our work with patients.

When I began my psychoanalytic training in 1968, we were taught that analysts were meant to be "blank screens." Patients could and would project their difficulties onto us. Who we were, our conflicts and character, were to have been smoothed out in our personal analyses and our personalities purged of the tendency to appear in our offices. Analysts were assumed to be interchangeable. I know this sounds like a parody of analysis. I also now know that many analysts even then were not like this, but it was what we were taught. I admit to having been incredulous. Really? Who we were as people would not enter our work with patients? Prior to my training, I had worked primarily with children and been relatively free in using myself intuitively in the work.

My classic analytic training did help to provide a discipline for my spontaneity that was useful, but the idea that I, or anyone, could be grayed down sufficiently to be a "blank screen" defied both my imagination and personal experience. The impression I got as a candidate was that an analyst should listen and understand but not influence the way an analysis proceeded apart from providing insight. This belief may explain why there was a period of time of the "silent" analyst—as though silence was a neutral state. The amount I spoke lessened, but I rebelled against the idea that who we are as people could be expunged from our work.

I thought then, and still do, that we can and should learn to curb our judgments about how to live a life. We will do better work with some people than with others because of who we are, especially when our conflicts and character mesh or clash. This is what I have called the patient-analyst match, which inevitably affects the nature and outcome of our analytic work. Since we are inevitably part of the process, we need to find a way to be mindful about our influence without becoming constricted by arbitrary rules.

The psychoanalytic world changed. In the early 1980s, James McLaughlin (1981) wrote about analysts' transferences to their patients; Irwin Hoffman (1983) proposed that patients were interpreters of their analysts' conflicts, not just the other way around. I performed a pilot study (Kantrowitz at al1989) that showed the patient-analyst match—the effect of overlap in character and/or conflict—was the variable most related to the analytic outcome. By the 1990s, there were many psychoanalytic papers about what we called the analyst's countertransference and the inevitability of the analyst's personal characteristics as contributing to what transpires in analysis. The pendulum swung. Soon, the person of the analyst rather than the patient became the center of psychoanalytic attention. Then postmodernist ideas frequently led to the "disappearance" of focus on either patient or analyst character and conflict as the concept of "the third" ascended, for example, reverie as a co-construction, washing out distinctions between self and other. The belief that one could stand neutrally outside of transference and countertransference faded.

This sort of dialectic seems inevitable in our thinking. We swing one way and then the other : a focus almost exclusively on the patient, then a central scrutiny of the analyst, and finally a merger of the two making them almost indistinguishable While we cannot obliterate who we are as people from our work, we need to be mindful that our characters and conflicts do not dominate our interactions. We need to try to catch our selves when our personal characteristics intrude and hone their expression when they threaten to disrupt what we and our patients are trying to understand. We, the analytic dyad, are two people, each with our own intrapsychic issues involved in an interpersonal relationship in a world that impinges on both of us, though how we perceive that world and our engagement with it may in some important way be different. Currently, many analysts—perhaps most—see a value in being more welcoming and transparent; some engage in a Ferenczi-style mutual analysis, the obverse of what I was taught in the 1970s. How do we negotiate these boundaries of self and other, keeping our patients as our focus, being real and humane while trying not to let our judgments and values intrude, as they try to find who they are and who they want to be. Who we are influences how we work. So following Ted Jacob's (1991) felicitous phrase, the use of the self, I will try to illustrate what I have understood about this concept in relation to my work with patients and in relation to the complexity of our intersubjective match.

How I use myself is something that has evolved over time. Always, it is the clinical interaction that stimulates my reflection. Rather than provide a single case example, I will present a number of brief illustrations reflecting different parts of me at different times in my professional life. My aim is to show a process of how I use my self and work through what is stimulated by my patients.

Early in my professional life, I think I would characterize myself as working intuitively. I tried to follow my patients' affect and thought and used my own (not always so clear or nameable) affects and thoughts that resonated to formulate what I was hearing. My analysis and analytic training supplied a discipline that helped me to achieve greater asymmetry, to stand back more, rather than automatically mirror the patient's state. Theory, when I found it meaningful, helped to organize my affect and broadened my thinking. I continued to learn a great deal about myself in the process of trying to understand my patients' conflicts and states. An example in Chapter 4, I now present again here to specifically illustrate work with a patient that lifted my own repression as well as his as I located similar conflicts. It was in the early 1970s, not long after I had terminated my training analysis, very early in my career. I repeatedly dreamed of a patient—just his image. My patient, when only age four, had been left to babysit for his two years' younger brother. His brother had fallen from a second story window and become permanently brain damaged. His mother accused my patient of pushing his brother out the window. My patient did not believe he had pushed him but suffered intense guilt ninetheless, as if he had. I tried to analyze my dream but seemed stymied about its meaning. My dream of him—his image—recurred until I imagined telling my former analyst about the dream and had an image of myself standing in front of a summer house when I was four; I also recalled the memory of my mother's miscarriage. At that moment, I had an intense awareness of how much I didn't want a sibling. Theses memories of my mother's miscarriage and the house were not new, but my associated thought and affect were. Until then, I had thought I only bemoaned being an only child. My guilt was buried in my reversing my wish. Following this realization, I could much more effectively address my patient's sense of guilt. I didn't dream about my patient again. My dreaming of the patient—an uncommon experience for me—had stimulated my self-scrutiny. My associations enabled me to find a similarity to my patient—our common sense of guilt in relation to fantasies of harming a sibling that occurred at a similar age. My guilt had not been conscious while his was, and I had been trying to lessen his guilt—focusing on his self-criticism—rather than analyzing it, until I discovered I was avoiding facing guilt in myself (see Racker 1957).. My patient had been ready to explore his guilt, but I had been defending and moving away from my experience of guilt. Once I was ready to inhabit mine, we shared a state of an affective distress that we could both explore. A different and increased focus on his guilt opened the way for exploring his aggressive fantasies (Kantrowitz, 2009).

Over the years, I learned more about my characterological tendencies—tendencies that were ones I would not welcome recognizing—stimulated by discoveries of overlapping character issues with my patients. Engagements involving patients' fury or perceptions of me as withholding and mean would lead to my own fury and intense feelings of experiencing myself as someone I would hate and fear. When these experiences first occurred, I did not think in terms of projective identification, though the experience could, of course, be conceptualized that way. My understanding of patients who stirred these intense affects in me is that they were externalizing one half of a relationship, in most cases a sadomasochistic one—most often with me as the sadistic abuser. I understood that I needed to tolerate being in this role for them to understand it. I didn't think of it as just providing a holding environment because I felt so acutely the intensity of the affect with my patients in our interactions. In order to contain what I felt, to find a resonance, I needed to understand what was stirred in me—an exploration of affective memories of being on both sides of the conflict.

For example, one patient was intensely preoccupied with me: She wished to call and share her daily experiences, to accompany me on vacations and professional trips, to have me read what she read, see what she saw. She had felt neglected by her busy professional mother. The problem for me in the treatment was that she would become depressed or paranoid in response to my interpreting her longings for more from me. She felt I was rejecting her when her literal wishes were not granted. I felt pressured; my reaction was an anxious, angry stiffening and wish to pull away. Though I manifestly contained these reactions, I am sure she sensed my feelings, and this increased her pressure on me. One day, she requested that I be the guardian of her children. She realized I might think of this as a conflict in my role, but since she would be dead, this would not be so. Who better than I would know her wishes? I felt the familiar stiffening in myself in response to her push for more from me, but having spent much time exploring in myself how it felt to be on either side of such conflicts, I invited her to do the same. After much exploration, getting nowhere, I asked her how she would respond if a patient asked this of her—my patient was a therapist. She became very thoughtful, then said she wouldn't want to say no, it would be hurtful. But it would be such a huge responsibility; she wouldn't really want to do it. But she would feel she had to or injure her patient. She wouldn't want me to say yes if I didn't want to. I said I knew she wished I would want to do this, but if I didn't and said no, she had put me in a position where she would experience me as being hurtful to her in a way she knew she didn't want to be. Following this interaction, she began to recognize her role in what she had experienced as others' meanness. I had used the discomfort I felt in being "the mean one" to find an empathic way to help her see her part.

It was Sandler's (1976) concept of role-responsiveness, more than the idea of projective identification that resonated because he was very explicit that there needed to be something in us that got hooked by the patient's conflict for this to occur. Enactments as compromise formations, sometimes more influenced by the patient's issues and sometimes more by our own, made a great deal of sense to me. Another example, previously presented in Chapter 2, I offer again to illustrate the recognition of my own struggles with feelings of helplessness and difficulties in accepting my own limits that emerged from my countertransference enactment. I vividly recall a time in the late 1980s when a patient was railing against the limits of reality, refusing to accept any possible solution to a situation that caused her acute narcissistic injury. I tried all the ways I could think of at the time, but I failed to provide any soothing or insight-promoting effect for my patient. Our time was up, or so I thought; however, I'd ended the hour ten minutes early. I don't want to leave the impression that I had earlier worked through my susceptibility to feeling guilty! But it wasn't only guilt I felt. I recognized that I had been unable to tolerate my own sense of helplessness, a feeling similar to my patient's. My patient had stimulated in me the very feeling she was experiencing. My patient dealt with feeling helpless by having a tantrum, while I, once out the door and realizing my error quickly, knew a familiar experience of feeling unable to master something and wanting to throw up my hands. I had dealt with my helplessness by walking out on it as I often fantasized doing, but didn't usually allow myself to do. Clearly containing both my own and my patient's sense of helplessness had been more than I could tolerate at that moment, and I abandoned both of us—a clear example of mutual, reciprocal impact.

In the last few decades, I would say that I have been more actively mindful about the way I offer myself to be used by patients. I welcome and embrace negative transferences, finding them a rich avenue for exploration, and am not usually thrown into states of self-criticism by them. I've come to appreciate that with some patients not only half of a conflict, but half of an internalized object relationship is externalized and extruded. When there is no representation for the patient of what is extruded, it is the analyst's capacity to contain and to empathize with both the patient's conscious experience and all that the patient disavows—including registration of the disavowed "other's" subjectivity—that enables the patient both to re-internalize the extruded, conflicted parts and to accept "otherness" itself.

This conceptualization emerged from work with traumatized patients whose distrust, fury, and sense of deprivation can make them unable to take in the point of view of others. When I have been able to find a place in myself that can resonate and tolerate the intensity of feeling unseen, deprived, frightened, or abandoned and a reactive emptiness, greed, fury, and neediness, we can find a place of subjective meeting and the work can deepen. But my conscious willingness to let myself participate with such malleability to my patient's needs is not always sufficient.

A severely traumatized patient resisted all work in the transference and experienced any observation about her as competitive and demeaning. Anything beyond empathy evoked her anger or withdrawal. I knew she was frightened and feared humiliation. Observations produced both of those responses; she dreaded and resisted this experience. I finally observed that she was willing to go places with her own patients that she was unwilling to go with me. She said she heard that as an invitation; I agreed it was. I can't really tell you what happened next, because for the following month she bombarded me in a way that my mind became paralyzed. I tried everything I knew how to do—took copious notes after hours to try to get perspective, talked with several colleagues about what was transpiring, tried to analyze my dreams. Nothing I learned or said to my patient changed her assault on me. The content seemed less relevant than the intensity and its unrelenting flow. Finally, I said I could only think that she was communicating to me what her own experience had been growing up. Not long after, she said, "Enough—being so rageful isn't good for me," and stopped her assault. Try though I did, I concluded we were not a facilitating match. I believe I was unable to tolerate the extent of her fury. To survive, I dissociated as she had done in childhood. I took on her state, and she became the abuser of her childhood. Since I was unable to offer her a place in myself of empathy and containment for her state, I was abandoning her to being someone she hated and feared and could not tolerate being. The split was repeated, but not repaired. I felt regretful but accepting of my limits. We worked together for a while longer, talking some but not adequately about what occurred between us, and ended the treatment several months later. We both recognized we could not work further on our experience. I have had no further contact with her.

Conceptualizations of conflict and affect states, any theories that increase appreciation of how and why people struggle, help our patients and us feel understood and contained—but they are not always enough. When theory helps, it is not just intellectual. The ideas become integrated as part of ourselves and then used in a more spontaneous fashion. I don't think I'm apt to be listening for a process of projective identification and projective counteridentification with patients, though I think for the most part I recognize it when it occurs. I'm sure all I do is influenced by what I've learned over the years about human psychology and disturbances in others and myself. So in a sense, I find myself less conscious of myself—still operating intuitively, but now having absorbed so much cognitively and having gained increased affect modulation. It feels seamless until there's a disruption. Then I return to self-scrutiny and try to untangle what has transpired between my patient and myself that has interfered with our work.

Another consideration in how we use ourselves concerns our attitudes about self-disclosure. I don't mean telling our patients about our private lives—though I realize some analysts find this is a productive way to work—but our willingness to use our own feelings about what happens between a patient and ourselves as a way to help the patient recognize the extrusion of the perception of another in order to help them access parts of themselves that they find unacceptable, and by so doing help them access those parts. The intimacy of the therapeutic situations permits patients, when they are able, to find a freedom of thought and expression. If I introduce my life, my pain, my fears, I believe that I distract them from themselves; they may hear or sense my revelation as an implicit request for a response; our contract is to focus on their needs, not my own. Disclosing deeply personal feelings in a presentation, or even a published paper, is different from disclosure directly to my patients—though, of course, disclosures in these formats if our patients learn of them will likely stir many reactions. When I was younger, I thought the actual information presented a potential interference in our work, but I no longer believe this is so. It is not the information itself that interferes with patients' transferences to us—though such information may delay the development of their fantasy use of us for their needs. But, of course, we do reveal personal things all the time. Our offices reveal our taste. It is apparent when we are sick, tired; we make slips. We may sometimes answer questions about why we go away, where we go, certainly we always tell for how long. And there are many ways in which we convey information about ourselves about which we are not aware. Anything a patient learns about us can be understood in terms of its meaning to the patient. We need to be able to explore together what the information has stimulated in them, how it has altered their perception of us, and if it has, how they believe this might change our work. Such inquiry is part of our work. The internet also has changed what personal information can be discovered. But I think that even without this easy source for finding personal facts, I would feel the same. We can explore the meaning of anything that is learned about me, but when the information comes from me, I have also introduced the meaning of my telling, a meaning that may not even be conscious to me at the time.

Answering personal questions when they arise in the course of our work together is a related matter. While there are occasions where answers may be necessary, or possibly desirable, answers can confuse patients about boundaries. I am not an affectively distant analyst, but I have both seen, as well as know of, too many patients whose therapists have not remained clear about their place in their patients' lives. They may assume multiple roles. No matter how such shifts in stance or role are rationalized at the time, entering into dual relationships is likely to have untoward reverberations over time, , such as when the analyst becomes a personal friend, or, most dramatically, when the analyst enters into a sexual relationship with a patient, I treat many patients who, were they not my patients, could have been my friends. But I feel very clear even when we end the treatment that my role remains as their therapist or analyst, someone to return to should they ever feel the need.

Although who I am in the world may not be so different from who I am in my professional roles, who I am to each patient is also influenced by who each patient needs me to be and so perceives me. If I consciously chose to introduce myself, my own needs and foibles, I believe this could complicate and confuse what my patients take away and what they need to mourn. My everyday, out of the office self can muddle this process. Who I am as a person is inevitably present to some extent in the work, but that is different from the choice to actively bring these personal aspects in. Over time, I have come to accept seeing how my own character and conflicts, when they inter-digitate with those of my patients, may be played out in ways I wish they hadn't. I regret when my ignorance about some issue or blind-ness to my conflicts complicates our work, but I feel less ashamed about such intrusions occurring. These disruptions seem inevitable from time to time, and while I am unlikely to reveal the content of my own issues, there are times when I feel it is important that I ac-knowledge with patients that I have introduced such complications. Sometimes, interferences that limited our work are not recognized until many years later.

Events in our own lives can have a powerful effect on our work with patients. In the mid-1990s I suffered a loss in my personal life that greatly affected me and my patients, My loss had reverberations both inside and outside my analytic work; it both disabled and enabled me. Twenty-one years ago, vacationing in the south of France, my husband and I returned to our hotel imagining many more glorious days ahead. As we entered our room, the phone was ringing. I picked it up to hear our twenty-six-year-old son say, "Mom, I have some bad news. I have a brain tumor."

We flew home the next day. Our older son was already by his side. Our daughter, who was on a safari in Africa, was not reachable for several days. Our son was operated on two days later. The diagno-sis was an Astrocytoma. The tumor was debulked, but could not be completely removed; it overlapped with his motor functions. When he reached us that night in France, my husband, who is a physician and very wise, said, "He will die." I knew it must be true, but I could not, would not, accept living emotionally with that reality. He was too young. We were too young. I had to have hope—for our son, for me, to go on living and finding pleasure in whatever time he had. I held dearly to the thought: "There has to be a time that someone will find a cure for this kind of brain tumor. Maybe it will be now. How can we know that it won't?" This is the doubleness of knowing and not accepting what you know: How do you sustain hope, optimism about a future, when reason tells you it won't exist?

It was early August. I was not scheduled to see my patients again until more than a month later. So I could attend visits to his doctors and be by our son's side as he began a course of radiation all with-out canceling patients' appointments or considering what I would tell or would not tell them. Surely, I tried to say to myself, the doctors wouldn't plan all this if there were no hope, even though I knew—you always do what you can—that the doctors were proceeding as if what I clung to was true: a possibility might still exist that he could be cured.

In the weeks that followed, I began to think about my patients and disruptions in my schedule. What, if anything, would I tell my patients? I know, and still believe, that if I were the one who was ill, I would tell them of my illness. I have witnessed too many colleagues who did not inform their patients about serious, often life-threatening illnesses. Some of these analysts—many who were older, but not all— had died without any chance to say goodbye, leaving their patients shocked and bereft. Even when death is not the outcome, patients struggle with what they think they perceive as changes in their analysts, worrying if they could or should address it, burdened not only by their own concern and anxiety for their analyst, but also anxious that they might be intruding, exacerbating their analysts' concerns, especially as they age. I thought if I were the analyst who was seriously ill, I would want to deal with the effect of my illness and possible death on my patients. But would it be the same for them and for me facing my son's life-threatening illness? What would my patients perceive in me? How would it change our work together?

I thought about each of my patients—their histories, their vulnerabilities, their relationships, and transferences to me. I was fortunate at the time that most of my patients were people I'd worked with for a considerable period of time and were engaged in intensive work. I knew them well. As I thought about each one, I decided that there would be time in the future to deal with the meaning of my son's illness to them—again a reflection of my "knowing" the outcome of his illness while simultaneously refusing to accept it. But one patient made me pause. Her view of me was so often of my being distant and withholding, as she had experienced her mother. Would it be worse for her to find out from others rather than from me? But as I considered her response, I recognized that my thinking of telling her was a way of my protecting myself from her anger—which she'd likely try to hide, but I knew her well and thought I would be able to help her bring it to the surface if that occurred. But the more I thought about it, however, the more I thought I should try to protect all my patients' treatments for as long as I could. I knew I would need to be vigilant to attend to what they might not be conscious of or might not be willing to risk seeing or saying if they suspected something was wrong, or if they actually knew. Trying to protect my patients from the reality I was facing, to make it easier for them, for me, all, I realized were as impossible as saving a child. On some level, they inevitably would be registering my changed and upset state.

And then I began to recognize that I wanted and felt I needed to preserve my work space for myself. I wanted it to be a respite from the anxiety and grief that I was fending off by an illusion of hope. I could be there for our son, supporting and loving him, but I could not really be effective in helping him, in changing the heartbreaking reality that he was likely to die. I recognized my work as a place where I was not helpless, and where I could be effective in helping others. I could not know whether I could keep my patients from knowing the reality of our son's illness. I did not plan to keep it secret from my friends and colleagues. Relationships bring me comfort. Many of my colleagues' and friends' lives overlapped with my patients; I did not want to impose on them some sense of secrecy about our life—but would they preserve my privacy? What if they didn't? I would manage later. With these considerations, I decided I would not tell my patients. Throughout my career as a psychoanalyst, I have turned to a colleague-friend to be an ear for me, to process with me what went on in sessions with my patients, to listen for what I might be missing. Now, I felt a more acute need to be told if I were concealing from myself distress my patients might be perceiving in me or expressing themselves. Having an outside listener gave me a way to feel I could trust I would be less self-deceptive. I was grief-stricken about our son, but I was feeling more settled about how I would approach my work.

In my first hour of the first day back, a patient told me that she had been told about my son's illness in early August—so much for careful planning. The person doing the telling had no idea she was talking to a patient of mine; it was just a sharing of tragic reality about the life of someone who was part of the patient's community. My patient said to me, "I am SO sorry I have intruded on your life." I said, "On the contrary, my life has intruded on your analysis." But of course, it was not on the contrary. I realized that both were true and actually inseparable. I did not mind that she knew the information about my life, but I knew it was likely to be a burden requiring greater vigilance for me in our work. I quickly lost the illusion that I would be able to preserve my work as a place to escape my worries about my son. I knew my patient had a close enough relationship with another patient and anticipated that she soon would know my situation. So I impetuously told this other patient, thinking—but not really thinking it out—that it would be preferable to come as information from me. As it turned out, the first patient never told the second, so I had compounded my own need for extra scrutiny—now two patients, not just one, knew my son had a brain tumor and that they had an analyst who was in state of anxiety and grief, even if she (I) could try to put it aside in the context of analytic work. Trying to work, putting my distress asid, was my way of managing my grief.

I had adult analytic children who were physically healthy, whom I hoped I could help to grow, and develop into their best selves. I wanted, I needed, to bring my best, most effective self to our analytic work, to not be thinking and feeling about the dread of impending loss of our son. I knew I had to be alert for signs that my patients would try to avoid their worries about me and my worries about my son, but that I must also avoid reading into what they said or didn't say as thoughts about me or him when they were not present. I had complicated their transferences and their treatments. When the second patient ended analysis, I apologized for having added this burden to our work.

After a period of remission, our son's tumor recurred. I continued to try to keep my work as a respite. I talked with (now two) colleague-friends about what was going on with my patients and me. I was trying to be self-scrutinizing but would not have trusted myself not be self-deceptive. Not only did I want to continue believing against all the odds that our son could survive, I also wanted to, needed to, believe I could still be effective in my work. I analyzed my dreams where fears and grief intruded, disrupting my need for mastery. My husband respected my defenses and did not continue to impose his realism on me, and sometimes, I think, he was comforted by joining me in thinking/hoping that the next treatment would work. My close friends—some of whom are colleagues, others not—provided nurturance in so many ways, staying attuned to my mood, what I wanted to talk about, what I didn't. But of course, some did not maintain this sensitivity and so a few friendships did not survive the stress of my son's illness. These were other losses. But mostly my friendships provided me a source of support, helping me stay available for our son and for my work with my patients.

Our son died a little less than four years from the time of his diagnosis, a week after he turned 31. When you have a brain tumor, unlike other cancers, there is no pain. He became increasingly diminished and spent the last month of his life in a nursing home near us where we visited multiple times a day. Our son was a journalist, so when he died, my patients were informed not only by people in the analytic community, but by a lengthy obituary in the *Boston Globe*, the most prominent of the Boston papers, telling the facts of his all too brief but adventurous life. His funeral was a celebration of his life, people recounting stories of his antics—like taking ten round trips on the air shuttle from Boston to New York in the course of a single weekend to earn a free trip to Europe. He was a character, and our memories of him still make us laugh and bring us joy. Apart from the two patients who knew about his illness, it turns out that none of the others had known. My colleagues had protected my privacy—patients, me, and our work—and yet... I don't know what they may have known without consciously knowing.

When I returned to work a few weeks later, all my patients knew the reason for my absence—informed by a colleague about the reason for my absence. They expressed their sadness for me. But the death of a child defies expectations; responses are different from the death of an elderly parent, a more emotionally expectable sequence. With each patient, I felt the continued need to remain vigilant to what might be avoiding, while also trying not to read in this focus when it wasn't there. I believe for some of my patients my son's death made it harder for them to terminate. Perhaps they felt a need to stay with me, possibly, as replacement children—and I tried to be vigilant about monitoring my wish to keep them.

When I am distressed, unhappy, confused—any state of emotional disturbance—I write. Writing helps me clarify what's going on with me. Dreams bring unconscious facets of myself to my attention. Writing helps me sort them out. But I didn't write about my son then. I told myself I didn't want to use him that way: surely I could have written just for myself. But I didn't. Instead, I continued to plunge myself into my work, and my husband did the same. We talked about our son a lot together, retold stories about him that made each of us laugh—we missed him a lot and this was a way we kept him present. I talked about him with others so it wasn't that I moved away from feelings or thoughts about him. But I didn't turn to writing.

Mourning, grieving takes so many different forms. I began a project exploring how analysts thought about and chose to write about their patients. I interviewed 140 analysts, and it took me several years to put the material together (Kantrowitz, 2006). Then a colleague-friend asked, "So why did you do this project? It's not what you usually think or write about." I hadn't asked myself this question; I was just doing it. Instantly, I knew the answer: My son was a reporter, by preference an investigative reporter. I had unconsciously been continuing his life, living out his role in my research. I had found another way of keeping him alive and returning to writing. The realization brought tears to my eyes.

About eight years after our son's death, a former patient of mine returned. She had been in analysis with me as a young adult in her late 20s and early 30s—the age of my son's illness and death. There had been occasional check-ins over the years, but now she returned because she was frightened by the emergence of hostility she did not consciously experience. She found herself unable to modulate her anger. We worked for several years putting together pieces of herself, her relationships, of affects that she had split and knew of in what she described as "separate stripes." Our work was intense and demanding—gratifying to each of us. We had begun to talk about ending when she was suddenly diagnosed with pancreatic cancer, a disease that had a statistical likelihood of limiting her life to two more years. I was grief-stricken. My analytic child, who I had known over 30 years—how could she die? She had worked so hard, was so vital, so alive, so much younger than myself! How could this be? And while I knew her expected lifetime was just a statistic, it was now difficult for me to again wholeheartedly throw myself into a hope for a medical cure. But there was work for us to do—and I think I wanted to keep her close, to help where I could. We had explored the vicissitudes of her aggression and her fear of being destructive, and now she was terrified that she had brought this illness on herself. I kept at our task of untangling her fantasies about her power and powerlessness, to try to help her live as fully as she could while she could. Although my patient had not been in treatment at the time of my son's illness, she knew he had died and now his death was alive in her treatment. She was frightened she would drive me away, that she would make me think of him and his death, of my own death, and that I would not want to be with her, to work with her. She feared all she would bring to me would be memories of pain and, much as she wished it, she did not really believe I could protect her from dying. If I had those powers, I would have saved my son. So what was the point? Yet she knew she wanted to be with me, to express her fear, her anger, her regrets. She had a good marriage, and her children came to be with her, showing their concern and love. She wept with a newfound sense of intimacy. She had felt unseen by her mother and was intensely self-critical for her not attending enough to her own children. It was only in her hours with me that she felt free to say all this.

Her fears and thoughts about dying did reawaken for me the hope and despair of those years of accompanying our son through his treatment. I struggled to keep my focus on her, but of course, it was inevitably also on him, my lost child. My grief was revived and intensified. Loss compounds loss. And now I was, of course, older too. Although healthy and energetic, I also thought of my own dying.

Before each three-month scan, my patient was overcome with anxiety; she could not help anticipating a recurrence. I felt as if I were reliving my son's course of treatment; I knew I had to contain my anxiety if I were to help her contain her own. She did well, resumed teaching part time, and began an ambitious and meaningful research study. The scan frequencies were decreased to every six months. We were working hard together in her analysis Whatever happened, we both knew we were living this work as fully as we could. In the background for me, though there was sadness as well as this pleasure, for I could not let myself fully believe that with her it could end differently, that she would not die while I still lived on.

But over time, as her scans were clear, her energy was restored—three years from the end of her treatment, it seemed she was cured. It felt miraculous to both of us. We wondered if she were ready to think about ending treatment. First she said no, but then reconsidered; perhaps it was time. We had done this before, but this time it was different. We were both so much older now. She couldn't be sure I'd still be there if she wanted to come back. I am more than ten years her senior. She really knew now that anything could happen. And if she was not here with me, how could she be sure I was okay? And of course, someday I won't be, and how could she know? How could she leave me? And how will I bear not to know about her ongoing health and life? She is my analytic child, but she is not mine to keep. How do we ever end with our patients who have grown in our presence? With our real-life children, when we are lucky, we know and can share in their adult lives, but our patients we have to let go and may never know of their futures. But she has asked a question of me: If she was not here with me, how could she be sure I was okay? I tell her I have a list of my patients and their contact information that I leave with a colleague, and she is on it. If—when—something untoward happens to me, my colleague would let her know. "But if you were ill?" she asks. "I'd want to know. Would you call me?" Tears are now behind my eyes. I say, "If I am able to." She cries. The realism brings the poignancy home to both of us.

When we, when our patients, end a meaningful treatment, we grieve the loss of ongoing contact, but we do not lose what we have found in ourselves and in the other: how the relationship has changed each of us. When a beloved person in our ongoing life dies, the ripples of what we lose are more far-reaching. For me, and for my husband, our work, our ability to be helpful to others, to focus on them rather than ourselves, seemed our ways to cope. Yet I realize that in being an analyst, I was also keeping my son with me, initially by working against the grain of my own preoccupying sadness through the immersion in others struggles, trying to monitor how and when my grief limited my participation, to recognize when my patients were trying to protect me and limiting themselves; later, I more fully reentered my experiences of anxiety, grief, and the fear of impending death with my patient's life-threatening illness.

When I presented this chapter as a paper on the occasion of the seventy-fifth anniversary at the William Alanson White Institute in the context of her discussion of the paper, Ruth Imber wondered whether my 2014 book, *Myths of Termination: What Patients Can Teach Analysts about Endings*, was also part of my mourning process. Similarly when my colleague's question had made me aware of the link of my book, *Writing about Patients*, to my grieving son's death, I was immediately aware that, of course, she was correct. Interviewing former patients about ending analysis and ramifications over time enabled me to vicariously enter their experiences of grief and assimilation of the meaning of this important relationship held for them, what they kept alive in themselves after their analyst was no longer part of their daily lives—what they kept and what they had to relinquish and mourn. The experience of loss of a loved one is simultaneously a unique and universal experience. We can find comfort in bridging our existential aloneness. My work with patients and my writing both provided this comfort for me. I feel fortunate and grateful to have found a profession that satisfies so much.

In analytic work, the personal and professional self cannot always be clearly divided in the way I was taught 50 years ago, but I do believe that keeping our patients' needs, distress, and conflicts as central in our attention, and trying to maintain a neutrality when our own conflicts, attitudes, and values are challenged, in order to understand another without imposing ourselves, is an analytic responsibility. That we gain personally—grow emotionally through our analytic work with patients—is an added benefit, but we need to be careful not to let this self-benefit dominate our work.

In this chapter, I have tried to convey my understanding of the analyst's role in the process of analytic work: conscious decisions about what and what not to reveal, awareness of the inevitability of preconscious and unconscious intrusions, and a commitment to keep the focus on the patients' needs and conflicts. Yet, even while we are trying to find ways to both modulate and make use of our intrusions when they occur, we know the inevitably that what is personal will encroach. Having an external observer, such as a peer supervisor, adds to what we can see. That is the best one can do, but it doesn't erase our potential blindness. So the pleasure and pain in our work inevitably continues, as does our responsibility to remain both inside and outside the process.

Follow-up of psychoanalysis five to ten years after termination

The relation between the resolution of the transference and the patient-analyst match[1]

In the first chapter, I presented the development of my idea about the patient-analyst match. Here I will describe the research I undertook in order to demonstrate that what I saw clinically as the effect of the patient-analyst match is more than a unique perception of my own. As clinicians, we each have our individual experiences. Despite attempts to view psychoanalysis as similar to a natural science where results can, and need to, be replicated, what transpires between each patient and analyst has its unique aspects—though certainly there are principles we adhere to. As analysts, we now learn many theories and techniques; we are supervised by other analysts, who are experienced in doing this intense, intimate analytic work. How we apply what we learn, I maintain, looks slightly different for each of us and for each of us with each patient. I would never have undertaken doing clinical research had I not needed to do so to be able to become a psychoanalyst-clinician. But I would have believed as the later projects I undertook indicated (Kantrowitz, 1996, 2006, 2014) that having the views and experiences of many other analysts was essential for us as a field. Psychoanalysts can see only a limited number of patients in their lifetime and will inevitably know only how treatments take place under their purview—even supervised cases are influenced by their views and personhood. So I value the idea that we can see and study psychoanalytic work that is not our own. But how to do that and make it meaningfully related to what we really do?

In the 1970s when I began this project, the kind of empirical rigor required of most research was unsuitable for the study of the psychoanalytic process and its outcome. An exception to this observation was the Menninger study (Wallerstein, 1986) following the treatment and lives of 42 people. I had neither the experience nor resources to undertake such a project, but by the time I was ready to undertake the follow-up part of my CORST project, I knew I wanted to explore more than the predictor variables of reality testing, level and quality of object relations, and affect availability, tolerance, and motivation for psychoanalysis; I was convinced that psychoanalysis was a two-person process, and that the nature of its outcome depended on the character and conflicts of both participants as well as the analyst's skill, and I wanted to see if I could find a way to demonstrate it. As noted in my introduction, when I first submitted my paper, proposing this thesis, to the major psychoanalytic journals, it was rejected. I was told I had to choice a theory based on making the unconscious conscious or something about the relationship. By the time I undertook the follow-up of my project, the psychoanalytic climate in North America had begun to change. The appendix summarizes the part of my research that was directly related to exploring the impact of the patient-analyst match on the outcome of psychoanalysis.

In recent years, analysts have increasingly viewed psychoanalysis as a two-person situation (Cooper, 1986; Kantrowitz, 1986; Sandler, 1976; Shapiro, 1976; Tartakoff, in Panel, 1981), in which the characteristics and conflicts as well as skills and talents of both participants play a role in determining the ultimate outcome of the treatment. I have defined patient-analyst match along a spectrum of compatibility and incompatibility between patient and analyst that is relevant to, and may facilitate or impede, the analytic work (Kantrowitz, 1986; Kantrowitz et al., 1989). The concept of match examines contributions from both the patient and the analyst and their interaction. From the side of the analyst, it includes countertransference reactions to the patient, but also encompasses other attributes. Reactions to patients that reflect the analyst characteristic responses to particular styles, qualities, values, and attitudes are likely to be derived in large part from the analyst's own dynamic history, but not necessarily countertransference manifestations. Our view of countertransference is less inclusive than the view that all inadvertent expressions of personal characteristics are countertransference (Blum, 1986). On the other side of the match, the patient's reactions to the analyst are shaped not only by the patient's own history and dynamics which lead to transference responses, but also by the analyst's style, qualities, and attitudes, and how these are manifested in the analyst's responses to the patient.

Contributions from the analyst may come into play in several ways. First, the analyst has personal characteristics that are relatively enduring, such as tendencies to be warm or distant or relatively intellectual or emotional in style. Second, the analyst has reactions that are personal but more transient, arising in response to attributes of the particular patient or, in a reverberating way, to the patient's reaction to the analyst. The intensity of the patient's reactions to the analyst, the degree to which they are an outgrowth of transference or reality, and the extent to which the analyst makes these reactions a focus of analytic inquiry vary for each patient-analyst pair. Third, there may be events in the analyst's life, such as illness, marriage, pregnancy, or achievements, leading to changes in the analyst that are likely to have an impact on the patient.

Cooper (1986) states that it is an analyst's responsibility to recognize when a patient's resistance is expressed either by compliance with or opposition to what the patient perceives to be the analyst's needs. It is also necessary for the analyst to be aware when his or her reaction to the patient is excessively positive or negative. Such intense reactions to patients sometimes make treatment impossible. Cooper cites cases where the transference remains unresolved at termination. He points out that analysts have personal limitations; his focus is on factors within the analyst's consciousness. Other analysts stress the less conscious aspects of the analyst's response to patients.

All these authors emphasize the analysts' lack of awareness of their particular reactions and subsequent behavior toward the patients.

In a survey of analytic candidates regarding their training analyses, Shapiro (1976) found that the majority of the candidates who believed their analyses were limited or unsuccessful attributed the difficulty to personal qualities or conflicts of their analysts. Tartakoff (Panel, 1981) places considerable importance on the "fit" between the particular patient and analyst. While she views transference and countertransference as central factors in the analytic process, she does not believe they account for all the analyst's cognitive and emotional responses to the patient. In addition to the self-understanding gained through the analyst's own analysis, she believes that the analyst's personal attributes are crucial in determining what the analyst responds to and communicates when treating a patient.

Since analysis invites the patient to project his or her experience of past and present conflicts onto the analyst, it is often difficult to view the patient's perspective on the analyst as reliable or valid. The subjectivity of patients' impressions is still significant, even when the transference appears to have been resolved and a more objective view of the analyst has been achieved. Given the patient's subjectivity, we must nevertheless respect and take seriously the patient's experience of the analytic treatment.

To my knowledge, no systematic study has been undertaken to assess the impact of patient-analyst match on psychoanalytic outcome. Outcome studies of psychoanalytic treatment have focused primarily, if not solely, on the analysand's psychological characteristics and the change in those characteristics during the course of analysis (Applebaum, 1977; Bachrach & Leaff, 1978; Kantrowitz et al., 1986, 1987a, 1987b; Wallerstein, 1986; Weber, Solomon, & Bachrach, 1985a, 1985b).

I assume that all analysts do better work with some patients than with others. I also assume that all analysts retain some areas of only partially resolved conflict and some attitudes, values, styles, and reactions of which they are not completely aware. The analysand's reaction to the analyst, beyond elements of the transference neurosis per se, is also influenced by the analysand's experience of the analyst's style, attitudes, values, and conflicts (to the extent to which these are apparent). The analysand will react to the analyst's characteristic reactions. Although it may become the focus of inquiry, the resulting interaction often escapes the notice of both parties.

My interest in investigating the impact of the two-person interaction on the analysis evolved from a prospective, longitudinal study of psychoanalytic outcome that focused on both suitability for and response to psychoanalytic treatment. The study sample consisted of all patients who applied for institute analysis and were assessed by senior analysts as suitable for supervised psychoanalysis in a given calendar year. These patients were then independently rated[2] prospectively for capacities thought to be critical to the psychoanalytic process: reality testing, level and quality of object relations, affect availability and tolerance, and motivation for treatment (Kantrowitz, Singer, & Knapp, 1975). I was surprised to find that the degree to which an analysand gave evidence of these capacities, both as determined by clinical interview and psychological test findings, was not predictive of successful outcome (Kantrowitz, 1986). Our inability to predict outcome using such measures has been confirmed by other studies (Weber, Solomon, & Bachrach, 1985a). Such dimensions of psychological strength may be necessary, but are not sufficient prerequisites for successful outcome. Various factors, including limitations of the assessment process, could account for the failure to predict outcome; nonetheless, it seems likely that a particularly important omission might have been consideration of the effect of the match in shaping the two-person psychoanalytic interaction.

When analysts' characteristics that remain outside their awareness are confluent with difficulties of the patient has either kept out of awareness or deliberately avoided in treatment, such difficulties or characteristics will go undetected and, therefore, will remain unanalyzed. If this difficulty is central to the patient's pathology, the analysis will not have a successful outcome. If the overlapping "blind spot" exists in an area that is peripheral to the central issues, the analysis may be seen as successful overall, but no change will occur in this particular area. If an analyst's character or style, as manifested in the analysis, provides a quality or dimension that has been absent or limited in the history of the patient and is centrally related to the patient's difficulties, then the personal characteristic will have a facilitating effect on the outcome of the treatment (Kantrowitz, 1986).

In undertaking an exploration of the patient-analyst fit from the data I collected, several very significant limitations were confronted. The pre-analysis data had not been collected with this question in mind. The limitations of the data include: (1) small sample size, (2) lack of comparable data for the patients and analysts, (3) lack of experience of the treating analysts, (4) inability to take into account the effect of supervision on the analyst, and (5) lack of comparability of the analysts' interviews in terms of openness and completeness.

My original research project was begun at the Boston Psychoanalytic Society and Institute in 1972. Twenty-two patients, accepted for supervised psychoanalysis, became the subjects of this longitudinal study. The methodology and results of this study have been reported in a series of papers describing the initial study design and outcome changes in the predictive variables of reality testing, level and quality of object relations and affect availability, and tolerance and motivation for psychoanalysis (Kantrowitz, 1986; Kantrowitz, Singer, & Knapp, 1975, 1986, 1987a, 1987b).

Only 17 of the 21 patients who had participated in the one-year follow-up were available for follow-up interviews. In the previously reported study, one year after termination, pre- and post-analysis psychological tests were compared, and post-analysis interviews were conducted with both patients and analysts to assess the nature and extent of change.[3] The post-analysis interviews with the analysts, although not initially designed for this purpose, were then used to illuminate the analysts' personal characteristics, styles, attitudes, values, and particular reactions to their analysands. Independent judges reliably rated these qualities from a subtext found in the analysts' interviews. The methodology and design for this assessment has been previously reported (Kantrowitz et al., 1989).

For the purpose of this pilot study in relation to the factor of the match, the analysts' recorded, transcribed post-analytic interviews were reexamined. These interviews reviewed the course of the analytic treatment and the obstacles encountered within it. The research psychoanalysts independently assessed the treating analysts' more personal responses to their patients and the ways in which these reactions were manifest in their interactions with the patients. The data we used were found in the spontaneous comments that analysts made about their patients and about their own attitudes, reactions, and responses to them during the course of analysis.

A rating system was designed to codify our findings along dimensions related to the effect on the match. We labeled the first area Basic Attitudes. Here we noted any statements the analyst made which reflected (1) negative and/or positive value judgments about the patient, (2) reactions of liking or disliking the patient, and (3) sympathy or lack of sympathy toward the patient. The analysts' responses to the patients were evaluated in terms of the extent and the direction of deviations from a neutral analyzing position toward either gratification or distancing. Withholding and antagonism are examples of extreme distancing. The extent to which the analyst entered into and accepted the patient's psychic reality was assessed. Here the continuum ranged from the analyst who totally entered the patient's psychic world and only reflected its content and affect without interpretation or question, to the opposite end where the analyst contradicted and argued against the patient's expressed views and experiences. More subtle expressions of this latter position are seen in attempts to alter the patient's point of view and silent disagreement or disrespect for the patient's point of view without any open disagreement. The raters gave specific quotes from the treating analyst's interview to document the assessments.

The concordance of patient and analyst views, expressed in their post-analysis interviews, was assessed independently by the same judges. They then compared the patient's and the analyst's views. The judges compared patient's and analyst's (1) assessments of the patient's major issues, conflicts, strengths, and limitations; (2) accepting or unaccepting attitudes toward the patient's character structure, conflicts, behavior, and mood states; (3) views of the analyst's goals, intentions, and methods used in relation to the patient (e.g., increasing the patient's self-understanding, making conscious what has been unconscious, analyzing defenses and transference or modifying the patient's behavior); (4) agreement or disagreement about the goals of treatment; and (5) views of the methods that should have been used to attain those goals. Finally, whatever aspect(s) emerged as highly concordant or discordant for each patient-analyst pair was evaluated for both centrality in the analysis and for the extent of the analyst's awareness, acceptance, neutral exploration, or lack of acceptance in this area.

The researchers showed a high degree of agreement in their assessments of the interviews. A profile for each analyst was constructed in which the views of all judges were incorporated. In the summary, the judges and I speculated about the important aspects of the analyst that emerged in relation to his or her patient and the possible effects these might have had on the analysis.

Another psychoanalytically trained psychologist, a psychoanalytic candidate[4] at the time, uninformed about any of the analysts' data or the patients' interviews, evaluated the pre- and post-analysis tests. A description of the central conflicts and concerns at the outset of treatment was made. Comparisons of pre- and post-analysis tests were used to assess the extent to which the patients had changed with regard to these presenting issues. In addition, any other areas that had improved or deteriorated were noted. Reliability of these pre- and post-analysis test evaluations was established by comparing these reports with the psychological assessments made at the time the test material was initially collected and evaluated.

All 21 cases were evaluated for the impact which match might have on the outcome of analysis. Two advanced psychoanalytic candidates independently[5] compared the analyst profile and the evaluation from the psychological tests for each patient-analyst pair. Their task was to assess whether or not the match of patient and analyst influenced the success of the patient's analysis. To do this, they listed the central characteristics and issues for the analyst as revealed in the profile, and the central problematic issues or areas for the patient as revealed in the test report. They were then asked which, if any, of these issues interdigitated for patient and analyst in a manner that they thought might influence the success of the analysis. They were asked to evaluate the amount of influence, the centrality, the direction (i.e., negative or positive), whether it impeded or facilitated the engagement in the analytic process, the course of the analytic work or the completion of the process, and the degree of certainty they had in their evaluations. The judges also grouped the cases into two broad categories of outcome, based on psychological test results: improved and little or no improvement. Next, they reviewed the actual interview with the analyst to corroborate or modify their impressions. They did not make major shifts in their assessments based on these reviews of the transcripts. Each judge wrote a summary paragraph describing, with documentation, his or her perception of the influence of the patient-analyst match on the outcome of treatment. While this method did not allow for formal tests of reliability, the agreement between the two raters was high. Differences were only in terms of emphasis.

Match seemed to play some role in all 21 cases; however, in 8 of the 21 cases we were unable to evaluate the extent of its importance because a preponderance of other factors seemed more central. These factors included: lack of skill on the part of the analyst, possibly due to lack of experience; severity of the patient's pathology, even to the extent of unanalyzability; lack of agreement between supervisor and analyst; and a traumatic experience which occurred between termination and retesting. This left 13 cases in which to try to study the role of the match. This sample size is suitable only for exploratory investigation. Given these data, our findings do not allow us to validate our hypothesis, but the patterns that emerge suggest we may have a concept that can be validated by future research using a similar strategy.

We[6] hypothesized that when an analyst's character or style provided a quality or dimension that was missing or limited for the patient during childhood development and was centrally related to the patient's conflicts or difficulties, it would have a facilitating effect on the outcome of analysis. We also hypothesized that when an analyst's unconscious reactions and responses overlapped with a central issue for a patient, and the analyst remained unaware of his or her reactions, the analysis would be impeded.

We found two kinds of impeding match. In one kind, which we called a match of similarity, the analyst and patient shared similar issues, traits, or expressions of conflicts or conflict derivatives. While the analyst might or might not be aware of these dimensions in him- or herself, the analyst did not notice the similarity with the patient. The shared area might or might not represent a major difficulty for the analyst; however, it was a central area of disturbance for the patient.

In the second kind of impeding match, which we called a match of complementarity, the analyst and patient employed different modes of expression for similar conflicts. The analyst, in this case, was unconsciously defending against the issue with which the patient was manifestly struggling. The shared problem area was central to the patient's disturbance, but might or might not be a central problem for the analyst.

We found one kind of facilitating match, which we called compensatory match. The analyst's character or style provided the patient with a quality or dimension with which to identify, or modified a previously negative or interfering identification that impaired the patient's functioning in a central area of disturbance.

Match was evaluated as playing a central role in the outcome of psychoanalysis for 13 of the 21 patients based on the one-year post-termination evaluations. Seven cases were rated as impeding, five as facilitating, and one as mixed. In several cases, factors that were at first facilitating later in the analysis became impediments to progress. The pilot study defined types of matches.

The present paper more fully describes the relation of match to the outcome of treatment. In this paper, we (1) examine the patient's retrospective view of the analytic experience, (2) reassess whether a transference was established, understood, and at least partially resolved, which had been assessed on the one-year post-termination interviews, and (3) determine the relation between resolution of the transference and the match between patient and analyst. In our interviews, we asked patients about the impact of the match on their treatment. Based on our earlier findings, we believed that the interdigitation of the personal characteristics of the analyst with the particular difficulties and characteristics of the patient was a crucial factor in the outcome of the analysis (Kantrowitz et al., 1989). As stated above, we hypothesized that limitations in the analyses might be related to an interaction of personal characteristics, styles, or attitudes of the analyst that overlapped with difficulties of the patients.

Two researchers, who had not administered the interviews, independently rated the transcribed interviews for the presence of unresolved transference and the role of match in the treatment. Both ratings were made on a four-point scale (see the Appendix). Cohen's Kappa was used to establish the reliability of these ratings, which were statistically significant (K = 0.82; K = 0.75, respectively).

I will describe those cases that have been assessed as having unresolved transferences. I use the term transference rather than transference neurosis since the patients studied did not always have only clearly neurotic conflicts. Their transferences varied from neurotic conflicts to narcissistic and borderline pathology. There was also variation in the intensity or degree of formation of the transference. When a transference is unresolved, the patient continues to relive central conflicts and concerns in relation to the analyst without realizing that an earlier experience is being repeated. As a result, the patient fails to gain perspective on past and present experiences through the reworking of these issues with the analyst.

In certain cases where patients had unresolved transferences, the patient-analyst match appeared to contribute to the stalemate of the treatment. In other cases of unresolved transference, the match seemed to have played a role, but there is insufficient data to confirm or deny the importance of the match in the treatment difficulties. A case that had been successful until the termination phase illustrates a match that was initially facilitating, but became impeding in the closing phase of treatment. I offer illustrations of both impeding patient-analyst match in unsuccessful cases and facilitating patient-analyst match in successful cases.

Unresolved transferences

Based on their retrospective reports, 7 of 17 patients in this study enacted their neurotic conflicts and/or narcissistic or borderline pathology in the transference, but neither understood nor worked through these issues in the context of the analytic relationship. Two patients reported having intense negative feelings toward their analysts, which they now recognized as transference, but were unable to gain perspective on during treatment. It seemed to one patient that the analyst "really" was "hostile and angry," and to the other patient that the analyst was "non-giving and passive." Both patients experienced themselves reliving their historical responses to parental figures. The first patient was superficially compliant but underneath took, in his own words, "a rigid stance" that was "passive-aggressive," refusing to allow the analyst to do anything that would have an impact. The other patient also described "rejecting all help" from the analyst and then "breaking away in anger" in order to feel independent. At the time of termination, both patients felt responsible for the failure of the analysis, but reported no understanding of what had taken place. Subsequent treatment, an analysis in one case and intensive psychoanalytic psychotherapy in the other, enabled both patients to recognize their projections and externalizations, and to gain some insight and understanding of the psychological reasons for what they had lived out in their earlier treatment in analysis.

Two patients maintained intense idealizing transferences that had never been understood or analyzed. Almost ten years after the termination of their analyses, both these patients described their analysts in glowingly positive terms. One patient described the analyst as someone relied on for "guidance and acceptance," "a mentor" who was admired and emulated, whom the patient tried to be "just like." The other patient described the analyst as "exactly what I was looking for... patient, warm, nurturing, unqualified respect, full of integrity... intelligent... perceptive... my better mother." Both patients expressed unqualified enthusiasm for their analyses, believing themselves to be "saved" and transformed by the experience. They revealed great pride in having been analyzed, but neither of them demonstrated or described any insight into themselves or their relationships or showed any self-analytic ability. Both patients seemed to have a greater sense of well-being, apparently derived from feeling continuing connections to their former analysts whom they viewed as benign sources of power. Neither patient had returned to treatment since termination, but both had contacted their analysts at the time of significant life events. The analysts seemed to play ongoing and significant roles in their lives. Both patients describe therapeutic benefit, but not analytic insight, from their treatment.

Two patients described adapting themselves to what they believed their analysts wanted of them just as they had with their mothers. One of these patients, in the course of a second analysis, came to recognize a long-standing search for guidance, and "tried to please in hopes of getting love and care" just as he had with his parents, and again with his boss, following the termination of the initial analysis. The patient believed this transferred dependency was central to his difficulties, though it had not even been noted in the first analysis. The other patient had no subsequent treatment. She reported, and demonstrated, an ability for self-analysis. She described her analyst as "cool, self-contained, not responsive," but benign. She felt the analyst had left her on her own to figure things out for herself, but added, without conscious complaint, that she felt they "had not clicked as a match." She accepted this as the way analysis was supposed to be, and never explored her reactions to a lack of response on her analyst's part or to being poorly suited to the analyst. The patient described her mother in terms similar to those she applied to the analyst, and reported a history of having raised herself without receiving much warmth. There was a striking absence of complaint and bitterness in her account. She appeared to have made the best of her analysis just as she had of her life, taking what she could from her own efforts and not dwelling on what was not offered. This form of adaptation was never noted in the analysis. The analyst viewed the patient as unmotivated and poorly suited for analysis, and did not believe the analysis had had much impact on the patient. While the patient vividly demonstrated her ability to analyze herself, face conflicts, and modify her behavior in response to new understandings, she did not offer any perspective or apply her insight to her transference to her analyst.

Another patient, whose analysis was successful in many respects, became mired in an unresolved transference in the termination phase. The patient believed that termination had not been mutually agreed upon, but rather imposed on him by the analyst. Struggles around control, which had been analyzed during the treatment, reappeared and were reexamined at this time; however, the resentment and hurt, similar to that which the patient had experienced earlier in his life in relation to his family, were not fully enough examined for him to resolve his bitterness. The patient terminated with "residual hostility" which prevented him from feeling free to recontact the analyst at times of future difficulties. To quote the patient: "If you don't want to talk to me anymore, I don't want to talk to you anymore."

In all seven of these cases, patients enacted their earlier life experiences in the treatment. Other patients, however, also described instances of living out conflicts that had not been understood or resolved in the transference, though their reports were more fragmentary and the issues did not take the same prominence as in the seven cases described. For the seven patients, analysis reinforced earlier painful experiences rather than enabling them to understand and come to some resolution in relation to the past. We cannot be sure how much the analysts' inexperience contributed to the failure of these cases, but we suspect it was a relevant factor. The contributing factor for which we can offer data is the role of the match between the patient and the analyst and its impact on the outcome of the transference. In three of the seven cases described as having unresolved transferences, there was evidence that characteristics of the match between the patient and analyst interfered with the resolution of the transference in the treatment.

Match

For some patients who seemed to have relived their pasts in psychoanalysis more than to have understood them, the analyst's role in the reenactment took the form of apparent nonparticipation, for example, in the analyst's holding him- or herself relatively aloof from the patient. In other instances, a dynamic interplay seemed to exist between the issues of the patient and issues or characteristics of the analyst. In a previous paper (Kantrowitz et al., 1989), I described profiles of the analysts in this study in relation to the patients they analyzed. All these analyst profiles were written prior to conducting the five- to ten-year follow-up interviews. As I have defined match in previous papers (Kantrowitz, 1986; Kantrowitz et al., 1989), the analyst's characteristic personality, styles, and attitudes as well as specific countertransference reactions which interdigitate with central conflicts of the patient are all considered aspects of match. The researchers' evaluations found match was a factor in the outcome in 12 of the 17 cases reviewed. For the purpose of illustrating the influence of the match on the outcome of analysis in terms of resolution of the transference, I have divided the cases into two categories: unsuccessful cases, that is, with primarily unresolved transferences, and successful cases, that is, with primarily resolved transferences. I offer four illustrations of the role of patient-analyst match in unsuccessful outcomes and four illustrations in successful outcomes.

Unsuccessful cases

Three cases, cited previously in the description of unanalyzed transferences, have specific features where we can observe the contribution of the analysts' characteristics and the patient-analyst match to the outcome. In the case of the patient who felt left on her own and who had not felt she "clicked" with the analyst, the patient's presenting complaint was sexual inhibition. The patient described bringing the analyst a dream with "naked" women and wondering about homosexual impulses. According to the patient, the analyst deflected her attention from the sexual aspects and focused on the "maternal" aspects of breasts. The profile of this analyst described a rigid, moralistic analyst who did not seem at ease personally and professionally. This analyst subsequently gave up the practice of analysis.

The patient who felt such a strong need to please and be accommodating had an analyst who similarly seemed to desire to keep things pleasant. In a summary about the analyst's work, the two researchers who had independently assessed the role of match state:

> There is a huge discrepancy between what the analyst presents as an overview of the work with the patient and what the analyst actually describes doing. Everything is portrayed as smooth and under control. The analyst recognizes the patient's anger and its intensity, feels the patient could not tolerate not being gratified at times, but none of this is analyzed. The analyst is neutral, seemingly benevolent, but non-analyzing.

The researcher added the speculative notes, "Does the analyst share the patient's difficulty with dealing with aggression? Everything seems to be kept so pleasant... almost as if the interview were designed for a supervisor's approval." This analyst is also no longer seeing analytic patients.

One of the patients who had maintained an unanalyzed idealizing transference had an analyst who seemed to place special value on the "special and unusual" (analyst's words) qualities of the patient, especially the patient's creativity and high intelligence. The summary from our earlier study states:

> The analyst is very committed to mastery and tries to help the patient master intellectually, which this patient seems to value and use positively. Analyst and patient seem to share a wish to replace being judgmental and critical of others with being fair-minded and honorable. For both, a tinge of reaction formation seems apparent as well as their commitment to self-improvement. They work hard and one would expect therapeutic benefit, but not the unfolding of an analytic process.

In this case, there is a suggestion of a mutual "idealization" of the intellect and integrity that may have "blinded" the analyst to the patient's idealizing transference. While I do not have data on any other patients this analyst has treated, this analyst has continued to maintain an active analytic practice.

Another patient, while gaining therapeutic benefit from analysis in the increased availability and modulation of his affects, was aware that he had both an unanalyzed narcissistic transference and unaddressed sexual concerns. He believed the failure to confront his sexual problems was due to an unfortunate fit between his issues and the analyst's. The patient commented in the follow-up interview:

> A mutual avoidance... it's difficult what you say to certain people. I felt at some level it was awkward for both and I think that was a pity; I could see another therapist nudging it along a little bit more. I was inhibited... sex was not talked about... I suspect her problem too. I could label her the problem, that she probably had similar inhibitions. I was shy, awkward... one time she

raised a reference to sex and I said I didn't think it had to do with that. I think it's this kind of thing where the ball got dropped in retrospect. We didn't get beyond that point... I think that could have been more directly addressed toward the end. I felt she was more awkward around these things than I was... Having made the venture of that interpretation, I think she pulled back a bit too rapidly because I felt that even at the time it was more her pulling back for her own reasons, not [for] me... I still have sexual shame.

With regard to narcissism, the patient said:

I continued to have a certain narcissism about me. I believe I'm right and others are wrong, that kind of confidence. I've got these grandiose ideas of what I should be, the little Prince... I think I always felt special... insights from marriage, professional training, supervision, being exposed to a whole mish-mash of things. I think I did the whole process in an objective way... there was a certain lack of curiosity, and I think that's what I call the narcissistic side of me... in a sense I didn't care about this person, I could use this person, in terms of her being hard-working, self-disciplined, a scientist.

The researchers' summary states:

The patient seems very intelligent and articulate. The analyst joined and admired this style. The analyst said they never reached a deeper level, but the analyst did not push for this. The two of them recognized but did not analyze areas of narcissism and aggression, especially sadism. The psychological testing reveals undifferentiated sexual/aggressive impulses that are poorly contained. The analyst describes the patient's primitive aggressive fantasies as a rich fantasy life. The analyst seems to be in collusion with the patient. She seems to conclude that the patient sees himself as special because he is special. High intellectual achievement is very prized by both of them. Is there a blind spot around aggression per se, or could it be that a mutual investment in seeing and keeping him as special causes her to view him so benignly? If this case is assessed as having a successful analytic result by the analyst, we must hold some suspicion.

The analyst did assess the patient as having a successful, though limited, analytic result.

The avoidance of the sexual material had not been apparent to the two researchers who made the independent assessment of the role of match, since they had been more impressed by the pre-oedipal difficulties, but one of the original interviewers and the psychological test results do allude to this issue. The patient was aware of and troubled by the mutual avoidance of sexual material and aware, at least in retrospect, of his narcissistic issues. The analyst retrospectively acknowledged, but did not analyze, the sexual or narcissistic issues according to both patient and analyst accounts of the treatment. Again, this is the only patient on whom we have data from this analyst's practice. The analyst maintains an active analytic practice as well as being a teacher and supervisor of psychoanalysis.

Successful cases

Several of the successful cases have been described in our pilot study of the effects of the patient-analyst match on the psychoanalytic process (Kantrowitz et al., 1989). In some of these cases, the match between analysand and analyst was at first facilitating to the process. Later in the treatment, however, the match seemed to have had an influence in preventing the completion of the analytic work. While we assessed these cases as having successfully completed considerable analytic work, the extent of resolution varied from case to case.

In one case, according to the researchers who evaluated the analyst's interview:

> the analyst was careful and thoughtful with the patient, while also being distant and somewhat rigid in style. The analysis was characterized by many affective storms, loss of accurate reality testing, and an intense negative transference throughout most of the treatment. Despite the analysand's fragile state, no parameters were used. The analyst remained calm and neutral, while rather remote. While calm acceptance would be considered good analytic technique, the researchers perceived these qualities to be particularly characteristic of this analyst's style and manner when describing his work. Post-analysis testing revealed

improved reality testing and better modulation of aggression, but difficulties with sexuality now emerged as a central concern. The analysis ended when the analysand said his analytic relationship conflicted with his real-life love relationship; he could not be involved with two people at the same time. The analyst seems to have accepted his wish to stop rather than to have analyzed it. Thus, the analyst's attitude of calm acceptance, while previously facilitating in helping the patient to contain, reexamine, and eventually modify both his perceptions of the world and his experience and management of affect, later in the analysis presented a barrier to exploring what appeared to be oedipal material and conflicts. The analyst viewed the analysand as successful in analysis. Although the analyst may not have believed the patient could work through these issues, since these conflicts were not even addressed, it appears more likely that the analyst failed to perceive them as requiring analysis. Perhaps the analyst had residual conflicts around sexual issues; we have no data to deny or confirm such a speculation. There was no awareness on his part of a 'blind spot.' Our hypothesis is that whatever its origin, the detachment of the analyst, which was so enormously beneficial during most of the analysis, was an impediment to doing this next piece of analytic work.

In the five- to ten-year follow-up interview, this patient made the following observations about his analysis:

> a pretty good outcome... the relationship was a little on the rigid side... maybe in some ways it was good for me and worked for me... but it didn't help me get to some issues... in response to his loosening up a little, I probably might have loosened up in certain ways too. I think that's true, but I also don't know what kind of resistance there was then. I dealt only a very little with sexual issues... still a troublesome area for me, so we didn't get to it... something I could work on but won't. [The analyst] was accepting and gentle. I thought he was rigid and so was I, so the two of us didn't get out of that one. Well if he's not going to give anything away, then this is how far I'm going... and I got stuck there, maybe we both did.

Another patient, whose initial fearfulness and poorly differentiated sense of herself had shown much improvement on post-analytic psychological tests, had an analyst whom the researchers had described as "nonjudgmental and gentle." They commented further:

> The analyst's gentle patience seemed to have helped her to separate from a mother she perceived as critical and terrifying. However, sexual anxiety not present initially emerged in the later part of the treatment. The analyst recognized the development of increased sexual concerns, but felt that the analysand was not able or ready to deal with them. Termination took place at this point. In the post-analytic interview with the analyst, the analyst expressed concern about being gentle and patient and not frightening this easily intimidated person.

The researchers speculated that the analyst's gentleness in this context was operating in the service of defense. "The very gentle approach which had facilitated the extensive work they had accomplished now served as an impediment, since the analyst failed to actively pursue a particular area, which the patient was reluctant to pursue as well."

In the five- to ten-year follow-up interview, this patient said:

> I never did well in my inhibition about talking about sex, particularly to men. [The analyst] was fairly passive. He was actively involved, and I always felt he was very interested and engaged in the process, but he was exceptionally good at avoiding being directive, and I used to try to get a lot of direction, especially with men.
>
> There's a part of me that would like to avoid and be passive... he was patient, gentle, accepting. If anything, he didn't put enough limits on me. I made hay with his acceptingness and gentleness. [His lack of directiveness] may have slowed down the process. I could get into a lot of struggles around control and not work on a lot else, but he probably could have been a little more assertive himself.

The patient, who was described previously as having had an unresolved transference and "residual anger" about the non-mutually planned termination which precipitated a retaliatory withdrawal, had an analyst who described himself in the post-analysis interview as "very formal and very distant." The researchers' summary and speculation about the analysis was:

> The patient demands that his needs be met, but has some recognition that he is doing with the analyst what he did with his mother. He wants to stay and work out his difficulties, but needs his shame and rage to be tolerated. The analyst recognizes that these are issues for the patient, but keeps failing to understand that the patient's withholding is a mirrored expression of his experience and responds to it exclusively as a resistance. The analyst becomes 'bored' and frustrated. The patient says to the analyst, you don't give enough, and the analyst implicitly says to the patient, you don't give enough either. The patient feels not responded to with enough warmth and caring, and the analyst feels not appreciated, valued, or liked by the patient.

Although this patient and this analyst previously accomplished a great deal of analytic work, especially around issues of control, they came to a stalemate. The analyst decided it was time to terminate and announced this to the patient. We wonder, as did the evaluators of the one-year follow-up interview, if:

> the analyst had too fully joined the patient in despair and been unable to maintain his sense of esteem as an analyst in the face of the patient's demands and criticisms; he withdrew just as the patient had... Both analyst and patient agree that although there have been many positive changes, the treatment has been a disappointment. Analyst and patient have distanced from each other, both feeling somewhat a failure. The analyst's inability to perceive and contain his reactions seemed to make the patient and analyst poorly suited for each other at this phase of their work.

At the time of the five- to ten-year follow-up interview, this patient was much more positive about the analytic experience:

> It was clearly a valuable experience, no doubt about it. In retrospect, I think I probably didn't quite appreciate what it was about

at the time. It made me, through widening self-awareness, able to deal with who I am, able to live more richly and perhaps more efficiently.

The patient commented about the analyst:

> I respected him; he clearly took his work seriously, and it was pretty no-nonsense... a master of being neutral... I knew what analysis was all about and yet I wanted him to be conversational with me... I felt that the ending of analysis should have been something mutual, and perhaps my decision and the way it came down was that I had no control over it at all. [He] prepared me months in advance [for termination], so it wasn't that he didn't handle it correctly.

Nonetheless, the patient "made a conscious decision after analysis not to contact him for ten years," and understood that this was a retaliation, in addition to an attempt to counter the dependency that had existed. The patient summarized this situation, "You don't want to talk to me anymore, I don't want to talk to you." Both patient and analyst had focused on the anger and control issues; neither had addressed the sadness and hurt in the ending. At the time of the second follow-up interview, almost ten years after termination, the patient was experiencing intense feelings of conflict and much unresolved guilt. Despite positive regard for the analyst and great appreciation for the work they had done, the patient had not returned to see the analyst nor sought consultation with anyone else, though at the conclusion of the follow-up interview, the patient was considering doing so.

Another patient, assessed by the analyst as having a successful analytic result, reported considerable disappointment with the analytic outcome. She did not report any working through of the transference relationship, did not achieve the ability to do self-analytic work following analysis, and had not been able to establish the kind of intimate relationships she had hoped an analysis would free her to establish. Nevertheless, she believed there had been significant gains from analysis. Her treatment had helped her to accept and consolidate a professional identity, to feel more confident, and to tolerate her feelings without becoming overwhelmed, though she felt more depressed. In describing this patient-analyst pair in the pilot study on match, the researchers noted that this "analysand began analysis feeling isolated and depressed and was strongly defended against rage. Difficulties with separation-individuation were paramount. The analyst's style was forceful and energetic, and often confrontational." The analyst's interview suggested that the analyst was less comfortable with sad, depressive affects. These characteristics of the analyst may reflect both more enduring characterological traits and countertransference reactions to this particular patient. These factors seem to make this analyst poorly suited to treat this patient. It may be that this analyst is poorly suited to treat all patients who struggle with deeply dysphoric affects, but data from one patient is not a sufficient basis for this generalization. According to the post-analysis psychological test results, this patient emerged from analysis as more differentiated, responsive to others, and less worried about aggression. Depression persisted, however. We hypothesize that the analyst's comfort with aggression along with the analysis of related unconscious issues in the patient enabled the patient to explore her rage and made it seem less frightening. Since her difficulties in separation-individuation were tied to her rage and related conflicts, her development in this area was facilitated. In the follow-up interview, the analyst's tone was impatient in describing the patient's sadness. While the patient brought up these issues, they did not seem to have become the focus of analytic inquiry. "The analyst's active, assertive style may have been a disadvantage when it came to analyzing dysphoric experiences."

In the five- to ten-year follow-up interview, this patient said about her analyst:

> She was a smart, very driven woman... she was a model for me... concerned about career... she said I made assumptions, and that was very helpful... but not very empathic... times I felt she didn't give a damn... opening her files. I never trusted her. I don't think she helped me with the issues burning for me now. Biggest mismatch was her difficulty in acknowledging her part in things. My problem is in being right, and her style didn't facilitate getting out of that position.

The patient's feelings of being embattled and depressed apparently had not been analyzed; yet the patient had mobilized and integrated her aggression in more than a superficial way in the process of analysis and had become more confident and successful in her work. These gains had been sustained. The patient described the analyst as a model, and it is our hypothesis that even though the transference remained largely unresolved, this patient identified with her analyst's assertiveness, a capacity she was able to maintain.

Discussion

In part I of my study (Kantrowitz, Katz, & Paolitto, 1990a,b), I reported that many of the patients in this study retained the therapeutic gains they made in analysis years after termination. The material I report in this chapter indicates that in many instances where therapeutic gains did not occur by the time of termination, patients had relived but not understood in the context of the transference earlier troublesome relationships in their lives. The analysts' failure to recognize, interpret, and free the patient from these transference binds may have been due to lack of experience or lack of talent on the part of the analyst. In fact, two analysts with unsuccessful cases are no longer practicing analysis. In some instances, the patients may not have been suitable for an analytic process. However, as I have suggested, a crucial variable in the limitation of many analytic results is the match between patient and analyst.

All analyses remain incomplete in some ways. Patients may be ready to work on certain issues only at certain junctures in their lives. Similarly, analysts may not see or respond to certain issues at particular stages of their careers or lives, while they may be able to be more perceptive about and responsive to these issues at later stages. I suspect that these developmental aspects of the match may be less of an impediment for experienced, older analysts than for those who are less experienced and younger. The data also suggest that when the analyst has blind spots, unresolved conflicts, or personal styles or characteristics that interdigitate with the patient's problems, these issues are likely to be areas that are not recognized, explored, or worked through in the patient's treatment. The importance of the patient-analyst match for the treatment has been given support by the views of patients themselves, five to ten years after the termination of their analyses. Many of the patients, those with both unsuccessful and successful analyses in terms of resolution of the transference, recognized and described characteristics and issues of their analysts which corresponded to those the researchers independently identified in their previously collected and assessed interviews with these analysts. Given that analysts strive to maintain a certain anonymity with their patients and that patients' perceptions of their analysts are greatly shaped by the complexity and depth of transference reactions, it is especially striking that patients' perceptions of their analysts as real people often have considerable reliability when compared with more "objective" evaluations.

I have distinguished among analyses in which the transferences are primarily resolved and those where the transferences are unresolved, and have seen that the match between the patient and the analyst may contribute to determining the analytic outcome. Termination may occur when there is a patient-analyst impasse due to a lack of recognition of some hindrance stemming from the patient-analyst match. Even when the transference is largely resolved, however, there may remain aspects of the transference that have not been fully understood or worked through. In every analysis, even those that are highly successful, there are unexamined issues. We believe that the match between the patient and the analyst may influence which issues remain unexplored at termination.

Some patients are easier to analyze than others and bring to the work greater capacities. Some analysts are more talented than others and work in greater range and depth. The more easily analyzed patient may require only the talented-enough analyst. The more talented analyst is more likely to be successful with a wider range of patients, including those who present greater difficulties in treatment. Even given the most analyzable patients and gifted analysts, however, the particular match between patient and analyst seems likely to exert facilitating and limiting influences on the treatment. Difficulties in analysis stemming from a poor match are less likely to arise as analysts increase their experience and skills and better understand themselves in the context of their analytic work.

One major limitation of the present investigation is that we have evaluated only one patient for each analyst. While we have no data on how these analysts worked with other patients, we do have information on how some of these patients fared with other clinicians. In subsequent treatment, some patients revealed a greater capacity for emotional growth than could be predicted from the initial analysis. This later growth might have been due to the patient's continued reliance on insight and change gained in the previous analysis, the patient's having arrived at a different stage of life, various external factors offering increased support, use of a different treatment modality, or a better match with a subsequent therapist. For the analyst, we have no comparable information. Were it available to us for observation, the analyst's work with other patients might or might not reveal similar facilitating or impeding characteristics. In the future, it would be useful to study experienced analysts working with several patients to determine the impact of match on the outcome of analytic work.

Appendix

Scales

Transference neurosis

1. Understood and at least partially resolved
2. Enacted and understood only with later treatment
3. Enacted and not understood. No evidence of the meaning of the relationship except for support

Match

Presence of issues, characteristics, attitudes, or styles that interdigitate for the patient and the analyst that have an impact on the outcome of the treatment:

1. Mainly facilitating match
2. Facilitating, but at end aspect of match impedes
3. Impeding match recognized by patient
4. Impeding match not recognized by patient

Notes

1 Partially funded by a grant from the Boston Psychoanalytic Society and Institute.
2 Judith Singer, PhD, and I independently rated the original psychological test material.
3 Frank Paolitto, MD, Jerome Sashin, MD, and Leonard Solomon, PhD, all graduate members of the Boston Psychoanalytic Society and Institute independently rated the pre- and post-analysis patient material.
4 Ann Katz, PhD, now a Training and Supervising analyst at the Boston Psychoanalytic Society and Institute.
5 Deborah Greenman, MD, and Humphrey Morris, MD.
6 Here, "we" refers to me and the analysts who did the reliability ratings.

References

Abend, S. M. (1982). Serious illness in the analyst: Countertransference considerations. *Journal of the American Psychoanalytic Association*, 30, 365–379.

Abend, S. M. (1986). Countertransference, empathy, analytic ideal: The impact of life stresses on analytic capability. *Psychoanalytic Quarterly*, 55, 563–575.

Adams-Silvan, A. (1994). "That darkness—is about to pass": The treatment of a dying patient. *Psychoanalytic Study of the Child*, 49, 328–348.

Adler, E., & Bachant, J. L. (1998). Intrapsychological and interactive dimensions of resistance: A contemporary perspective. *Psychoanalytic Psychology*, 15, 461–479.

Agger, E. M. (1993). The analyst's ego. *Psychoanalytic Inquiry*, 13, 403–424.

Alexander, F., & French, T. M. (1946). *Psychoanalytic therapy: Principles and application*. New York: Ronald Press.

Almond, R. (1999). The patient's part in the analytic process: The influence of the analyst's expectations. *Journal of the American Psychoanalytic Association*, 47, 519–541.

Almond, R. (2013). Varieties of psychoanalytic experience: Lessons from returning patients. *Journal of the American Psychoanalytic Association*, 61, 957–976.

Applebaum, S. A. (1977). *The anatomy of change*. New York: Plenum.

Arlow, J. A. (1963). The supervisory situation. *Journal of the American Psychoanalytic Association*, 11, 576–594.

Arlow, J. A., & Brenner, C. (1964). *Psychoanalytic concepts and the structural theory*. International Universities Press.

Aron, L. (1991). The patient's experience of the analyst's subjectivity. *Psychoanalytic Dialogues*, 1, 29–51.

Aron, L. (1992). Interpretation as expression of the analyst's subjectivity. *Psychoanalytic Dialogues*, 2, 475–507.

Aron, L. (1996). *A meeting of minds: Mutuality in psychoanalysis*. Hillsdale, NJ: Analytic Press.

Aron, L. (1999). Clinical choice and the relational matrix. *Psychoanalytic Dialogues*, 9, 1–30.

Asch, S. (1952). *Social psychology*. New York: Prentice-Hall.

Atwood, G. E., Orange, D. M., Stolorow, R. D. (2002). Shattered worlds/psychotic states: A post-cartesian view of the experience of personal annihilation. *Psychoanalytic Psychology*, 19(2), 281–306.

Bacal, H. (2010). *The power of specificity in psychotherapy: When therapy works and when it doesn't*. Lanham, MD: Jason Aronson.

Bachrach, H. M., & Leaff, L. A. (1978). "Analyzability": A systematic review of the clinical and quantitative literature. *Journal of the American Psychoanalytic Association*, 26, 881–920.

Bass, A. (2003). Enactments in psychoanalysis: Another medium, another message. *Psychoanalytic Dialogues*, 13, 657–676.

Bass, A. (2014). Three pleas for a measure of uncertainty, reverie, and private contemplation in the chaotic, interactive, nonlinear dynamic field of interpersonal/intersubjective relational psychoanalysis. *Psychoanalytic Dialogues*, 24, 663–675.

Bass, A. (2015). The dialogue of unconsciouses, mutual analysis and the uses of the self in contemporary relational psychoanalysis. *Psychoanalytic Dialogues*, 25, 2–17.

Baudry, F. (1991). The relevance of the analyst's character and attitude to his work. *Journal of the American Psychoanalytic Association*, 39, 917–938.

Beebe, B., & Lachmann, F. M. (1998). Co-constructing inner and relational processes: Self and mutual regulation in infant research and adult treatment. *Psychoanalytic Psychology*, 15, 480–516.

Beiser, H. (1984). Example of self-analysis. *Journal of the American Psychoanalytic Association*, 32, 3–12.

Benjamin, J. (1993). *Like subjects, love objects: Essays on recognition and sexual difference*. New Haven, CT: Yale University Press.

Benjamin, J. (2004). Between doer and done to: An intersubjective view of thirdness. *Psychoanalytic Quarterly*, 73, 5–46.

Benjamin, J. (2017). *Beyond doer and done to: Recognition theory, intersubjectivity and the third*. London: Routledge.

Berman, L. (1949). Countertransference and attitudes of the analyst in the therapeutic process. *Psychiatry*, 12, 159–166.

Bibring, G. L. (1936). A contribution to the subject of transference resistance. *International Journal of Psychoanalysis*, 17, 181–189.

Bion, W. R. (1971). *Second thoughts: Selected papers on psychoanalysis* (S. Lederman, Ed.). London: William Heineman.

Bion, W. R. (2013). Attacks on linking. *Psychoanalytic Quarterly*, 82, 285–300.

Bird, B. (1972). Notes on transference: Universal phenomenon and hardest part of analysis. *Journal of the American Psychoanalytic Association*, 20, 267–301.

Blatt, S. J., & Behrends, R. S. (1987). Internalization, separation-individuation, and the nature of therapeutic action. *International Journal of Psychoanalysis*, 68, 279–297.

Blum, H. P. (1979). Curative and creative aspects of insight. *Journal of the American Psychoanalytic Association*, 27, 41–70.

Blum, H. P. (1986). Countertransference and the theory of technique: Discussion. *Journal of the American Psychoanalytic Association*, 2, 309–328.

Boesky, D. (1982). Acting out: A reconsideration of the concept. *International Journal of Psychoanalysis*, 63, 39–55.

Bromberg, P. M. (1998). *Standing in the spaces: Essays on clinical process, trauma, and dissociation*. Hillsdale, NJ: Analytic Press.

Bromberg, P. M. (2001). The gorilla did it: Some thoughts on dissociation, the real, and the really real. *Psychoanalytic Dialogues*, 11, 385–404.

Bromberg, P. M. (2003). One need not be a house to be haunted: On enactment, dissociation, and the dread of "not-me"—a case study. *Psychoanalytic Dialogues*, 13, 689–709.

Buie, D. (1993). *Discussion of case vignettes by Drs. Steckler and Demos*. Paper presented at Boston Psychoanalytic Society and Institute Symposium: First relationships—later therapies: Implications of infant research for theory and treatment.

Cabaniss, D. L., Glick, R. A., & Roose, S. (2001). The Columbia supervision project: Data from the dyad. *Journal of the American Psychoanalytic Association*, 49, 235–267.

Calder, K. T. (1980). An analyst's self-analysis. *Journal of the American Psychoanalytic Association*, 28, 5–20.

Chused, J. F. (1991). The evocative power of enactments. *Journal of the American Psychoanalytic Association*, 39, 615–639.

Chused, J. F. (1992). The patient's perception of the analyst: The hidden transference. *Psychoanalytic Quarterly*, 61, 161–184.

Civitarese, G. (2005). Fire at the theatre: (Un)reality of/in the transference and interpretation. *International Journal of Psychoanalysis*, 86, 1299–1316.

Civitarese, G. (2010). *The intimate room: Theory and technique of the analytic field* (P. Slotkin, Trans.). London: Routledge.

Colarusso, C. A., & Nemiroff, R. A. (1981) Adult development, a new dimension in psychodynamic theory and practice. New York: Plenum Press.

Cooper, A. M. (1986). Some limitations on therapeutic effectiveness: The "burn-out syndrome" in psychoanalysis. *Psychoanalytic Quarterly*, 55, 576–598.

Cooper, A. M., & Wittenberg, E. G. (1985). The "bogged-down" treatment: A remedy. *Contemporary Psychoanalysis*, 21, 27–41.

Cooper, S. H. (1998). Analyst subjectivity, analyst disclosure, and the aims of psychoanalysis. *Psychoanalytic Quarterly*, 67, 379–406.

Davies, J. M. (1994). Love in the afternoon: A relational reconsideration of desire and dread. *Psychoanalytic Dialogues*, 4, 153–170.

Davies, J. M. (1996). Linking the pre-analytic with the postclassical: Integration, dissociation, and the multiplicity of unconscious processes. *Contemporary Psychoanalysis*, 32, 553–576.

Dewald, P. A. (1982). Serious illness in the analyst: Transference, countertransference and reality response. *Journal of the American Psychoanalytic Association*, 30, 347–363.

Doehrman, M. J. G. (1976). Parallel process in supervision and psychotherapy. *Bulletin of the Menninger Clinic*, 40, 3–104.

Dorpat, T. (1974). Internalization of the patient analyst relationship in patients with narcissistic disorders. *International Journal of Psychoanalysis*, 55, 183–188.

Dorpat, T., & Miller, M. (1992). *Clinical interaction and the analysis of meaning*. Hillsdale, NJ: Analytic Press.

Eagle, M. N. (2000). A critical evaluation of current conceptions of transference and countertransference. *Psychoanalytic Psychology*, 17, 24–37.

Eagle, M. N. (2001). The postmodern turn in psychoanalysis: A critique. *Psychoanalytic Psychology*, 20, 411–424.

Ehrenberg, D. B. (1992). *The intimate edge: Extending the reach of psychoanalytic interaction*. New York: Norton.

Ehrenberg, D. B. (2005). Working at the "intimate edge": Intersubjective considerations—Comments on "A case study of power and eroticizes transference-countertransference. *Psychoanalytic Inquiry*, 25, 342–358.

Eifermann, R. R. (1987). Germany and the Germans: Acting out fantasies and their discovery in self-analysis. *International Review of Psychoanalysis*, 14, 245–262.

Eifermann, R. R. (1993). The discovery of real and fantasized audiences for self-analysis. In J. W. Barron (Ed.), *Self-analysis: Critical inquiries, personal visions* (pp. 171–194). Hillsdale, NJ: Analytic Press.

Eissler, K. R. (1953). The effect of the structure of the ego on psychoanalytic technique. *Journal of the American Psychoanalytic Association*, 1, 104–143.

Ekstein, R., & Wallerstein, R. S. (1958). *The teaching and learning of psychotherapy*. New York: Basic Books.

Engle, G. L. (1975). Death of a twin: Mourning and anniversary reactions. *International Journal of Psychoanalysis*, 56, 23–40.

Feinsilver, D. B (1999). Counteridentification, comprehensive countertransference, therapeutic action: Toward resolving the intrapsychic-interactional dichotomy. *Psychoanalytic Quarterly*, 68, 264–301.

Ferenczi, S. (1931). *Final contributions to the problems and methods of psychoanalysis*. London: Karnac Books, 1994.

Ferro, A. (2002). Some implications of Bion's thought: The waking dream and narrative derivatives. *International Journal of Psychoanalysis*, 83, 597–607.

Ferro, A. (2009). Transformations in dreaming and characters in the psychoanalytic field. *International Journal of Psychoanalysis*, 90, 209–230.

Ferro, A., & Basile, R. (2004). The psychoanalyst as individual: Self-analysis and gradient of functioning. *Psychoanalytic Quarterly*, 73, 659–682.

Friedman, M. (1993). When the analyst becomes pregnant—twice. *Psychoanalytic Inquiry*, 13, 226–239.

Freud, A. (1936). *The ego and the mechanisms of defense*. New York: International Universities Press, 1966.

Freud, A. (1954). The widening scope of indications for psychoanalysis: Discussion. *Journal of the American Psychoanalytic Association*, 2, 607–620.

Freud, A. (1965). *Normality and pathology in childhood: Assessments of development*. New York: International Universities Press, 1965.

Freud, S. (1895). Project for a scientific psychology. In J. Strachey (Ed. & Trans.), *The standard edition of the complete psychological works of Sigmund Freud* (Vol. 1, pp. 283–387). London: Hogarth Press, 1966.

Freud, S. (1910a). The future prospects of psychoanalytic therapy. In J. Strachey (Ed. & Trans.), *The standard edition of the complete psychological works of Sigmund Freud* (Vol. 11, pp. 139–162). London: Hogarth Press, 1957.

Freud, S. (1910b). "Wild" psychoanalysis. In J. Strachey (Ed. & Trans.), *The standard edition of the complete psychological works of Sigmund Freud* (Vol. 11, pp. 219–230). London: Hogarth Press, 1957.

Freud, S. (1912). Recommendations to physicians practicing psycho-analysis. In J. Strachey (Ed. & Trans.), *The standard edition of the complete psychological works of Sigmund Freud* (Vol. 12, pp. 109–120). London: Hogarth Press, 1957.

Freud, S. (1915a). Observations on transference love (Further recommendations on the techniques of psycho-analysis III). In J. Strachey (Ed. &

Trans.), *The standard edition of the complete psychological works of Sigmund Freud* (Vol. 12, pp. 157–171). London: Hogarth Press, 1957.

Freud, S. (1915b). On transience. In J. Strachey (Ed. & Trans.), *The standard edition of the complete psychological works of Sigmund Freud* (Vol. 14, pp. 303–308). London: Hogarth Press, 1957.

Freud, S. (1916–17). Introductory lectures on psychoanalysis. In J. Strachey (Ed. & Trans.), *The standard edition of the complete psychological works of Sigmund Freud* (Vol. 15–16, pp. 15–463). London: Hogarth Press, 1957.

Freud, S. (1921). Group psychology and the analysis of the ego. In J. Strachey (Ed. & Trans.), *The standard edition of the complete psychological works of Sigmund Freud* (Vol. 18, pp. 67–143). London: Hogarth Press, 1957.

Freud, S. (1937). Analysis terminable and interminable. In J. Strachey (Ed. & Trans.), *The standard edition of the complete psychological works of Sigmund Freud* (Vol. 23, pp. 209–253). London: Hogarth Press, 1957.

Friedman, R. J., & Natterson, J. M. (1999). Enactments: An intersubjective perspective. *Psychoanalytic Quarterly*, 68, 220–247.

Gardner, M. R. (1983). *Self inquiry*. Hillsdale, NJ: Analytic Press.

Gediman, H., & Wolkenfeld, F. (1980). The parallelism phenomenon in psychoanalysis and supervision: Its reconsideration as a triadic system. *Psychoanalytic Quarterly*, 49, 234–255.

Gedo, J. (1979). *Beyond interpretation*. New York: International Universities Press.

Gerson, S. (2004). The relational unconscious. *Psychoanalytic Quarterly*, 73, 63–98.

Ghent, E. (1989). Credo: The dialectics of one-person and two-person. *Contemporary Psychoanalysis*, 25, 169–211.

Gill, M. (1981). Discussion of: Schwaber, E. 1981. Empathy: A mode of analytic listening. *Psychoanalytic Inquiry*, 1, 357–392.

Gill, M. (1982). *Analysis of the transference: Volume I*. New York: International Universities. Press.

Gitelson, M. (1962). The curative factors in psychoanalysis: The first phase of psychoanalysis. *International Journal of Psychoanalysis*, 43, 194–205.

Glover, E. (1937). Symposium on the theory of therapeutic results in psychoanalysis. *International Journal of Psychoanalysis*, 18, 125–132.

Goldberg, A. (1979). New meanings and hidden meanings: Toward a developmental line of meanings. *Journal of the American Psychoanalytic Association*, 27, 627–642.

Goldberger, M. (1993). "Bright spot," a variant of "blind spot." *Psychoanalytic Quarterly*, 42, 270–273.

Grand, S. (1997). On the gendering of traumatic dissociation: A case of mother-son incest. *Gender and Psychoanalysis*, 2(1), 55–77.

Gray, P. (1973). Psychoanalytic technique and the ego's capacity for viewing intrapsychic activity. *Journal of the American Psychoanalytic Association*, 21, 474–494.

Gray, P. (1990). The nature of therapeutic action in psychoanalysis. *Journal of the American Psychoanalytic Association*, 38, 1083–1097.

Greenberg, J. (1995). Psychoanalytic technique and the interactive matrix. *Psychoanalytic Quarterly*, 64, 1–22.

Greenberg, J. (1986). Theoretical models and the analyst's neutrality. *Contemporary Psychoanalysis*, 22, 89–106.

Greenberg, J., & Mitchell, S. A. (1983). *Object relations in psychoanalytic theory*. Cambridge, MA: Harvard University Press.

Greenblatt, S. (2011). *The swerve: How the world became modern*. New York: W. W. Norton & Co.

Greenson, R. R. (1967). *The technique and practice of psychoanalysis*. New York: International Universities Press.

Harris, A. E. (2011). The relational tradition: Landscape and canon. *Journal of the American Psychoanalytic Association*, 59, 701–735.

Heimann, P. (1950). On countertransference. *International Journal of Psychoanalysis*, 31, 81–84.

Hirsch, I. (1993). Countertransference enactments and some issues related to external factors in the analyst's life. *Psychoanalytic Dialogues*, 3, 343–366.

Hirsch, I. (1996). Observing-participation, mutual enactment, and the new classical models. *Contemporary Psychoanalysis*, 32, 359–383.

Hirsch, I. (1998). Further thoughts about interpersonal and relational perspectives: Reply to Jay Frankel. *Contemporary Psychoanalysis*, 34, 501–538.

Hoffman, I. Z. (1983). The patient as interpreter of the analyst's experience. *Contemporary Psychoanalysis*, 19, 389–422.

Hoffman, I. Z. (1992). Some practical implications of social constructivist view of the psychoanalytic situation. *Psychoanalytic Dialogues*, 2, 287–304.

Hoffman, I. Z. (1994). Dialectical thinking and therapeutic action in the psychoanalytic process. *Psychoanalytic Quarterly*, 63, 187–218.

Hoffman, I. Z (1996). The intimate and ironic authority of the psychoanalyst's presence. *Psychoanalytic Quarterly*, 65, 102–136.

Houlding, S. (2013). When a patient dies. In A. Edelman & K. Malawista (Eds.), *The therapist in mourning: From the faraway nearby* (pp. 107–117). New York: Columbia University Press.

Howell, E. (2006). *The dissociative mind.* New York: Routledge.

Hurwitz, M. R. (1986). The analyst, his theory, and the psychoanalytic process. *Psychoanalytic Study of the Child,* 41, 439–466.

Isakower, O. (1938). A contribution to the patho-psychology of phenomena associated with falling asleep. *International Journal of Psychoanalysis,* 19, 331–345.

Jacobs, D., David, P., & Meyer, D. J. (1995). *The supervisory encounter.* New Haven, CT: Yale University Press.

Jacobs, T. J. (1973). Posture, gesture, and movement in the analyst: Cues to interpretation and transference. *Journal of the American Psychoanalytic Association,* 21, 77–92.

Jacobs, T. J. (1980). Secrets, alliances, and family fictions: Some psychoanalytic observations. *Journal of the American Psychoanalytic Association,* 27, 21–42.

Jacobs, T. J. (1983). The analyst and the patient's object world: Notes on an aspect of countertransference. *Journal of the American Psychoanalytic Association,* 31, 619–642.

Jacobs, T. J. (1986). On countertransference enactments. *Journal of the American Psychoanalytic Association,* 34, 289–307.

Jacobs, T. J. (1987). Notes on the unknowable: Analytic secrets and the transference neurosis. *Psychoanalytic Inquiry,* 7, 485–509.

Jacobs, T. J. (1991). *The use of the self: Countertransference and communication in the analytic situation.* New York: International Universities Press.

Kantrowitz, J. L. (1986). The role of the patient-analyst "match" in the outcome of psychoanalysis. *Annual of Psychoanalysis,* 14, 273–297.

Kantrowitz, J. L. (1992). The analyst's style and its impact on the psychoanalytic process: Overcoming stalemates. *Journal of the American Psychoanalytic Association,* 40, 169–194.

Kantrowitz, J. L. (1993a). Impasses in psychoanalysis: Overcoming resistance in situations of stalemate. *Journal of the American Psychoanalytic Association,* 41, 1021–1050.

Kantrowitz, J. L. (1993b). The uniqueness of the patient-analyst pair: Elucidating the role of the analyst. *International Journal of Psychoanalysis,* 74, 893–904.

Kantrowitz, J. L. (1993c). Outcome research in psychoanalysis: Review and reconsideration. *Journal of the American Psychoanalytic Association,* 41(Suppl.), 313–329.

Kantrowitz, J. L. (1995). The beneficial aspects of the patient-analyst match: Factors in addition to clinical acumen and therapeutic skill that contribute to psychological change. *International Journal of Psychoanalysis*, 76, 299–313.

Kantrowitz, J. L. (1996). *The patient's impact on the analyst*. Hillsdale, NJ: Analytic Press.

Kantrowitz, J. L. (1997). A different view of the therapeutic process: The impact of the patient on the analyst. *Journal of the American Psychoanalytic Association*, 44, 127–153.

Kantrowitz, J. L. (1998). Pathways to self-knowledge: Self-analysis, mutual supervision, and other shared communications. *International Journal of Psychoanalysis*, 80, 111–132.

Kantrowitz, J. L. (1999). The role of the preconscious in psychoanalysis. *Journal of the American Psychoanalytic Association*, 46, 65–89.

Kantrowitz, J. L. (2002). The external observer and the patient-analyst match. *International Journal of Psychoanalysis*, 83, 339–350.

Kantrowitz, J. L. (2003). Tell me your theory. Where is it bred? A lesson from clinical approaches to dreams. Charles Fischer Memorial Lecture. *Journal of Clinical Psychoanalysis*, 12, 151–178.

Kantrowitz, J. L. (2006). *Writing about patients: responsibilities, risks, and ramifications*. New York: Other Press.

Kantrowitz, J. L. (2009). Privacy and disclosure in psychoanalysis, plenary address Winter. *Journal of the American Psychoanalytic Association*, 57, 787–806.

Kantrowitz, J. L. (2013). The effect of postanalytic contact. *Journal of the American Psychoanalytic Association*, 61, 947–956.

Kantrowitz, J. L. (2014). *Myths of termination: What patients can teach psychoanalysts about endings*. London: Routledge Press.

Kantrowitz, J. L., Katz, A. L., Greenman, D., Morris, H., Paolitto, F., Sashin, J., & Solomon, L. (1989). The patient-analyst match and the outcome of psychoanalysis: The study of 13 cases. Research in progress. *Journal of the American Psychoanalytic Association*, 37, 893–920.

Kantrowitz, J. L., Katz, A. L., & Paolitto, F. (1990a). Follow-up of psychoanalysis five-to-ten years after termination: I. Stability of change. *Journal of the American Psychoanalytic Association*, 38, 471–496.

Kantrowitz, J. L., Katz, A. L., & Paolitto, F. (1990b). Follow-up of psychoanalysis five-to-ten years after termination: II. The development of the self-analytic function. *Journal of the American Psychoanalytic Association*, 38, 637–654.

Kantrowitz, J. L., Katz, A. L., & Paolitto, F. (1990c). Follow-up of psychoanalysis five-to-fen years after termination: III. The relationship of the transference neurosis to the patient-analyst match. *Journal of the American Psychoanalytic Association*, 38, 655–678.

Kantrowitz, J. L., Katz, A. L., Paolitto, F., Sashin, J., & Solomon, L. (1987a). Changes in the level and quality of object relations in psychoanalysis: Follow-up of a longitudinal prospective study. *Journal of the American Psychoanalytic Association*, 35, 25–46.

Kantrowitz, J. L., Katz, A. L., Paolitto, F., Sashin, J., & Solomon, L. (1987b). The role of reality testing in the outcome of psychoanalysis: Follow-up of 22 cases. *Journal of the American Psychoanalytic Association*, 35, 367–386.

Kantrowitz, J. L., Paolitto, F., Sashin, J., Solomon, L., & Katz, A. L. (1986). Affect and availability, tolerance, complexity, and modulation in psychoanalysis: Follow-up of a longitudinal study. *Journal of the American Psychoanalytic Association*, 34, 529–559.

Kantrowitz, J. L., Singer, J., & Knapp, P. (1975). Methodology for a prospective study of suitability for psychoanalysis: The role of psychological tests. *Psychoanalytic Quarterly*, 44, 371–391.

Karush, A. (1967). Working through. *Psychoanalytic Quarterly*, 36, 497–531.

Kernberg, O. F. (1965). Notes on countertransference. *Journal of the American Psychoanalytic Association*, 13, 38–56.

Kernberg, O. F. (1972). Summary and conclusions: The psychotherapy research project of the Menninger Foundation. *Bulletin of the Menninger Clinic*, 36, 181–195.

Kernberg, O. F. (1992). An ego psychology-object relations theory of structural change. O. F. Kernberg (Ed.), In *Aggression in personality disorders and perversions* (pp. 119–139). New Haven, CT: Yale University Press.

Kite, J. V. (2008). Ideas of influence: The impact of the analyst's character on the analysis. *Psychoanalytic Quarterly*, 77, 1075–1104.

Kohut, H. (1959). Introspection, empathy, and psychoanalysis—An examination of the relationship between mode of observation and theory. *Journal of the American Psychoanalytic Association*, 7, 459–483.

Kohut, H. (1965). Autonomy and integration. *Journal of the American Psychoanalytic Association*, 13, 851–856.

Kohut, H. (1971). *The analysis of the self.* New York: International Universities Press.

Kohut, H. (1984). How does analysis cure? University of Chicago Press, a Pilot Study. *Journal of the American Psychoanalytic Association*, 37, 893–919.

Kramer, M. K. (1959). On the continuation of the analytic process after psychoanalysis. *International Journal of Psychoanalysis*, 40, 17–25.

Kris, A. O. (1977). Either-or dilemmas. *Psychoanalytic Study of the Child*, 32, 91–117.

Kris, A. O. (1990a). Helping patients by analyzing self-criticism. *Journal of the American Psychoanalytic Association*, 38, 605–636.

Kris, A. O. (1990b). Resolution of conflict: Panel on therapeutic action. *Journal of the American Psychoanalytic Association*, 38, 777–780.

Kris, A. O. (1993). Support and psychic structure. *Journal of the American Psychoanalytic Association*, 23, 363–382.

Kris, E. (1950). On preconscious mental processes. *The Psychoanalytic Quarterly*, 19, 540–560.

Laub, D. (1992). Bearing witness or the vicissitudes of witnessing. In S. Felman & D. Laub (Eds.), *Testimony: Crises of witnessing in literature, psychoanalysis, and history* (pp. 57–74). London: Routledge.

Levenson, E. (1972). *The fallacy of understanding.* New York: Basic Books

Levine, H. B., & Friedman, R. J. (2000). Intersubjectivity and interaction in analytic relationships: A mainstream view. *Psychoanalytic Quarterly*, 69, 41–92.

Levine, H. B., Reed, G., & Scarfone, D. (2013). *Unrepresented states and the construction of meaning.* London: Karnac Books.

Levine, S. S. (2007). Nothing but the truth: Self-disclosure, self-revelation and the persona of the analyst. *Journal of the American Psychoanalytic Association*, 55, 81–104.

Lionells, M., Fiscalini, J., Mann, C., & Stern, D. (Eds.). (1995). *The handbook of interpersonal psychoanalysis.* Hillsdale, NJ: Analytic Press.

Loewald, H. (1960). On the therapeutic action of psychoanalysis. *International Journal of Psychoanalysis*, 41, 16–33.

Loewald, H. (1979). The psychoanalytic process and its therapeutic potential. *Psychoanalytic Study of the Child*, 34, 155–168.

Loewenstein, R. (1956). Remarks on some variations in psychoanalytic technique. *International Journal of Psychoanalysis*, 39, 202–210.

Maldonado, J. L. (1984). Analyst involvement in the psychoanalytical impasse. *International Journal of Psychoanalysis*, 65, 263–271.

Margulies, A. (1993) Contemplating the mirror of the other: Empathy and self-analysis. In J. W. Barron (Ed.), *Self-analysis: Critical inquiries, personal visions* (pp. 51–61). Hillsdale, NJ: Analytic Press.

Margulies, A., Orgel, S., & Poland, W. S. (2014). After the storm: Living and dying in psychoanalysis. *Journal of the American Psychoanalytic Association*, 62, 862–905.

Maroda, K. J. (1998). Enactment: When the patient's and the analyst's pasts converge. *Psychoanalytic Psychology*, 15, 517–535.

McLaughlin, J. T. (1975). Sleepy analyst: States of consciousness in the analyst at work. *Journal of the American Psychoanalytic Association*, 23, 363–382.

McLaughlin, J. T. (1981). Transference, psychic reality, and countertransference. *Psychoanalytic Quarterly*, 50, 639–664.

McLaughlin, J. T. (1991a). Clinical and theoretical aspects of enactment. *Journal of the American Psychoanalytic Association*, 39, 595–614.

McLaughlin, J. T. (1991b). *Retrospectroscope is 20/20: A perspective on psychoanalytic failures*. Paper presented at the spring meeting of the APA, New Orleans, LA.

Mclaughlin, J. T. (1993). Work with patients and the experience of self-analysis. In J. W. Barron (Ed.), *Self-analysis: Critical inquiries, personal visions* (pp. 63–81). Hillsdale, NJ: Analytic Press.

Meissner, W. A. (1989). Therapeutic action of psychoanalysis: Strachey revisited. *Psychoanalytic Inquiry*, 9, 140–159.

Mills, J. (2005). A critique of relational psychoanalysis. *Psychoanalytic Psychology*, 22, 155–188.

Mitchell, S. A. (1988a). The intrapsychic and the interpersonal: Different theories, different domains, or historical artifacts? *Psychoanalytic Inquiry*, 8, 472–496.

Mitchell, S. A. (1988b). *Relational concepts in psychoanalysis*. Cambridge, MA: Harvard University Press.

Mitchell, S. A. (1993). *Hope and dread in psychoanalysis*. New York: Basic Books.

Mitchell, S. A. (1998). The emergence of features of the analyst's life. *Psychoanalytic Dialogues*, 8, 187–194.

Mitchell, S. A. (2000). Reply to Silverman. *Psychoanalytic Psychology*, 17, 153–159.

Mitchell, S. A., & Aron, L. (Eds.). (1999). *Relational psychoanalysis: The emergence of a tradition*. Hillsdale, NJ: Analytic Press.

Modell, A. (1976). The holding environment and the therapeutic action. *Journal of the American Psychoanalytic Association*, 24, 285–308.

Modell, A. (1986). *Psychoanalysis in a new context*. New York: International Universities Press.

Modell, A. (1990). *Other times, other realities*. Cambridge, MA: Harvard University Press.

Modell, A. (1993). *Affects and the agency of the self: Discussion of papers of Trevarthen, Field, and Stern*. Paper presented at Boston Psychoanalytic Society and Institute Symposium: First relationships—later therapies: Implications of infant research for theory and treatment.

Modell, A. (2006). *Imagination and the meaningful brain*. Cambridge, MA: MIT Press.

Modell, A.H. (1970). The Transitional Object and the Creative Act. *Psychoanal Q.*, 39:240–250.

Myerson, P. (1973). The meanings of confrontation. In G. Adler & P. Myerson (Eds.), *Confrontation in psychotherapy* (pp. 21–38). New York: Science House.

Natterson, J. M., & Friedman, R. J. (1995). *A primer of clinical intersubjectivity*. Lanham, MD: Jason Aronson.

Norman, H. F., Blacker, K. H., Oremland, J. D., & Barrett, W. G. (1976). The fate of the transference neurosis after termination of a satisfactory analysis. *Journal of the American Psychoanalytic Association*, 24, 471–498.

Norton, J. (1963). Treatment of a dying patient. *Psychoanalytic Study of the Child*, 28, 540–560.

Nuland, S. (1993). *How we die: Reflections of life's final chapter*. New York: Vintage.

Nunberg, H. (1937). Symposium on the theory of therapeutic action. *International Review of Psychoanalysis*, 18, 161–169.

Ogden, T. H. (1994a). The analytic third: Working with intersubjective clinical facts. *International Journal of Psychoanalysis*, 75, 3–20.

Ogden, T. H. (1994b). *Subjects of analysis*. Northvale, NJ: Jason Aronson.

Ogden, T. H. (1997). Reverie and interpretation. *Psychoanalytic Quarterly*, 66, 567–595.

Ogden, T. H. (2004). The analytic third: Implications for psychoanalytic theory and technique. *Psychoanalytic Quarterly*, 73, 167–198.

Olinick, S. L., Poland, W. S., Grigg, K. A., & Granatir, W. L. (1973). The psychoanalytic work ego: Process and interpretation. *International Journal of Psychoanalysis*, 54, 143–151.

Orgel, S. (1990). The future of psychoanalysis. *Psychoanalytic Quarterly*, 59, 1–20.

Orgel, S. (2000). Letting go: Some thoughts about termination. *Journal of the American Psychoanalytic Association*, 48, 719–738.

Orgel, S. (2013). A patient returns. *Journal of the American Psychoanalytic Association*, 61, 835–846.

Orgel, S. (2014). Part 111 in after the storm: Living and dying in psychoanalysis Alfred Margulies, Shelley Orgel and Warren S. Poland. *Journal of the American Psychoanalytic Association*, 62, 877–880.

Petsky, I. (2000). *Discussion of Kantrowitz, "The vicissitudes of the patient-analyst match."* Paper presented at UNC-Duke.

Pfeffer, A. Z. (1961). Follow-up study of a satisfactory analysis. *Journal of the American Psychoanalytic Association*, 9, 698–718.

Pfeffer, A. Z. (1963). The meaning of the analyst after analysis: A contribution to the theory of therapeutic results. *Journal of the American Psychoanalytic Association*, 11, 224–244.

Pine, F. (1993). A contribution to the analysis of the psychoanalytic process. *Psychoanalytic Quarterly*, 62, 185–205.

Pizer, S. A. (1998). *Building bridges: The negotiation of paradox in psychoanalysis*. Hillsdale, NJ: Analytic Press.

Poland, W. S. (1984). On the analyst's neutrality. *Journal of the American Psychoanalytic Association*, 32, 283–299.

Poland, W. S. (1988). Insight and the analytic dyad. *Psychoanalytic Quarterly*, 57, 341–369.

Poland, W. S. (2000). The analyst's witnessing and otherness. *Journal of the American Psychoanalytic Association*, 48(1), 17–34.

Poland, W. S. (2013a). The analyst's approach and the patient's psychic growth. *Psychoanalytic Quarterly*, 82, 829–847.

Poland, W. S. (2013b). Discussion of Orgel's "A patient returns." *Journal of the American Psychoanalytic Association*, 61, 835–846.

Poland, W. S. (2016). Slouching towards mortality: Thoughts on time and death. *Journal of the American Psychoanalytic Association*, 64, 795–802.

Racker, E. (1957). The meanings and uses of countertransference. *Psychoanalytic Quarterly*, 26, 303–357.

Rando, T. A. (1993). *Treatment of complicated mourning*. Champaign, IL: Research Press.

Reich, A. (1960a). Further remarks on countertransference. *International Journal of Psychoanalysis*, 32, 25–31.

Reich, A. (1960b). Empathy and countertransference. In *Psychoanalytic contributions* (pp. 344–360). New York: International Universities Press, 1973.

Renik, O. (1993). Analytic interaction: Conceptualizing technique in light of the analyst's irreducible subjectivity. *Psychoanalytic Quarterly*, 62, 559–571.

Rosen, V. H. (1967). Disorders of communication in psychoanalysis. *Journal of the American Psychoanalytic Association*, 15, 467–507.

Rycroft, C. (1956). The nature and function of the analyst's communication to the patient. *International Journal of Psychoanalysis*, 37, 469–472.

Sachs, D. M., & Shapiro, S. H. (1976). On parallel process in therapy and teaching. *Psychoanalytic Quarterly*, 45, 394–415.

Sander, L. (1962). Issues in early mother-child interaction. *Journal of the American Academy of Child Psychiatry*, 1, 141–166.

Sandler, J. (1976). Countertransference and role-responsiveness. *International Review of Psychoanalysis*, 3, 43–47.

Schafer, R. (1959). Generative empathy in the treatment situation. *Psychoanalytic Quarterly*, 28, 342–373.

Scharfman, M. A., & Blacker, K. H. (1981). Insight: Clinical conceptualizations. *Journal of the American Psychoanalytic Association*, 29, 659–671.

Schlessinger, N., & Robbins, F. P. (1974). Assessment and follow-up in psychoanalysis. *Journal of the American Psychoanalytic Association*, 22, 542–567.

Schlessinger, N., & Robbins, F. P. (1975). The psychoanalytic process: Recurrent patterns of conflict and changes in ego functions. *Journal of the American Psychoanalytic Association*, 23, 761–782.

Schwaber, E. A. (1981). Empathy: A mode of analytic listening. *Psychoanalytic Inquiry*, 1, 357–392.

Schwaber, E. A. (1983). Perspectives on analytic listening and psychic reality. *International Review of Psychoanalysis*, 10, 379–392.

Schwaber, E. A. (1987). Models of the mind and data gathering in clinical work. *Psychoanalytic Inquiry*, 7, 261–276.

Schwaber, E. A. (1990). *Elucidating patients' particular experienced psychic reality*. Paper presented at a pane on therapeutic action.

Schwaber, E. A. (1992). Countertransference: The analyst's retreat from the patient's vantage point. *International Journal of Psychoanalysis*, 73, 349–362.

Searles, H. F. (1955). The informational value of the supervisor's emotional experience. *Psychiatry*, 18, 135–146.

Shapiro, D. (1976). The analyst's own analysis. *Journal of the American Psychoanalytic Association*, 24, 15–42.

Shapiro, L. (1973). Confrontation with the "real" analyst. In G. Adler & P. Myerson (Eds.), Confrontation in psychotherapy (pp. 342–369). New York: Science House.

Silber, A. (1996). Analysis, reanalysis, and self-analysis. *Journal of the American Psychoanalytic Association*, 44, 491–509.

Silverman, M. (1985). Countertransference and the myth of the perfectly analyzed analyst. *Psychoanalytic Quarterly*, 54, 175–199.

Skolnikoff, A. Z. (1993). The analyst's experience in the psychoanalytic situation: A continuum between objective and subjective reality. *Psychoanalytic Inquiry*, 13, 296–309.

Smith, H. F. (1993). Engagements in the analytic work. *Psychoanalytic Inquiry*, 13, 425–454.

Smith, H. F. (2004). The analyst's fantasy of the ideal patient. *Psychoanalytic Quarterly*, 73, 627–659.

Sonnenberg, S. (1991). The analyst's self-analysis and its impact on clinical work: A comment on the sources and importance of personal insights. *Journal of the American Psychoanalytic Association*, 39, 687–704.

Spillius, E. (1994). On formulating clinical fact to the patient. *International Journal of Psychoanalysis*, 75, 1121–1132.

Spitz, R. A. (1956). Transference: The analytic setting and its prototype. *International Journal of Psychoanalysis*, 37, 380–385.

Spruiell, V. (1984). The analyst at work. *International Journal of Psychoanalysis*, 65, 13–30.

Stein, M. H. (1981). The unobjectionable part of the transference. *Journal of the American Psychoanalytic Association*, 29, 869–920.

Stern, D. B. (1983). Unformulated experience: From familiar chaos to creative disorder. *Contemporary Psychoanalysis*, 19, 71–99.

Stern, D. B. (1997). *Unformulated experience: From dissociation to imagination in psychoanalysis*. Hillsdale, NJ: Analytic Press.

Stern, D. B. (2003). The fusion of horizons: dissociation, enactment, and understanding. *Psychoanalytic Dialogues*, 13, 843–873.

Stern, D. B. (2012). Witnessing across time: Accessing the present from the past and the past from the present. *Psychoanalytic Quarterly*, 81, 53–81.

Stern, D. B. (2013). Field theory in psychoanalysis, part 2: Bionian field theory and contemporary interpersonal/relational psychoanalysis. *Psychoanalytic Dialogues*, 23, 630–645.

Stern, D. B., Kantor, S., Mann, C. N., & Schlesinger, G. (Eds.). (1995). *Pioneers of interpersonal psychoanalysis*. Hillsdale, NJ: Analytic Press.

Stern, D. N. (1985). *The interpersonal world of the infant: A view from psychoanalysis and developmental psychology*. New York: Basic Books.

Stern, D. N. (1990). *Diary of a baby*. New York: Basic Books.

Stolorow, R. D., & Atwood, G. E. (1992). *Contexts of being*. Hillsdale, NJ: Analytic Press.

Stolorow, R. D., & Atwood, G. E. (1997). Deconstructing the myth of the neutral analyst: An alternative from intersubjective systems theory. *Psychoanalytic Quarterly*, 66, 431–449.

Stolorow, R. D., Atwood, G. E., & Lachman, F. M. (1988). *Psychoanalysis of developmental arrests: Theory and treatment*. Hillsdale, NJ: Analytic Press.

Stolorow, R. D., Brandchaft, B., & Atwood, G. E. (1987). *Psychoanalytic treatment: An intersubjective approach*. Hillsdale, NJ: Analytic Press.

Stone, L. (1961). *The psychoanalytic situation: An examination of its development and essential nature*. New York: International Universities Press.

Stone, L. (1962). *Psychoanalytic situation*. New York: International University Press.

Strachey, J. (1934). The nature of therapeutic action of psychoanalysis. *International Journal of Psychoanalysis*, 15, 127–159.

Strean, H. S. (1991). Colluding illusions among analytic candidates, their supervisors, and their patients: A major factor in some treatment impasses. *Psychoanalytic Psychology*, 8, 403–414.

Stuart, J., & Haseley, D. (2000, January). *The influence of candidate status on analytic process.* Presentation at meeting of the Psychoanalytic Association of New York.

Sullivan, H. S. (1953). *Conceptions of modern psychiatry* (2nd ed.). New York: W. W. Norton & Co.

Taylor, E. (1996). Discussion of J. L. Kantrowitz, "A different view of the analytic process: The impact of the patient on the analyst." Paper presented to the American Psychoanalytic Association, Los Angeles.

Thomas, D. (1952). A refusal to mourn the death, by fire, of a child in London. In J. W. Goodby (Ed.), *The poems of Dylan Thomas* (p. 221). New York: New Directions, 2003.

Thompson, C. (1938). Notes on the psychoanalytic significance of the choice of analyst. *Psychiatry*, 79, 23–28.

Tower, L. E. (1956). Countertransference. *Journal of the American Psychoanalytic Association*, 4, 224–255.

Tyson, R. L. (1986). Countertransference evolution in theory and practice. *Journal of the American Psychoanalytic Association*, 34, 251–274.

van Dam, H. (1987). Countertransference during an analyst's brief illness. *Journal of the American Psychoanalytic Association*, 35, 647–655.

Vaughan, S. C., & Roose, S. P. (2000). Patient-analyst match: Revelation or resistance? *Journal of the American Psychoanalytic Association*, 48, 885–900.

Viederman, M. (1976). The influence of the person of the analyst on structural change: A case report. *Psychoanalytic Quarterly*, 45, 231–249.

Viederman, M. (1991). The real person of the analyst and his role in the process of psychoanalytic cure. *Journal of the American Psychoanalytic Association*, 39, 451–490.

Wallerstein, R. S. (1986). *Forty-two lives in treatment: A study of psychoanalysis and psychotherapy.* New York: Guilford Press.

Weber, J. J., Solomon, M., & Bachrach, H. M. (1985a). Characteristics of psychoanalytic clinic patients. *International Journal of Psychoanalysis*, 12, 13–26.

Weber, J. J., Solomon, M., & Bachrach, H. M. (1985b). Factors associated with the outcome of psychoanalysis. *International Journal of Psychoanalysis*, 12, 127–141.

Weinshel, E. (1993). Psychic structure and psychic change: A case of inconsolability. In M. Horowitz, O. Kernberg, & E. Weinshel (Eds.), *Psychic structure and psychic change: Essays in honor of Robert S. Wallerstein* (pp. 251–262). Madison, CT: International Universities Press.

Weisman, A. (1973). Confrontation, countertransference and context. In G. Adler & P. Myerson (Eds.), *Confrontation in psychotherapy* (pp. 97–146). New York: Science House.

Winnicott, D. W. (1965). *The maturational processes and the facilitating environment*. New York: International Universities Press.

Winnicott, D. W. (1969). The use of an object and relating through identification. In *Playing and reality* (pp. 86–94). New York: Basic Books, 1975.

Index

Note: Page numbers followed by "n" denote endnotes.